Manual for the identification of medical bacteria

COWAN AND STEEL'S

Manual for the identification of medical bacteria

SECOND EDITION
REVISED BY

S. T. COWAN

M.D., D.Sc., F.R.C.Path.

Formerly Curator, National Collection of Type Cultures
Administrative Director, Central Public Health
Laboratory, Colindale, and
Deputy Director, Public Health Laboratory Service
England and Wales

CAMBRIDGE UNIVERSITY PRESS

Published by the Syndics of the Cambridge University Press
Bentley House, 200 Euston Road, London NW1 2DB
American Branch: 32 East 57th Street, New York, N.Y.10022

© Cambridge University Press 1965, 1974

Library of Congress Catalogue Card Number: 73–90651

ISBN: 0 521 20399 6

First published 1965
Second edition 1974

Printed in Great Britain
at the University Printing House, Cambridge
(Brooke Crutchley, University Printer)

Contents

CONTENTS

Preface to the first edition

Our 'Diagnostic Tables for the Common Medical Bacteria' were originally published in the *Journal of Hygiene*. The tables seemed to fill a need and the demand for reprints was so great that Cambridge University Press reprinted them in pamphlet form.

Many inquired about the technical methods, and there were constant complaints that the methods were not described and that the text lacked details of the taxonomic problems. We resolved, therefore, to expand the original paper and to prepare a book which would give sufficient detail of media and methods to justify its description as a laboratory manual.

Although designed for medical workers we hope that others will use it.

The value of a laboratory manual was impressed on one of us in 1935 at the British Postgraduate Medical School. Dr A. A. Miles had prepared a loose-leaf mimeographed manual to supplement (and improve on) a popular laboratory handbook. With this example in mind a manual suited to the special needs of the National Collection of Type Cultures was prepared, and contributions were made by other members of the Collection staff, particularly Mrs P. H. Clarke, Miss H. E. Ross, Miss C. Shaw, and Mr C. S. Brindle. The National Collection Manual in turn became the basis for the appendices to the present *Manual*.

In compiling the tables we sought information from various sources, including authoritative works such as the Reports of the Enterobacteriaceae Subcommittee of the International Committee on Bacteriological Nomenclature, and monographs such as Kauffmann's (1954) *Enterobacteriaceae*, Edwards & Ewing's *Identification of Enterobacteriaceae* (1962), and Smith, Gordon & Clark's (1952) *Aerobic Sporeforming Bacteria*. We found large gaps in published works, and in many instances our own data have been the only source of information. While we have taken great care in compiling and checking the tables, we are sure that the *Manual* is unlikely to be free from error. When such errors are detected we hope that the finders will let us know. We will also welcome data to fill up the few gaps in the tables.

It is with pleasure that we acknowledge our indebtedness to many friends and colleagues at home and abroad for facts and discussions that have helped to clarify our ideas. It is impossible to name them all but we could not have planned or written the *Manual* without the help of Dr R. E. Gordon, Dr P. R. Edwards, Dr W. H. Ewing, Dr T. Gibson, Dr Joan Taylor, Mrs P. H. Clarke, Miss C. Shaw, and Miss H. E. Ross. We also wish to thank Miss B. H. Whyte and Miss A. Bowman, the Colindale librarians, Miss M. I. Hammond who dealt skilfully with the manuscript, and Mr W. Clifford who made the figures.

London   S.T.C.
1964   K.J.S.

POSTSCRIPT

My colleague, Dr K. J. Steel, died suddenly on 25 September 1964, between the completion of the manuscript and the proof stage of the book. His death at the age of 34 is a great loss for he seemed destined to reach the highest branches of bacteriology. In this *Manual* he was responsible for the whole of Appendices A to D and F and for much of Chapter 3; and he played a big part in revising and recasting the tables that form the heart of our work. I hope that the book will serve as a fitting memorial to a great collaborator and friend.

London   S.T.C.
1965

Preface to the second edition

The first edition of this *Manual*, judged by its spread around the world, seems to have been useful to hospital bacteriologists. It was translated into Japanese by Dr Riichi Sakazaki, who will also translate this edition.

It has not been easy to prepare a worthy successor; not only have I been unable to discuss and argue every sentence with my colleague, but I have missed the ready access to libraries that one has when working in a large research institution. However, I have been greatly helped by the Librarians at Colindale (Miss B. H. Whyte) and the Royal Society of Medicine (Mr P. Wade) and their staffs.

In this edition Chapter 2 and Appendices A, B, C and E, originally written mainly by Dr Steel, are little changed; most of the other chapters have been completely rewritten. Chapters 8 and 9 are entirely new, as are appendices D, F, G and H. I must thank Mr A. Waltho, of the Medical Research Council's Central Store, who gave me great help in preparing the list of firms which supply media and chemicals (Appendix H) and, together with Dr O. M. Lidwell, suggested and drafted what became Table 2.1.

I am also grateful to many other colleagues who gave me information and advice; while it is impossible to mention all by name, I am particularly indebted to G. I. Barrow, W. B. Cherry, E. A. Dawes, N. E. Gibbons, R. E. Gordon, R. M. Keddie, S. P. Lapage, H. Lautrop, J. Midgley, M. J. Pickett, R. Sakazaki, R. Whittenbury and S. A. Wright.

On behalf of the Executive Committee of the International Association of Microbiological Societies (IAMS), Dr N. E. Gibbons gave permission for the reproduction of the Introduction to the proposed revision of the Bacteriological Code (Appendix G), and I should like to express my thanks to the IAMS Executive.

In a book with so many tables and cross-references it is inevitable that some errors and inconsistencies are still undetected; I hope that these will be drawn to my attention so that corrections can be made in later impressions.

For the proof reading I am grateful for help from former colleagues, Miss H. E. Ross, Dr G. I. Barrow and Dr A. F. B. Standfast. Checking the numerous and large tables in the manuscript and proof stages has been an onerous task which I could not have done without the co-operation of my wife, who also helped to check the references, which must now number about a thousand.

With all this help, I hope the book will continue to be a worthy memorial to my much missed young colleague, Dr K. J. Steel.

Queen Camel   S.T.C.
1973

Introduction

While all essential detail is given in the Appendices, it is assumed that the reader has some knowledge and experience of bacteriology and elementary chemistry and that the basic principles are understood. Thus we do not describe how to find the pH value of a medium, or how to make a normal solution; we do not give details of the use of anaerobic jars or microscopes. Serology is not discussed but we describe methods commonly used in the preparation of extracts for grouping streptococci, as the grouping finds a place in Table 6.3*b* and *c*. We give details of sterilization temperatures and times as these so-called standard procedures vary from one laboratory to another.

This *Manual* is intended to help those who have isolated a bacterium and want to identify it. We do not describe in detail the methods used by clinical bacteriologists to isolate organisms from specimens sent to the laboratory; to do so would lead us into ever-changing fields where we do not now wander, and our recommendations might well be out of date, but *Clinical Bacteriology* (1960; 1968*a*) by E. Joan Stokes will be found useful. We must stress, however, that before an identification is attempted the organism must be obtained in pure culture, and we give some advice on how to recognize that a culture is impure and the steps to be taken to purify it.

Our tables developed in three phases: the originals (Cowan & Steel, 1961) were based mainly on the results of tests carried out on our strains in the National Collection of Type Cultures (NCTC) between 1948 and 1960; in tables of the first edition of this *Manual* the NCTC information was supplemented by surveys of the literature up to the end of 1963, while the third (present) phase includes the results of further literature surveys up to the end of 1972. It follows that in this edition

we are less often able to indicate the value of the different technical methods to obtain the characters shown in the tables. Once again our survey revealed discrepancies between the results of different workers and these, we think, were more often due to differences in method than to variation between strains of the same species. When we bear in mind the older pathologist's adage that 'anything can happen anywhere at any time' we are tempted to try to cover every possibility in the tables; but this is self-defeating, for either we multiply the columns (species or varieties) or we increase the number of dee entries (d or D), the equivalent of the descriptive 'often', 'some(times)', 'not infrequently', so that a clear positive or negative character becomes a rarity and the tables become confusing and unhelpful. We have tried to be definite and in our reading have treated such phrases as 'occasionally', 'occasional strains' and 'a few strains' as exceptions not worthy of notice. Perhaps this will give our tables a sense of unrealism, but it is the users who must be realistic and bear in mind that the bacteria they are trying to identify have not read this book or, if they have, have enough Irish in them to be 'agin the government' (i.e. the tables).

Intelligent use of the tables demands technical skill and sensitive but specific methods for the individual tests. As in all determinative bacteriology a true identification must be based on careful work, and our tables will not help the man who is in too much of a hurry to carry out the tests needed, which does not mean all the tests in a table. We considered cutting down the tables to the smallest possible size, to show only those characters that had immediate value in distinguishing a species from others in the table. But we decided against that course because conditions vary in different laboratories and in different countries. We do not expect all the tests in our tables to be carried out; we know that each bacteriologist has his preferences and his dislikes, that all laboratories are not equally well (or badly) equipped, and we include many more characters than are necessary to make identifications. At one time we intended to indicate the more important characters in bold type, but this would merely reflect our own preferences and we decided against it, leaving the user to pick those tests that seem to him to be most discriminating and to choose those that can be performed with the equipment and media available. Because the tables were constructed from information from many sources we do not stipulate particular methods, but those given in the Appendices should be found satisfactory. In this edition we omitted many of the micromethods described in the first edition; those that we retain are included in Appendix C with methods using larger volumes – and often taking a longer time.

Three points should be emphasized about the tables. (i) They should not be considered in isolation; other evidence such as colony form or experimental pathogenicity that cannot be included in them should also be taken into account. (ii) The tables do not characterize an organism, though they give more detail than corresponding tables of the first edition; they are intended to focus attention on tests and characters most valuable in differentiation. (iii) The tables do not form part of any classification but they may draw attention to similarities and relations that are not otherwise apparent. Unfortunately we have not been able to avoid completely the jargon of taxonomy and taxonomists, but we try to make amends for our lapses by providing a brief glossary in Appendix F.

Names of species are not shown in the table headings but as numbered footnotes, and these include common synonyms (limited to names most often used in the last twenty years) so that, with the Index, it should be possible to trace the main characters of many named species. The older generic names *Bacterium* and *Bacillus* (except for the aerobic sporeformers) are not included in the brief synonymies.

In general the tables make possible the identification of species that can often be broken down into serotypes and phage types. However, users of the *Manual* will seldom have all the sera needed to work out the detailed antigenic structure of the species they isolate; this is a task for a reference laboratory. Those who aspire to do this work themselves should consult the excellent practical manual by Edwards & Ewing (1962, 1972) which spotlights the problems and, for the Enterobacteriaceae, gives the essential details.

Our tables seldom mention sensitivity or resistance to antibiotics; our view is that in this era of antibiotic therapy and feeding, the organisms we isolate are the survivors resistant to the enthusiasm of clinicians and farmers. If the predictions of E. S. Anderson (1966) are correct – and the work of J. D. Anderson, Gillespie & Richmond (1973) suggests they are – the genetic effects of antibiotics may affect more characters than sensitivity to antibiotics.

We have added many more references and by so doing are able to refer readers to pertinent literature in which fuller details of methods are given; in this way we are able to keep this *Manual* free from detail unnecessary for the diagnostician, and from the more theoretical aspects of taxonomy and nomenclature.

In plan the *Manual* falls into two parts: the first, divided into chapters is discursive; the second, made up of appendices, is instructive, written tersely, and there is free use of abbreviations (which conform to Ellis, 1971), chemical formulae, and prescription-like recipes for media. The heart of the book is in Chapters 6 and 7, which are made up of the diagnostic tables and notes on the different genera. In this edition we have included more little-known genera, many of them incompletely worked out; it may seem to readers that we have wandered outside the medical field, but if we have it is to the fresh pastures and waters of the food microbiologists that we have strayed.

We have also given a practical example of the application of our diagnostic tables and the information they contain to the preparation of punched cards for easy sorting and identification.

1
Classification and nomenclature

Taxonomy is not every man's meat, neither is it everyone's poison; but what needs to be said of it now should not be indigestible. For those interested in taxonomy Chapters 8 and 9 will form a more stimulating diet, even if they are not found to be particularly appetizing or palatable. By diverting the taxonomist to the later chapters we hope to encourage others to look upon identification as one of the most interesting fields of bacteriology, the orchard into which the fruits of taxonomic work will fall when mature and ripe, for the benefit of the rich (taxonomists) and poor (clinicians) alike.

Taxonomy can be likened to a cocktail; it is a mixture of three components skilfully blended so that the outsider relishes the whole and cannot discern the individual ingredients. In taxonomy the ingredients are: (i) *classification*, or the orderly arrangement of units, (ii) *nomenclature*, the naming or labelling of units, (iii) *identification* of the unknown with a unit defined and named by (i) and (ii). The subdivisions should be taken in the order indicated, for without adequate classification it is impossible to name rationally, and without a system of labelled units it is impossible to identify others with them and communicate the result to a third person.

1.1 Classification

Before discussing identification, the subject of this *Manual*, we must first deal briefly with the principles of classification and nomenclature; but since this book is essentially a practical manual, theoretical considerations of the validity of bacterial species (Lwoff, 1958; Cowan, 1962a) have no place here.

For a book of this kind we must accept the bacterial species as a convenient unit, but as it so obviously has different values in different groups of bacteria we do not attempt to define it, or repeat

our attempt to analyse the qualities that distinguish one species from another or determine whether the taxon (taxonomic group) is a species, a variety or subspecies, neither do we try to estimate the value or importance of different kinds of character (Cowan, 1968b, 1970b). We dislike subspecies but recognize subdivisions of species either as varieties (biotypes) or as serotypes; we cannot accept Kauffmann's (1959a, b; 1963b) contention that the serotypes or the phage types of the various members of the Enterobacteriaceae should be equated with species. The collection of similar species into larger groups (genera), and similar (we do not say related) genera into families, are convenient groupings and have found common usage.

However, we do not believe that these are phylogenetic groupings and we are not willing to combine families into even larger groups (orders) which we regard as artificial and highly speculative. The different kinds of bacteria are not separated by sharp divisions but by slight and subtle differences in characters so that they seem to blend into each other and resemble a spectrum (Fig. 1.1a and b). The spectrum-like intergrading of different kinds of bacteria is confirmed by newer methods of grouping, such as the base composition of the deoxyribonucleic acid (DNA) of the bacterial cell (Vendrely, 1958). The DNA of a bacterial group should be homogeneous (Rolfe & Meselson, 1959), and different groups often have different DNA compositions. Marmur, Falkow & Mandel (1963) and Hill (1966) collected the results of numerous workers and summarized in tables the DNA-base composition of many bacteria. These techniques are not applicable to day-to-day diagnostic work but the results are of fundamental importance to the taxonomist.

A theoretical classificatory scheme divides the

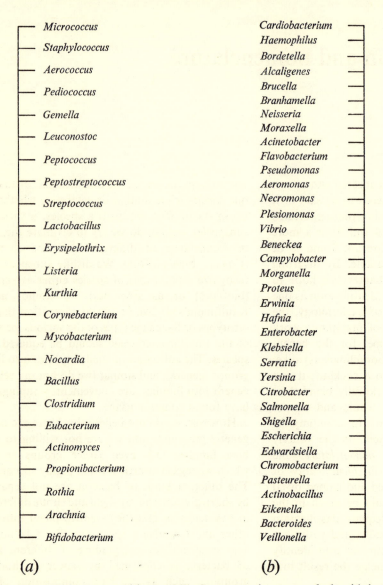

Micrococcus	Cardiobacterium
Staphylococcus	Haemophilus
Aerococcus	Bordetella
Pediococcus	Alcaligenes
Gemella	Brucella
Leuconostoc	Branhamella
Peptococcus	Neisseria
Peptostreptococcus	Moraxella
Streptococcus	Acinetobacter
Lactobacillus	Flavobacterium
Erysipelothrix	Pseudomonas
Listeria	Aeromonas
Kurthia	Necromonas
Corynebacterium	Plesiomonas
Mycobacterium	Vibrio
Nocardia	Beneckea
Bacillus	Campylobacter
Clostridium	Morganella
Eubacterium	Proteus
Actinomyces	Erwinia
Propionibacterium	Hafnia
Rothia	Enterobacter
Arachnia	Klebsiella
Bifidobacterium	Serratia
	Yersinia
	Citrobacter
	Salmonella
	Shigella
	Escherichia
	Edwardsiella
	Chromobacterium
	Pasteurella
	Actinobacillus
	Eikenella
	Bacteroides
	Veillonella

(a)   (b)

Fig. 1.1(a) Gram-positive, and (b) Gram-negative genera dealt with in this *Manual*.

higher ranks into two or more kinds of a lower rank; for example, *Bergey's Manual* (1923–57) divides the kingdom Bacteria into orders and continues the breakdown through families, tribes, genera, and species; however, the latest edition (1974) does not attempt to produce a complete hierarchy.

We suggest that a pragmatic classification should be built up from the basal unit (species); basal units which share a number of characters are combined to form the next higher unit (genus), and the common characters become those which are important in the definition or characterization of the genus. The stressing of certain characters (which we say are important characters because they are significant in identification), differs from the Adansonian concept (that it is proper to apply to orthodox theoretical classification (Sneath, 1957a)), in which each character has equal merit in the eyes of the taxonomist.

2

What we call 'important characters' may be of three kinds: (i) *specific*, as the ability to produce coagulase by *Staphylococcus aureus*; (ii) *distinguishing* characters which, while not specific, are useful in separating organisms that are otherwise very similar. An example is indole production by *Proteus vulgaris*, one of the characters that distinguishes it from *P. mirabilis*; (iii) characters *shared* by all members of a group; thus, acid fastness is an important character of mycobacteria (since all members are acid fast) but not of the nocardias (only some of which are acid fast).

Needless to say, there are degrees of importance and it would be feasible to continue the list; but we think that we have said enough to illustrate the point that characters can have an importance in a pragmatic scheme that they are denied in an Adansonian classification.

Taxonomists use and put much weight on what are called 'fermentation tests' without paying much attention to the type of carbohydrate breakdown; this is characteristic of an organism and of great informative value to the diagnostician. In this connexion we follow Hugh & Leifson (1953) and use the terms 'oxidative' and 'fermentative' though it is not at all certain that these words describe accurately what is happening in the test, which we shall refer to as the Oxidation–Fermentation (OF) test.

We think that a practical classification should be based on characters that are easily determined; consequently we cannot use features that demand difficult techniques or special apparatus. Thus, cytological details of the bacterium such as cell walls, septa, nuclei, and fimbriae do not find a place in our scheme although we are well aware of their importance and know that to add them would increase the weight of our arguments and support our general conclusions.

Again, because it is difficult, even with an electron microscope, to obtain an accurate picture of the arrangement of flagella on bacteria, we have placed little weight on this character which, in all except the most rigidly Adansonian taxonomy, is given a very important place.

The scheme we use is built on a wide range of characters; the identification of each unit is based on the same characters and it is not necessary to

make the hypothetical (and sometimes absurd) assumptions of classical taxonomy.

By omitting the type of flagellation we do not need to postulate that *Shigella* species, if they had any, would have peritrichous flagella.

We do not use any formal classificatory scheme but, because of the need to label recognizable taxonomic units (usually at the level of species), we take advantage of the specific epithets and generic names that are parts of formal systems. We shall discuss labelling more fully in Chapter 9; here we deal only with the problems that immediately concern the identification of bacteria, and how the organisms are to be described in reports to clinicians and health officers.

It is convenient to divide bacteria into two large groups based on the reactions of the organisms to Gram's method of staining, but we do not give latinized names to these groups. In formal schemes most genera are made up of bacteria that are either Gram positive or Gram negative, so that we can distribute them according to the Gram reaction of the majority of species they contain. We can arrange the genera in some order whereby adjacent genera show some similarities but the more distant ones have less in common (Fig. 1.1*a, b*); the arrangement resembles a series of pigeon-holes (or two series, one for Gram positives, the other for Gram negatives), and we can imagine that the partitions between the individual pigeon-holes can be removed so that the contents of adjacent holes will be in contact with each other. But although we look upon bacteria as a series of gradually intergrading forms and liken them to a spectrum, we do not imply that the sequences shown in Fig. 1.1*a, b* are the best that can be devised to show relationships, if existent, between the genera. The sequences have some merit in that they do not violate too severely the order that might be presented in a classification made on orthodox lines. A point that we should stress is that the lists of names in Fig. 1.1*a, b* are those of taxa that are normally regarded as having generic rank; they are not an attempt at a classification. Most of the names have been in use for a long time and are generally accepted; to change them is not our wish.

With some bacteria the Gram reaction is regarded as variable, indeterminate, and occasionally misleading. Many cocci and some rods may be positive in young cultures and become negative as the culture ages; in such cases it is usual to treat the reaction of the young culture as correct. Occasionally the opposite sequence of reactions is observed; Acinetobacter strains may acquire a slight Gram positivity in cultures several days old and some workers (e.g. Thornley, 1967) describe them as Gram variable; this is a phenomenon better known outside the medical field, as in the genus *Arthrobacter*. Gemella strains are unusual in that when stained they seem to be Gram negative, but in the chemical nature of the cell wall they resemble the Gram-positive bacteria. Although cell wall analysis is far from being a routine procedure we have shown the genus *Gemella* in Fig. 1.1*a* (i.e. among the Gram-positive bacteria) but show the characters of the species in tables dealing with both Gram-positive (Table 6.3) and Gram-negative (Table 7.3) cocci.

Because we do not start with an orthodox classification in a hierarchical system it may be objected that we cannot present the identifying characteristics of bacteria in a logical manner. On the contrary, we believe that by avoiding a formal classification we can display the characters in a manner that is both logical and orderly; that similarities and differences shown by the tables will point the way to a more orderly arrangement of the different taxa. And, as orderly arrangements are the essence of all classifications, our tables may lead to a logical classification, which completes this circular argument.

It is essential that the reader should understand that there is not one classification (made by God, Nature, or by man) but any number of classifications, all made by men, each with a particular purpose in mind. The main difficulty created by the omission of a classification relates to the labelling of the taxa; we get over this difficulty in our tables by using the name(s) by which each taxon (usually a species) is generally known, irrespective of the rightness of the name(s) in terms of the Bacteriological Code. The taxa listed in Fig. 1.1*a, b* are groups approximating to genera (*Chromobacterium* might represent two genera), and the components of these groups will be species whose characters are shown in the secondary (and tertiary) tables in

Chapters 6 and 7. Usually the acceptable name for a group will be obvious and well known. Names such as *Clostridium welchii* are not used in American- and French-speaking countries but are understood, just as English-speaking bacteriologists understand what is meant by *Serratia marcescens*.

The Gram-positive and Gram-negative bacteria can each be considered as a continuous series. Some of the genera shown in Fig. 1.1*a, b* are dealt with only summarily in this *Manual* but they are mentioned because they may be met either as contaminants or as suspected pathogens. We could not fit into our scheme such organisms as Leptospira and other spirochaetes that are diagnosed on morphological and serological grounds, or on their pathogenicity for various animals. Neither do we deal with mycoplasms, though we make passing reference to them (Section 7.10.5). Our purpose is to identify bacteria isolated in medical laboratories, commonly, if incorrectly, called the medical bacteria. They are mainly from clinical material (hospital laboratories) but may be from apparently healthy individuals (public health laboratories), and from water, sewage, and foodstuffs. Apparently identical bacteria may produce infection in animals other than man, so our survey must cover the fields of medical and veterinary science, and it will impinge on plant pathology and industrial processes.

1.2   Nomenclature

In this *Manual* emphasis is put on the characterization of organisms, for it is a waste of time to work out carefully the characters of the unknown and then compare these with vague descriptions. We have not made any great point about nomenclature, believing that a simple label, as long as it is unique, is adequate for communication. In the tables of Chapters 6 and 7 the columns of characters of a taxon are numbered and the name(s) by which the taxon is known will be found in numbered footnotes. The first name, usually in bold type, is what we regard as the most acceptable name; this is often, but not necessarily, the nomenclaturally correct name. What is important is that everyone concerned – the bacteriologist, the clinician, and the health official – should all understand what organism is being reported; in our more academic days we found that the nomenclaturally correct name often meant little outside the laboratory and those in charge of patients could be blissfully unaware of the nature of the organism reported; on the other hand, the common name in English was always understood. In our tables we give, for good measure, other names used in English- and American-speaking countries; these synonyms appear in the footnotes without further explanation. Our schooldays have left such permanent scars that Latin and latinized names in the text are avoided as far as possible; similar scars affect most Englishmen, who seem to be less literate than Americans, who revel in latinization.

We do not propose to discuss in this chapter the problems and principles of nomenclature, but we must point out now that, as nomenclature is dependent on classification, there may be more than one correct name for a bacterium. Nomenclature is subject to the Rules and Recommendations of the Bacteriological Code; there are not, and never can be, any rules for classification. Classification is subjective and a matter of opinion, and it is within the rights (if not the competence) of each worker to classify bacteria as he will. The classification adopted determines the names to be appended to the organisms, and the rules of nomenclature should be a guide to the choice of correct names. If a worker believes that all rod-shaped organisms are to be grouped together in one genus, he is entitled to name the diphtheria organism *Bacillus diphtheriae*, but if he thinks that rod-shaped bacteria can be split into different groups he can use a name such as *Corynebacterium diphtheriae*; each name is correct within its own taxonomic scheme or classification, and would be wrong in the other scheme. Regrettably, the application of the Rules of the Code is subjective and different workers may draw quite different conclusions from reading the Rules and may interpret them in contrasting and even conflicting ways.

One of the aims of the Bacteriological Code is to stabilize nomenclature; this is an impossibility for nomenclature is itself dependent on ever-changing ideas on classification. The rediscovery and application of an old or the development of a new technique may act on taxonomists as a blood transfusion.

Sometimes, an organism remains unclassified for decades after its discovery and characterization. Morgan's no. 1 bacillus (Morgan, 1906) needed the insight of Rauss (1936) and the discovery that under the right conditions it could be made to swarm, to recognize it as a species of *Proteus*. It was the rediscovery and application of the phenylalanine test that made Singer & Bar-Chey (1954) see that Stuart's 29911 (Stuart, Wheeler & McGann, 1946) or Providence group was a species of *Proteus*.

It is often easier to create a new genus or species than to do the comparative work necessary to put an organism into its rightful place in an existing genus or species. The temptation to designate a new genus or species should be resisted; it would be if people realized that the ability of a taxonomist is judged as inversely proportional to the number of new taxa he has created.

Many workers use common names (in the vernacular of the country) in preference to scientific names that are subject to change. Since English is now the language of science, common English names are widely understood, but French or German equivalents may present difficulty to English-speaking people (e.g. Bacteridie de charbon = der Milzbrandbazillus = the anthrax bacillus = *Bacillus anthracis*). The great advantage of the latinized binomial is that it is accepted throughout the world and the same word should have the same meaning everywhere. Although printed in the same way, even in journals using pictorial characters, the sound is not always the same as is apparent when the different pronunciations of the epithet 'anthracis' are compared.

Nomenclature often presents difficulties because a change in name may be necessary when an organism is moved from one group to another. Sometimes the nomenclatural difficulties arise because the Rules, first published in 1948 (Buchanan, St John-Brooks & Breed, 1948), revised and annotated in 1958 (Buchanan *et al.* 1958), revised again in 1966, were made retroactive. This means that we should apply them to names first used in the last century, long before a Bacteriological Code was thought of, and in some instances, before the organism named had been isolated and characterized. The Code is undergoing further revision and, we hope, simplification; if some of the suggestions

5

that have been made are approved, the International Committee on Systematic Bacteriology (the successor to the International Nomenclature Committee) will make lists of approved names and after 1 January 1980 the petty squabbles on priority of names should be abolished. Such a day cannot come too soon.

Another source of confusion is due to the well-intentioned efforts of workers to give a meaning to the specific epithet, and to make the epithet appropriate. In the 1930s one of us was concerned with an ill-conceived attempt to apply an appropriate epithet 'pyogenes' to the generic name *Staphylococcus* because the legitimate epithet 'aureus' was inappropriate when applied to strains that produced white colonies. In more recent times Foster & Bragg (1962) suggested that various specific epithets for *Klebsiella*, correctly proposed (by the Rules), should be transposed (which would

greatly add to confusion) because, as originally proposed, they seemed to them to be inappropriate.

Another source of confusion is the re-use of a discarded name for a newly described genus or species. An example is the use of *Aerobacter* (a later synonym of *Klebsiella*) for a group of motile organisms which share several characters with non-motile organisms formerly named *Aerobacter aerogenes*. This confusion was remedied by its authors (Hormaeche & Edwards, 1960) who withdrew their proposal and substituted the new generic name *Enterobacter*. Unfortunately so many authors continued to use the name *Aerobacter* for both motile and non-motile organisms that the problem was submitted (Carpenter *et al.* 1970) to the Judicial Commission for an Official Opinion on the validity of the name *Aerobacter*; the Commission ruled (Opinion 46, 1971) against the use of the generic name *Aerobacter* because its application was uncertain.

2
Media: constituents and sterilization

In a Postgatian introduction to a *Good Food Guide* for bacteria, Miles (1965) described most media formulations as 'frankly kitchen recipes, written ... by increasingly sophisticated cooks'. There are two entirely different kinds of media and the distinction is between defined media and those of undefined composition, usually containing peptone. Defined media have disadvantages for the diagnostician because the characters of the organisms grown in them may differ from those developed in undefined media (Meynell & Meynell, 1965). In general, published descriptions of bacteria are those found after growth in complex, undefined media, and the results of biochemical tests do not always correspond with those obtained in defined media.

Media preparation seldom receives the attention it deserves; moreover, the media room is often overcrowded and understaffed, and the conditions in which media-makers work are usually the worst in the laboratory.

Complaints about media, both commercial and home prepared, are so common that some laboratories have opened a control department adequately staffed to be able to watch media making in all its stages and to test the final products.

In this chapter we shall discuss the general aspects of media making; formulae for the different media will be found in Appendix A, beginning on p. 137.

The majority of the commonly used culture media are now commercially available as dehydrated products which are reconstituted by the addition of distilled water and then sterilized in the conventional manner. The manufacturers' directions for reconstitution should be followed for best results. The advantages of dehydrated media include ease of preparation without the necessity of pH adjustment or phosphate removal, batch to batch uniformity which is often greater than with laboratory prepared media, convenience for the preparation of small quantities, ease of storage, and economy especially in saving time and labour. Against these must be set certain disadvantages: primarily, the absence of control by the user. Most of the dehydrated products are hygroscopic but this can be overcome by the use of plastic or foil sachets containing sufficient for one batch of medium. Dehydration is not suitable for media containing blood, other thermolabile components, or egg. An important consideration where dehydrated media are widely used is that technical staff are not adequately trained in media preparation.

While ordinary media may be used for the growth of strict anaerobes, better growth will be obtained when the media are reduced before inoculation rather than after inoculated plates and slopes have been put in an anaerobic jar. Ideally, reduction should be made during preparation of the media, reduced conditions maintained during storage and, as far as possible, during inoculation. The techniques used are quite specialized and are described fully in the *Anaerobe Laboratory Manual* (1972) of the Virginia Polytechnic Institute. There are three essential steps in the preparation of reduced media, unnecessarily termed 'prereduced anaerobically sterilized' or PRAS media, namely: (i) driving off dissolved oxygen by boiling, (ii) addition of cysteine, and (iii) flushing with oxygen-free gas and storing in stoppered bottles containing oxygen-free gas. These media contain an Eh indicator (resazurin) which is colourless when reduced; if oxidation occurs the contents of the bottle becomes pink, indicating that it should not be used. Oxidized reducing agent may be toxic. Cysteine inhibits some proteolytic enzymes, so should not be added to media for tests of this property.

2.1   Media for a purpose

Not all media are intended to encourage the growth of all bacteria; media are tailored to the organism(s) they are to encourage, and sometimes made unsuitable for the growth of certain (specified) organisms.

2.1.1   Media for isolation

may be simple nutrient media containing all essential constituents for growth; in medical laboratories the commonest general purpose medium is blood agar, but often chocolate agar may be more successful in the isolation of fastidious bacteria. We generally know the nature of the specimen we are to examine and, by exercising an intelligent anticipation of the probable bacterial flora, we choose a medium or media to suit the nutritional requirements of the organisms we can reasonably expect to find. For some bacteria the medium is made from constituents of known composition (that is, a defined medium) but most organisms isolated from clinical material are exacting and need the basal nutrient medium to be enriched or supplemented by ill-defined substances such as serum, ascitic fluid, or blood. Thus media used in medical and veterinary laboratories are rich in unspecified protein and encourage the growth of both wanted and unwanted organisms.

2.1.2   Selective or inhibitory media.

When the specimen is from a part of the body (skin, throat, mouth, nose, intestine, vagina) that has a natural microbial flora, growth of the normal inhabitants may be inconveniently profuse and the bacteriologist will want to limit or suppress them and at the same time encourage growth of the invaders which, in clinical pathology, are the 'wanted' organisms. For this, selective or inhibitory media are developed, and as the inhibitory properties may be specific, the media must be chosen with some particular organism (or group of organisms) in mind. There is no such thing as a medium exclusively or universally selective for pathogens, and it might seem that the successful clinical bacteriologist must be one who can predict accurately which bacteria are to be inhibited and what are the requirements of those that are to be encouraged. Since prediction is not one of a bacteriologist's skills, most workers increase their chances of isolating the wanted organism by using several kinds of selective media.

2.1.3   Enrichment media,

which are usually both selective and inhibitory, are liquids into which a swab or specimen is placed; after incubation for 6 and 18 hours subcultures are made to plates of (i) selective, and (ii) nutrient, non-inhibitory media (nutrient agar, blood agar). After incubation these plates are examined and subcultures made from selected colonies to non-inhibitory media. This second plating is an important step in the isolation process; without it the chances are that the colony picked will produce a mixture of wanted and unwanted organisms. Whenever possible, bacteriologists* avoid selective media and prefer to work from repeated platings on non-inhibitory media, but we all know that this is a council of perfection, seldom satisfied by practice.

2.1.4   Media for maintenance

are simple and should not encourage too luxurious a growth; nutrient agar (in its many formulations) is the commonest (see Lapage, Shelton & Mitchell, 1970). For the preservation of serological characters, Dorset egg, in spite of its imperfections, seems to be the medium of choice. An all-round maintenance medium for anaerobes is Robertson's cooked meat medium.

2.1.5   Media for determining nutritional requirements or ability to use a substrate

are being used increasingly in diagnostic work. To avoid chemical contaminants agar of the highest purity (Table A5 footnote) should be used for solid media. When the nutritional requirements of an organism are unknown, omission of one component at a time and substitution by another may be used to find which substrates are essential and which can be replaced by a substitute. This is a time-consuming process not used in routine work. But in a simplified form, as in Koser's citrate medium, a test for the

* The difference between a bacteriologist and a microbiologist is most clearly seen in the media he uses; a microbiologist uses defined (the illiterate call them synthetic) media; the bacteriologist uses media as a means to an end, and doesn't worry too much about their composition.

8

ability to use citrate as a carbon source, is a useful characterizing test for enteric bacteriology.

For non-exacting bacteria a basal medium inadequate for the growth of the organism is used and to it one substrate at a time is added to find out whether the organism can use the substrate as carbon or nitrogen source. A suitable mineral base of this kind was described by Owens & Keddie (1969) and Cure & Keddie (1973). For the value of these tests see Snell & Lapage (1973).

Chemically clean glassware is essential for tests that are to determine the nutritional requirements of an organism; dirty glassware can provide nutrients; it may also be contaminated by inhibitors (see Section A 1.1).

2.1.6   Media for characterization generally consist of a simple (but nutritionally adequate) base to which the substrate under test has been added. Sometimes an indicator is included to show that a change in reaction has occurred; in other cases reagents are added after a set time of incubation, and the effect (colour change, precipitate formation, etc.) observed.

2.1.7   Media for screening are intended to show at a glance the reactions obtained with several substrates, hence the name multitest media; they can be relied upon only when pure cultures are used. Multitest media are popular in the USA but are less frequently used in Europe. The Knox (1949) plate, described as a screening plate, cannot be used for the original specimen. Some media intended for multitest usage find a better use as a standard, relatively insensitive method for one of the tests, as is seen in the use of TSI for H_2S production by enterobacteria.

2.1.8   Media for microbiological assay of vitamins and amino acids need stringent control to ensure freedom from impurities; commercial sources (Appendix H) supply such media. The assay of antibiotics and the sensitivity testing of micro-organisms do not need media of rigid specification and can be carried out on ordinary nutrient media, with or without indicator.

2.1.9   Non-nutrient basal media. Occasionally a clear solidifying medium without nutrient properties is wanted. Such a medium is needed for the top layer of chitin agar; the insoluble chitin is suspended in water- or salt-agar.

Saline agar has other uses. As physiological saline solidified with agar it may be used to line tubes into which rabbit blood is shed. After the blood has clotted the agar lining retracts with the clot, and the serum, expressed through the agar, is water clear. Such serum is anti-complementary.

2.2   Media constituents

A fuller account of peptone, meat extract, yeast extract, gelatin, agar, and bile salts is given in the Special Report of the Society for General Microbiology on constituents of bacteriological culture media (Report, 1956a); the design and formulation of media is reviewed by Bridson & Brecker (1970).

2.2.1   Agar can be obtained as shreds, flakes, granules or powder and is made from certain types of seaweed. The usefulness of its unusual gelling properties for bacteriological work was recognized by Frau Hesse, who suggested its use to her husband, Walther Hesse, an early colleague of Robert Koch (Bulloch, 1938; Hitchens & Leikind, 1939).

When mixed with cold water agar does not go into solution; as a consequence it can be washed to free it from soluble impurities. The concentration to be used depends on the geographic source or species of the seaweed from which the agar is made, and on the purpose for which the medium is intended (Table A5, p. 141). In the formulae for media described in this *Manual* the concentration of agar relates to the product from Japanese seaweed.

In addition to the agar concentration other factors will affect gel strength; for example, repeated melting of the medium or sterilization at a low pH value will decrease it.

2.2.2   Peptone is a product of varying composition made by acid or enzymic hydrolysis of animal or vegetable protein, such as muscle, liver, blood, milk, casein, lactalbumin, gelatin, and soya bean. The exact composition will depend on the raw material and the method of manufacture.

No two batches of peptone are exactly alike, but commercial firms now try to produce peptones in which the measurable constituents are present within certain defined limits. For many kinds of media the make or type of peptone is immaterial, but for certain tests a particular type may be specified (e.g. Eupeptone no. 1 for British Standard 541: 1934). This does not mean that all other types are unsuitable, more often than not it means that other peptones have not been tried. Certain batches of peptone, however, may be quite unsuitable for a particular purpose, and before being taken into use a peptone should be tested. In Appendix A in the section on media control we discuss this problem in more detail and give examples of fallacious results due to the use of unsuitable peptones. Our own experience of peptones is limited to English products such as Evans, Oxoid and Benger's, and American such as Difco and BBL, but we are assured that other peptones (e.g. the Danish Orthana) are equally good.

2.2.3   Meat. Beef heart, muscle, and liver are commonly used but calf brain, veal, spleen, and placenta also have a place in media preparation. The quality of meat and other tissues varies with the age and health of the animal and with the conditions under which it was slaughtered. As far as we know the effect on media of using meat 'tenderized' by papain has not been investigated. To minimize variations the preparation of meat media requires extensive quality control, and this may be impracticable for small laboratories. In these circumstances, commercial meat extracts or dehydrated meat media are often more convenient. When meat media are to be used as the basis for fermentation studies, they should be tested for the absence of fermentable carbohydrate.

2.2.4   Meat extract. Commercial meat extracts contain soluble organic bases, protein degradation products, vitamins, and minerals. As these extracts are readily available and easy to use they have largely superseded fresh meat infusions which are both time-consuming to prepare and variable in quality.

2.2.5   Yeast extract is made from bakers' or brewers' yeast and is a rich source of amino acids and vitamins of the B-complex. In culture media it is used to supplement or replace meat extracts. In our laboratory we replaced beef extract (1 %) by yeast extract (0.3 %) in nutrient broth without significant change in the growth-promoting capacity.

2.2.6   Blood. The choice of blood is often a matter of convenience and depends on the animals kept by a laboratory. When bought from a commercial source we commonly use horse blood, but the blood of other species (man, goat, rabbit, sheep) may be used for special purposes. Sheep blood agar can be used for detecting the different haemolysins of staphylococci (Elek & Levy, 1954); sheep and goat blood are said to be lysed by el Tor vibrios, but human blood may also be used. Sodium citrate is said to be inhibitory to staphylococci (Rammell, 1962) and Liquoid to anaerobic cocci (Holdeman & Moore, 1972). Our preference is for defibrinated horse blood; it should be relatively fresh and should not be used when haemolysis is obvious. Blood must be stored in a refrigerator but should not be allowed to freeze; all blood products must be tested for sterility.

2.2.7   Plasma is used for demonstrating coagulase activity. In medical bacteriology human plasma is preferred but rabbit plasma may be used. As some bacteria utilize citrate, oxalated plasma is better but citrated plasma may be used when heparin is added (Harper & Conway, 1948). Plasma may be obtained by removing the supernatant of blood + anticoagulant in which the red cells have settled. Blood samples obtained for biochemical examination and containing sodium fluoride or ethylene-diaminetetra-acetic acid ('sequestric acid') are to be avoided. Liquid plasma is an unstable product liable to coagulate or to form particles which cause a turbidity or deposit. It should not be filtered. Plasma should be stored in a refrigerator but should not be frozen. Dehydrated plasma is available commercially.

2.2.8   Serum is prepared from blood, collected without addition of an anticoagulant, by removal of the liquid which separates when the clot contracts. Alternatively it may be citrated plasma clotted by calcium. Serum should be sterilized by filtration. Horse serum may contain a maltase and an amylase and it is essential that these be inactivated by heat before addition to maltose- or starch-containing media (Goldsworthy, Still & Dumaresq, 1938). Hendry (1938) reported that the maltase was inactivated at 75 °C for 30 minutes but not at 55 °C for 4 hours; Goldsworthy *et al.* (1938) recommended heating serum at 65 °C for 1 hour. Horse serum kept at 0–4 °C for a month or longer may show a deposit, believed to contain calcium, lipids and protein (Roche & Marquet, 1935) and this deposit may be mistaken for bacterial contamination.

2.2.9 **Ascitic** and **hydrocele** fluids are preferred to serum by some workers in hospitals. Most laboratories do not use them because they are not generally available.

2.2.10 **Bile** contains several bile acids as compounds conjugated with amino acids; bile acids can also form addition compounds with higher fatty acids and other substances. Bile also contains the pigments bilirubin and biliverdin. Fresh ox bile (ox gall) has been superseded either by bile extract, dehydrated bile or bile salts. Bile extract, a dark yellowish green plastic material, is prepared by concentration of fresh bile, extraction with 90% ethanol, and evaporation of the ethanolic extract. A 10% solution of the dehydrated product is equivalent to fresh bile.

2.2.11 **Bile salts.** Commercial bile salts are prepared by extracting dried ox or pig bile with ethanol, decolorizing the extract with charcoal, and precipitating the bile salts with ether to form a water-soluble yellowish-brown hygroscopic powder. When prepared from ox bile the salts consist mainly of sodium taurocholate and sodium glycocholate with smaller amounts of the sodium salts of taurodeoxycholic and glycodeoxycholic acids. The bile acid conjugates may be hydrolysed by alkali, and it is possible to prepare sodium cholate or deoxycholate but these substances are not chemically pure. Several workers (Mair, 1917; Downie, Stent & White, 1931) showed that in bacteriology deoxy-

cholic acid is the most active component of bile and its effects were studied by Leifson (1935).

2.2.12 **Gelatin** is the protein obtained by extraction of collagenous material, and is available as sheets, shreds, granules or powder. A gelatin of pharmaceutical or edible grade should be used for culture media. When immersed in water below 20 °C, gelatin does not dissolve but swells and imbibes 5–10 times its weight of water. Solution is effected by heating and the solution gels on cooling to about 25 °C. Gelatin has little nutritive value but is used in culture media as a substrate for detecting gelatinase activity. As with agar gels, excessive heating is detrimental and destroys the setting properties.

2.2.13 **Carbohydrates.** The bacteriologist uses carbohydrates (collectively called 'sugars') to enrich media for growth, pigmentation, and to determine whether the organism can produce acid or acid and gas from them. The carbohydrates generally used are listed in Table A2 (p. 139), which also includes glycosides and polyhydric alcohols, with concentrations of aqueous solutions suitable for addition to media. The concentration of carbohydrate in oxidation and fermentation studies is usually 0.5–1%; we prefer 1% carbohydrate as reversion of the reaction is then less likely. Some carbohydrate solutions may be sterilized by autoclaving whereas with others decomposition may occur. Durham (1898) recommended steaming for 'sugars' but Mudge (1917) found that maltose and lactose suffered greater hydrolysis when steamed on three days than when autoclaved at 121 °C for 15 minutes. Smith (1932) showed the adverse effect of heat and the accelerated decomposition of glucose and maltose in the presence of phosphate.

Although Whittenbury (1963) found that some lactic acid bacteria differed in oxygen requirements for fermentation in media (i) made up with carbohydrate before sterilization, and (ii) with filtered or autoclaved carbohydrate solution added to previously autoclaved basal medium, he could not detect any significant difference in the ability of the organisms to utilize the substrate sterilized by the different methods. Solutions are often sterilized by momentary autoclaving or by steaming but we think it is better to sterilize them by filtration.

We have deliberately omitted dextrin from the list of carbohydrates. White dextrin is generally prepared by heating starch, which has been moistened with a small volume of dilute nitric acid and dried, at 100–120 °C; it contains up to 15% of starch, the remainder consists of erythrodextrin. Inferior grades are prepared by roasting starch without acid at 150–250 °C, and have a yellow colour; they are hydrolysed to a greater extent than white dextrin and may contain appreciable quantities of maltose. Because of its variable composition, we do not recommend the use of dextrin. Soluble starch is prepared by treating potato starch with dilute hydrochloric acid until, after washing, it forms a limpid, almost clear solution in hot water; it is insoluble in cold.

2.2.14 Defined media for studies of bacterial nutrition and CSU (carbon source utilization) tests are solutions of mineral salts to which the substrate being tested is added. For nutritionally exacting organisms, e.g. the coryneforms, media such as mineral salts medium E (Owens & Keddie, 1969) need to be supplemented with 0.02% yeast extract and $2 \mu g$ vitamin B_{12} per litre (R. M. Keddie, personal communication).

2.3   Indicators
pH indicators are incorporated in some culture media and give visual evidence of pH changes occurring during the growth of bacteria. Indicators for this purpose must be non-toxic in the concentrations used; some samples of neutral red may inhibit growth of *Escherichia coli* in MacConkey broth (Childs & Allen, 1953). With some bacteria (e.g. *Actinomyces israelii*) we have observed better growth in media containing ethanolic than in media with aqueous indicator, showing that the solvent was being used as a readily available carbon source. Where the indicator is prepared as its sodium salt it is preferable to use water as the solvent. Table A1 (p. 138) lists the pH indicators commonly used; the concentrations recommended are for the purpose of adding concentrated indicator solutions to culture media and are not necessarily suitable for the colorimetric determination of pH

values. Many indicators and mixtures now used in chemistry have not yet been applied to bacteriology.

Indicators of oxidation–reduction potential (redox indicators) have limited use in culture media. Examples are methylene blue or resazurin in thioglycollate media and methylene blue in milk (Ulrich, 1944).

The use of tetrazolium compounds (e.g. 2:3:5-triphenyltetrazolium chloride) as indicators of bacterial growth has been advocated, for example in motility media (Kelly & Fulton, 1953) and in KCN broth (Gershman, 1961). As bacterial growth occurs the colourless reagent is reduced to an insoluble red formazan.

2.4   Sterilization by heat
Sterilization may be a misnomer when it is applied to the processes to which media or media constituents are subjected. In some cases, Tyndallization for example, the heat applied is sufficient only to kill vegetative bacteria. Again, media that appear to be sterile may contain viable spores of thermophils that are incapable of growing at the temperatures at which sterility tests are normally carried out (37 °C). Labile media constituents that are normally kept at about 4 °C may contain organisms that grow at room temperature but not at 37 °C; such material will pass the usual sterility tests. However, we do not think that we should attempt to qualify the words sterility or sterilization, for to write of partial sterility is a contradiction in terms.

For the safety of those who work in a laboratory, all discarded cultures (even those from water examinations), infected glassware, and plastic containers must be sterilized in the strictest sense, even although some of the material will ultimately be destroyed by incineration. The use of bowls of disinfectant for the disposal of cultures in Petri dishes and test tubes cannot be tolerated, and it should be an inviolable rule that all discarded cultures are sterilized by heat.

The lethal action of heat depends both on the temperature and the time for which it is applied; the higher the temperature the shorter the time needed to destroy micro-organisms. Sporing bacteria are more resistant to heat than vegetative bacteria, but all sporing forms are not equally resistant. Some, such as *Bacillus subtilis* spores, are killed by a short exposure to 100 °C; others, such as those of *B. licheniformis* and *B. stearothermophilus*, may resist boiling for hours or survive autoclaving at low pressures for short times. Heat, the only safe method for sterilizing discarded cultures, must reach all the plates in the discard bin, and to ensure adequate heat penetration, autoclaving must be at higher temperatures than those used for the sterilization of culture media; we use a time–temperature combination of 20 minutes at 127 °C (1.5 kg/cm²).

2.4.1   Autoclaving. An autoclave is a pressure vessel and must be regarded as potentially dangerous. When air has been expelled and the vessel is filled with saturated steam there is a relation between temperature and pressure (Table 2.1); if air is present, the temperature will be lower than that corresponding to the steam pressure.

Table 2.1 *Relation between temperature and pressure of saturated steam*

Temperature	Excess pressure above standard atmosphere*		
°C	kN/m²	kg/cm²	lb/in²
100	0	0	0
105	19	0.20	2.8
108.5	35	0.36	5.1
110	42	0.43	6.1
115	68	0.69	9.8
115.5	**71**	**0.72**	**10.2**
120	97	0.99	14.1
121	**104**	**1.06**	**15.0**
125	131	1.33	19.0
127	**146**	**1.50**	**21.2**
130	169	1.72	24.5
134.5	207	2.11	30.0

* 103 kN/m², 14.7 lb/in².
  Commonly used temperatures and steam pressures are shown in heavy type. These values are approximate only but are sufficiently accurate for all normal sterilizing techniques.
NOTE: 1 lb/in² = 6.89 kN/m²; 1 kg/cm² = 98.1 kN/m².

Overheating is detrimental to most media, but autoclaving is the most satisfactory method of sterilizing material or media that will withstand temperatures over 100 °C, the routine temperature–

time combination being 115.5 °C (0.72 kg/cm²; 10 lb) for 20 minutes. The rate of heat penetration into large containers is slow, especially when they contain agar. When the volume of medium exceeds 1 litre the time, but not the temperature, should be increased to ensure that the whole contents are maintained at the required temperature for the correct time. The temperature inside the autoclave should be allowed to fall to 90 °C or below before opening it to remove the contents.

Containers such as test tubes, flasks and bottles should be of a capacity sufficient to allow a generous head space; an exception is the container of Stuart's (1959) transport medium, which is completely filled.

2.4.2   'Momentary autoclaving' (Davis & Rogers, 1939). Heat or steam is turned off as soon as the autoclave reaches the required temperature (e.g. 121 °C), the valve opened when the temperature falls to 100 °C, and the medium is taken out between 80–90 °C.

2.4.3   Steaming is the process of exposing the medium to the vapour of boiling water, but the medium itself seldom reaches 100 °C. It is carried out in a non-pressurized vessel, a steamer. Sterilization by steaming may be carried out once only, or on three successive days when it is a high temperature form of fractional sterilization. Sterilization by boiling or steaming is clearly a misnomer, as these processes cannot be relied upon to ensure sterility. They may be necessary when media cannot be autoclaved without detriment to their constituents, for example those containing selenite or tetrathionate. Many of the media that cannot be sterilized by autoclaving are enrichment or selective media for isolating particular organisms from a mixed flora, and in these sterility is not essential.

2.4.4   Tyndallization (or fractional sterilization) has limited use in the media department and is only suitable for nutrient media in which spores can germinate. It is used for litmus milk which is heated at 80 °C for one hour on three successive days, but our experience shows that this time-consuming process is unnecessary and that autoclaving at 115 °C for 10 minutes does not damage the milk.

2.4.5   Inspissation is fractional sterilization carried out at a temperature sufficiently high to coagulate serum or other heat labile constituents (e.g. egg-white) and consists in heating at 75–80 °C for one hour on three successive days. An alternative method of inspissation using the autoclave will be described in Section A2.1.9. Other methods were described by Levin (1943), Foster & Cohn (1945), Spray & Johnson (1946), and Brown (1959).

2.5   Sterilization by filtration

Sterilization by filtration has the advantage that it is a process suitable for solutions of thermolabile materials; its disadvantages include the possibility of hidden defects in the filtration apparatus, the need for sterilization of the apparatus before use, the possibility of adsorption from dilute solutions and of pH changes, and difficulty in cleaning filters after use. Filtration is not only a mechanical sieve-action depending on porosity and thickness of the filter but is also a complex physico-chemical procedure involving the charge on the filter and the pH of the solution.

Bacterial filters may be made of porous porcelain, kieselguhr (diatomite), asbestos, sintered glass, or cellulose esters. Doulton and Pasteur–Chamberland candles or cylinders are made of porous porcelain and are available in varying porosities, not all of which are suitable for bacterial filtration. Berkefeld and Mandler filters are made from kieselguhr.

Asbestos pads have the advantage that the pad is used once only and then discarded, but their many disadvantages should make us consider whether their continued use is justifiable. Asbestos pads often impart an alkaline reaction to the filtrate and this cannot always be prevented by washing the pad before use; however this alkalinity is not significant with well buffered media. Release of calcium and magnesium ions from the pad may produce incompatibilities and induce the clotting of plasma. Adsorption phenomena are not uncommon and some pads tend to shed fibres into the filtrate. Asbestos, kieselguhr, and porcelain filters carry a negative charge.

Sintered or frittered glass filters are available in varying porosities, no. 5 being suitable for bacterial filtration; it is usually available as a 5/3 filter consisting of a no. 5 supported on a no. 3 for mechanical strength. Sintered metal filters are not widely used in bacteriology as they are not completely inert to the action of materials likely to be found in culture media.

Collodion filters have largely been replaced by the more convenient membrane filters composed of cellulose esters which are stored in the dry state, and although somewhat brittle they have good wet strength and may be sterilized by autoclaving.

3
Principles of isolation

With the possible exception of fluorescent antibody techniques, all diagnostic methods require that the unknown micro-organisms be isolated in pure culture.
Steel (1965)

3.1 Isolation methods

Isolation begins at the bedside with the collection of the specimen. Normally the clinician takes the specimen and sends it to the laboratory but there are occasions when the bacteriologist, his microscope, and the patient should meet so that fresh specimens can be examined while 'hot'.

3.1.1 Microscopy.
Since amoebic and bacillary dysentery cannot be distinguished clinically, it is essential when amoebic dysentery is endemic or is suspected, to examine a freshly passed stool on a warmed stage to see the characteristic movements of vegetative *Entamoeba histolytica*; even better specimens may be obtained at sigmoidoscopy. Only by seeing the movements of *E. histolytica* can it be distinguished from *Entamoeba coli*; the differences between the encysted forms are not sufficiently great or constant to be diagnostic. Other material that is examined unstained is the serous fluid of a chancre (collected in a capillary) which yields to the microscopist an interesting and varied reward. Stained material from the throats of victims of Vincent's angina shows a plethora; when spirochaetes are few they can be ignored, for small numbers occur in the throats of the healthy. Lesions from leprosy show a heavy infection which, as yet, defies the usual cultural methods.

It is a waste of time to stain blood films for bacteria, but in hot countries the bacteriologist knows that bacteria are not the only causes of fever and always looks for malaria parasites and other blood-borne protozoa. Pus, cerebrospinal fluid (centrifuged deposit), pleural effusions, and other transudates may show bacteria when stained by Gram's method; when none is seen a Ziehl-Neelsen stained film may show acid-fast rods. Failure to find bacteria is not conclusive and, like other negative results, may indicate merely that the method used was not sensitive enough; Corper (1928) estimated that 100 000 acid-fast bacilli per ml of sputum was the minimum concentration that could be detected microscopically. A negative microscopial result could indicate that the infecting agent was a virus or a mycoplasm. Apart from films stained by Ziehl-Neelsen, microscopic examination of sputum is unlikely to be helpful and stained films of faeces are seldom worth examining. Urethral smears, on the other hand, may be more successful than cultures, and after seeing Gram-negative diplococci treatment can be started before the results of culture are available. When treatment is started before the specimen is taken, cultures are unlikely to give a growth of gonococci.

To summarize: microscopic examination of all specimens except blood (in temperate climates), faeces, and rectal swabs are always worth making but prolonged and exhausting searches for tubercle bacilli do not justify the effort expended on them.

3.1.2 Cultural methods.
With knowledge of the site of origin of the specimen and observation of stained smears, the clinical bacteriologist is able to anticipate the kinds of organism he is likely to isolate and can attempt to match the culture media to the expected organism(s). Perhaps more than any other bacteriologist he knows what he is trying to isolate and the probability and kind of contaminating (and unwanted) organisms he has to meet and try to eliminate, but it is often only too true that he isolates what he is looking for and misses the unexpected or unsought organisms. Anaerobes should not be regarded as special cases and, apart from faeces and sputum sent for routine examination, should be looked for in most specimens.

In considering isolation procedures our strategy

15

must start from the nature of the specimen; it is important to know whether, as in pus or cerebrospinal fluid, it is likely to contain only one kind of organism, or, as in faecal material and throat swabs, it has a natural flora that, on culture, will yield a background from which the one species of pathological interest has to be distinguished and separated. Specimens from blood and tissues that are normally sterile are inoculated on rich, non-inhibitory media, for it is our aim to isolate all kinds of organism present in such a specimen. And bearing in mind that not all bacteria grow in air, replicate plates should be made for incubation under increased CO_2 and under anaerobic conditions. The specialized techniques used for isolating anaerobes are described in detail in several monographs (Willis, 1964; Beerens & Tahon-Castel, 1965; Barnes, Impey & Goldberg, 1966; *Anaerobe Laboratory Manual*, 1972) which give useful laboratory tips based on years of experience. But the methods described in these monographs are different, and the characterizations given by them are incompatible, which creates difficulties in drawing up diagnostic tables such as our Table 6.8 (p. 67).

The non-specialist will probably do his anaerobic work in an ordinary laboratory, use ordinary media (in contrast to the reduced media used in the VPI Anaerobe Laboratory), and in anaerobic jars with a cold catalyst (Stokes, 1958). Most medical bacteriologists prefer plates to tubes, but a disadvantage of plates is that moisture may accidentally seal the lid to the dish; this can be prevented by notching the medium-carrying halves of plastic dishes (Stokes, 1968b). Those working in bigger institutions with more elaborate equipment may have a cabinet that can be flushed with oxygen-free CO_2 to produce anaerobic conditions (Leach, Bullen & Grant, 1971). It is probably looking too far ahead to think of the specialist anaerobiologist wearing oxygen-breathing apparatus and working in a wholly anaerobic (CO_2-conditioned) laboratory, but it may not be too extravagant a thought.

Even with the simplest of anaerobic methods about 10% of specimens will yield cultures of anaerobes and about a quarter of these will be in pure culture (Stokes, 1958). Holdeman & Moore (1972) regard the routine methods depending on

anaerobic jars and conventional (non-reduced) media as insufficiently sensitive and claim that if we exclude blood, throat, sputum, urine, and faeces routine specimens, about one-third of specimens should yield only anaerobes, another third both aerobes and facultative anaerobes, and the final third only aerobes.

A few organisms, notably the pathogenic mycobacteria, do not grow in Petri dishes incubated in air; they are slow-growing organisms and unless evaporation is prevented the medium will dry; normally they are grown in screw-capped containers (bottles in the UK, tubes in the USA). Some mycobacteria have not been isolated on lifeless media and our knowledge of their presence depends entirely on microscopial evidence (human leprosy) or is based on presumption after setting up a chronic infection in a susceptible animal (rat leprosy). Although our methods will not isolate viruses we shall, from time to time, isolate mycoplasms (*Mycoplasma* spp.) from specimens grown on media containing blood or serum in a closed – but not necessarily anaerobic – jar. When we suspect the presence of mycoplasms we can use special media (the so-called PPLO media) for their isolation and propagation; such media are available commercially.

Specimens from areas or sites that have a normal microbial flora cannot be treated so cavalierly. Look at the specimen with an appreciative eye, for it must be inoculated on to appropriate selective media; for example, a loose watery stool and faeces with flecks of blood and mucus should be inoculated on to different media. Experience is the best teacher but in its absence the tiro can compensate for his deficiencies by using several selective media. In all cases the repertoire should include the less inhibitory media such as MacConkey or EMB agar for faeces of adults; for stools from babies use blood agar on which the enteropathogenic strains of *Escherichia coli* can be successfully isolated and identified. When enrichment is used a large inoculum of the specimen (usually faeces) is placed in about 10 ml enrichment medium such as tetrathionate broth or selenite F medium; after incubation for a few hours subcultures are made to selective (inhibitory) media (deoxycholate citrate agar or SS agar) and to a basal or only slightly inhibitory medium (MacConkey or EMB). After

16

incubation overnight the plates are examined and colonies picked for subculture to non-inhibitory media. This selecting of colonies is not the end of the isolation process and further plating on non-inhibitory media may be necessary to procure a culture suitable for characterization tests. In the absence of good growth on the first batch of subcultures from the enrichment medium, further subcultures are made after longer incubation. Enrichment media such as tetrathionate broth can be used as transport media for faeces.

A few points need special attention.

(i) Blood should be inoculated into large volumes (at least ten times that of the specimen) of broth containing 0.03 to 0.05 % sodium polyanethol sulphonate (Liquoid) or other anticoagulant; incubation should be continued for a month and the broth subcultured at intervals to detect growth. Liquoid may inhibit growth of some anaerobic cocci and Holdeman & Moore (1972) recommend that blood cultures should be inoculated into media with and without Liquoid.

(ii) On first isolation most bacteria grow better in an atmosphere containing 5–10 % CO_2, but CO_2-inhibited mutants of *Escherichia coli* and *Salmonella typhimurium* have been isolated (Roberts & Charles, 1970).

(iii) Specimens from suspected gonorrhoea and meningitis should be inoculated on to freshly poured (and undried) blood agar plates; when the inoculation of plates cannot be made speedily, the swab specimen should be put into transport medium (Stuart, 1959).

(iv) Pathogenic mycobacteria grow slowly and usually not on the standard media used for pyogenic pathogens. *Mycobacterium bovis* may not grow on Lowenstein–Jensen medium but grows slowly on Dorset egg medium (Stokes, 1960). Egg media for tubercle bacilli can be replaced by blood agar made with blood from time-expired bottles from a local blood bank (Tarshis *et al.* 1953); as incubation will continue for several weeks the medium should be in screw-capped containers and have plenty of condensation (synæresis) water.

Specimens containing mycobacteria often have a mixed bacterial flora; to isolate the more slowly growing organisms the specimen must first be treated (with acid or alkali, to which mycobacteria

are unusually resistant) to destroy the more rapidly growing, and less acid/alkali resistant, bacteria; after treatment for a short time (usually about fifteen minutes) the acid or alkali can be neutralized before the specimen is inoculated on appropriate media.

3.2 Importance of pure cultures
Many difficulties in identification are due to the use of an impure culture as starting material. Before an organism can be identified it must be obtained in what we glibly describe as a 'pure culture'. By this we mean the descendants of a single colony obtained after plating the material in such a way that much of the growth consists of well-isolated colonies; it is only an assumption that these have developed from a single organism or a single clump of similar organisms. In routine diagnostic bacteriology a single plating may have to suffice but a replating can always be made with advantage, and, as will be explained below, is essential when highly selective and inhibitory media are used for the primary plating.

Our 'pure culture' is one that generally breeds true, that is, when replated the majority of the daughter colonies will be like the parent, but we know that occasionally (perhaps once in several million times) a bacterial cell will mutate and the colony developing from it will consist of organisms that have changed a character. Our 'pure culture' retains its original characters because the chances are, on an ordinary nutrient medium, millions to one against picking the mutant, and also because once satisfied that our culture is pure we stop picking isolated colonies (lest, perchance, the mutant is picked) and we subculture from a sweep (or pool) of several colonies.

When two organisms are grown together as in an impure culture, one of four things may happen: (i) each organism may grow independently; (ii) one may produce a substance that will enable the other to grow or grow better in the particular medium (synergy); (iii) one may produce a substance (bacteriocin) that inhibits the growth of the other; or (iv) one may grow faster than the other and deprive the second of some essential part of its food supply. In (i) and (ii) a characterization of the impure culture will probably yield a summation of

17

characters unless one organism produces say, acid and the other an equivalent amount of alkali to neutralize it. In (iii) and (iv) the characterization will be that of the organism which grows at the expense of the other. In (i) and (ii) an organism A (characterized as x+, y−, z−) growing with B (x−, y+, z−) in mixed culture (A+B), might be characterized as x+, y+, z−, which might be characteristic of a third organism C, and the mixture would inevitably be misidentified.

Often the bacteriologist is looking for a particular organism, e.g. a shigella in faeces or *Corynebacterium diphtheriae* in a throat swab, and many isolations are made on selective or differential media which contain substances that inhibit the growth of some (unwanted) organisms. The inhibitory substance(s) does not kill the unwanted organism but merely suppresses or retards its growth on that medium; when an inhibited organism forms part of a colony made up mainly of the suspected pathogen, subculture to another medium will result either in further suppression of growth of the unwanted, or, in the absence of its inhibitor, a resumption of growth in competition with the strain it is desired to isolate. From an inoculum of faeces on deoxycholate citrate medium a colourless colony (indicating a lactose non-fermenter) is likely to be made up of lactose non-fermenters and a few suppressed lactose fermenters. Subculture to lactose peptone water will allow the lactose fermenters to grow and produce acid from the lactose and, unless the colony is replated on a non-inhibitory medium, the presence of the lactose non-fermenters may be overlooked. A routine should be so developed that, before a culture is assumed to be pure, colonies picked from a selective medium are replated on a non-inhibitory and preferably an indicating medium. For, until a culture is known to be pure, it is a waste of time to attempt any characterization tests.

The reader may think that we have laboured the presence of mixed colonies, but experience has shown that many of the cultures that are difficult to identify are, in fact, mixed and came from colonies on inhibitory media, and we cannot stress too much the importance of obtaining a pure culture before attempting to identify it. While inhibitory media are the main source of impure cultures, other

causes are sufficiently common to warrant mention here. The presence of a 'spreader' on a plate may be difficult to detect; this spreading growth will also cover any discrete colonies on the plate. The most troublesome spreading organisms are members of two genera, *Proteus* and *Clostridium*, and different methods must be used to purify cultures contaminated by them.

Proteus species grow readily on most media but swarming can be inhibited by bile salts and by substances in some of the selective and inhibitory media on which Proteus organisms will produce discrete colonies. Thus, a culture contaminated by a *Proteus* species can be plated on MacConkey agar; if, however, the wanted organism will not grow on this medium the contaminated culture should be spread on plates of a richer nutrient medium in which the agar concentration has been increased to 7 % (Hayward & Miles, 1943).

It is much more difficult to purify a culture contaminated by a *Clostridium* species. This difficulty of freeing a culture from a clostridial contaminant applies also to separating one *Clostridium* species from another and explains why it takes so long to identify most cultures of this genus. Since more than one species of this genus may be found in the same material, it is not surprising that the original descriptions of many so-called species of *Clostridium* were based on mixtures of two or more species.

The separation of *Clostridium* species may entail a long series of platings and selection of colonies unless one of the mixture happens to be a pathogen with invasive properties. Such an organism might be isolated from a remote site (say the surface of the liver) when an animal dies after subcutaneous or intramuscular inoculation of the mixed culture in a hind limb. Separation may be achieved when the spores of the strains making up the mixture differ in their resistance to heat or when one of the strains is motile and the other non-motile. The separation of two pathogens may depend on the ability of the bacteriologist to recognize which species (or even toxin types) are present. Much information can be obtained from in-vitro tests, such as lecithinase production on egg-yolk medium, before going on to in-vivo tests in animals.

The contamination of bacterial cultures by

Mycoplasma species (pleuro-pneumonia-like organisms) is not believed to be a serious hazard, but our knowledge of these organisms is much less than that of ordinary bacteria, and their presence may escape detection. Mycoplasms grow slowly and generally only on media enriched with blood or serum, and if they are initially present as contaminants they are likely to be outgrown by the more hardy and less fastidious bacteria. However, they should be borne in mind and their presence suspected when bacterial cultures show inconsistencies on repeated testing. Bacterial cultures that have been isolated on media containing antibiotics or from patients treated with antibiotics, may show g, L or other aberrant forms, which may be confused with mycoplasms because they grow slowly and produce very small colonies.

3.3   Screening tests

Screening tests come in various forms and as improvements are constantly being made we intend to outline here only the development of different methods and to give a few references for those who propose to use these diagnostic aids. As the main objective of screening tests is economy of time and material, we can start with a statement applicable to all, namely that for quick results heavy inoculation is essential.

The tests are of two kinds: (i) *eliminating* – those intended to pick out unwanted and (believed to be) unimportant organisms; and (ii) *presumptive* – those tests that, by the use of media containing several substrates (multitest media), will indicate the major group into which an organism probably belongs. Both kinds of screening test rely heavily on the assumption that the test organism is in pure culture, and this assumption must be made at a time in the isolation and identification programme when the odds are against it.

Eliminating tests are usually quite simple as, when looking for salmonellas or shigellas, a tube of a urea medium is inoculated; if the urea is hydrolysed that particular culture can be discarded for it would be a most unusual salmonella or shigella that produced urease. Knox (1949) elaborated on this principle by using a multitest plate on which was spread a pure culture of the test organism and on its surface were placed coverslips (to detect gas

production) and impregnated test papers; from it, it was possible to detect H_2S production, mannitol, sucrose, and lactose fermentation, and swarming of the organism. In conjunction with a tube of urea medium the tests covered a wide range; some of the tests, when positive, suggested that the organism was unlikely to be a pathogen and that the culture could be discarded. Lányi & Ádám (1960) combined the impregnated paper disks of the Knox plate with a selective basal medium so that colonies from the primary plate could be used as inoculum; deoxycholate in the medium prevented interference by many organisms likely to be present in cultures of faeces.

The elimination of any culture involves the risk of loss of a rarely encountered organism or one that may be an unrecognized pathogen; this is the penalty that all must pay who discard their primary plates before they complete their investigations. The moral is never to discard the specimen or primary plate until all tests have been completed and the identification made satisfactorily; that this is not merely a counsel of perfection was known to the older bacteriologists and led to the discovery, among other things, of penicillin by Fleming.

Presumptive identifications can be made by inoculating media containing several substrates and one or more indicator(s). Some of these media contain inhibitory substances so that a colony from a selective medium can be used as inoculum, but most multitest media require the inoculum to be a pure culture. By a judicious choice of indicators and substrates, the originators of multitest media hope to show a sufficient range of colour or other changes to make a preliminary allocation of the test organism to a major group or subdivision. Multitest media and methods only justify themselves when they are both quick and accurate so that the bacteriologist can concentrate his efforts on cultures showing the reactions of established pathogens; to use multitest media to make the final identification is indefensible. But by eliminating unwanted organisms workers in busy laboratories should have time to investigate the presumptive pathogens by the more informative and reliable tests described in Chapter 4.

Because lactose fermentation was believed to be of paramount importance, Russell (1911) put ten

19

times more lactose than glucose in his double sugar medium. Kligler (1917, 1918) introduced lead acetate to the medium which was blackened when H_2S was produced in sufficient amount. In another variation, substituting mannitol for lactose, Kligler & Defandorf (1918) claimed to be able to distinguish the Shiga from the Flexner dysentery bacillus. To increase the differentiating power still further, Kendall & Ryan (1919) experimented with various combinations of sugars and ended with two double-sugar tubes which included glucose, lactose, sucrose, and mannitol. Other combinations and the addition of other substrates to bring in more characters have followed, and in more recent times another two-tube test (Kohn, 1954 as modified by Gillies, 1956) has become popular for the identification of intestinal pathogens. Kligler's iron agar (1917, 1918) formed the basis of TSI (triple sugar iron agar) which was apparently developed simultaneously by Sulkin & Willett (1940) and by workers in the Difco Laboratories (*Difco Manual*, 1953). Although TSI was introduced as a multitest medium it has become an unofficial standard for H_2S production at the low degree of sensitivity that has differential value among enteric bacteria.

Screw-capped containers, which do not allow volatile products to escape and so may affect the colour of indicators, are not suitable for multitest media (Marcus & Greaves, 1950).

Most multitest sloped media are intended for use in the identification of enterobacteria; others are aimed at picking out pathogenic vibrios (Hsu, Liu & Liao, 1964), and Chapman (1946, 1952) described some for identifying staphylococci. Multitest media have been exploited commercially especially for the identification of the enterobacteria, which are not only common and widely distributed but are easily identified and placed in their major groups by simple biochemical tests. So many schemes or systems have been marketed in the USA that some of the laboratory technology journals, with their trials and reports on these methods, read like publications of the consumer associations. Few of the systems have more than a fleeting popularity outside the home laboratory and recall the adage 'use a new drug while it works'.

We do not like identification methods that rely heavily on preliminary screening on multitest media;

we prefer to work from pure cultures on agar slopes and from these inoculate all the media needed to make an identification. In this we may be idealists, but we followed these principles when we did clinical bacteriology and we found that the methods worked not only to our satisfaction but even to that of clinicians. There are many disadvantages in multitest media, not least the possible interaction of one chemical reaction with another, as acid produced from fermentable sugar may inhibit the blackening of the iron indicator in TSI (Bulmash, Fulton & Jiron, 1965), or the ammonia produced from peptone may inhibit urease production (Stewart, 1965). There may also be interference in biochemical tests, as nitrite interferes with the detection of indole when tested by some of the older methods (Smith, Rogers & Bettge, 1972).

3.4 Single substrate and rapid tests

A different approach to identification, which although described as screening does not reject unwanted cultures, is to use rapid methods and to follow a flow chart or series of charts (Manclark & Pickett, 1961) but this seems to us to be an extension of the meaning of the term 'screening procedure' and to endow it with a new respectability. Pickett and his colleagues developed microtests in which the organism, after heavy inoculation, multiplied rapidly and briefly. We also developed a series of micromethods (Clarke & Cowan, 1952) in which there was little if any multiplication, and the constitutive and induced enzymes of heavy suspensions acted on buffered solutions of the test substrate. Both Pickett and ourselves believe that, as far as possible, bacterial characterizing tests should be carried out in such a manner that the organism acts only on one substrate in a test.

A variation of the single substrate principle is seen in a multitube, multitest method based on the work of Buissière & Nardon (1968); in a commercial form called the API system* tests are made in disposable plastic containers (Ivan Hall tubes) each holding one substrate, and at least one user (Nielsen, 1971) regards it as a means of carrying out fermentation tests in disposable containers. About

---

* Analytab Products Inc., Carle Place, New York 11514; API Laboratory Products Ltd, Philpot House, Rayleigh, Essex.

fifty characters can be determined by the API methods but only twenty tests seem to be enough for identifying enterobacteria; in these tests Washington, Yu & Martin (1971) obtained 88 %, and Smith, Tomfohrde, Rhoden & Balows (1972) 96 % agreement with conventional tests. The greatest discrepancy (about 10 %) was in the test for urease, but the tests were not strictly comparable; the conventional test (Christensen, 1946) used in the comparison was less exacting than the API test based on the method of Ferguson & Hook (1943), a buffered single substrate test with urea as the sole nitrogen source.

We prefer microtests and rapid methods with single substrates to multitest methods, but in diagnostic work rapid methods are useful only when the results are reproducible and agree with those of conventional methods. Because some of our micromethods gave different results (this applied particularly to tests involving carbohydrate breakdown) from those obtained with conventional peptone-containing media, we were faced with the choice of abandoning their regular use or preparing entirely new tables of sugar reactions. This seemed to be a very big undertaking and, as conventional methods would have to be run in parallel, did not justify the effort that would be expended. In this edition we have not included micromethods for sugar reactions but for other characters in which agreement with conventional tests is good, we retain micromethods and describe them in Appendix C.

Time-saving short cuts may be justified in the midst of an epidemic, when the infecting organism is known and further tests are merely confirmatory and when a quick, specific (usually serological) test is available. Under such circumstances a watch must be kept for the occurrence of other infections in the population being sampled, and any atypical organism investigated fully.

Some members of the enterobacteria are responsible for respiratory infections and similar isolation procedures are applied to sputum, aspiration juices, and blood cultures as to faeces and urine. Forty years ago it was important to know the source of a culture, for its identification might depend on whether it was isolated from above (*Klebsiella*) or below (*Enterobacter*, *Hafnia*, *Escherichia*) the umbilicus. Today we are not perturbed or surprised to isolate an intestinal organism from a respiratory site or vice versa.

Mention should be made of rapid methods using paper disks impregnated with substrate, test reagents and sometimes medium, used many years ago by Snyder, Donnelly & Nix (1951) and improved by Pickett, Scott & Hoyt (1955). Opinions about these impregnated paper disk methods are conflicting; Small (1968) and Prevorsek *et al.* (1968) gave them a general approval, but less enthusiasm was expressed by Narayan, Guinée & Mossel (1967) who found too many false positives, and by Martin, Bartes & Ball (1971) who gave only a qualified approval, 'reasonably accurate' for the best, and 'not recommended' for the other tests.

Another kind of impregnated paper test, intended for use with single substrates, was developed by Clarke & Steel (1966); these have not been applied to large-scale identification work, but Davies & Hoyling (1973) used them for VP tests on staphylococci and micrococci.

4
Characters and characterization

Features such as brightly coloured pigments may be characteristic of a few species and the bacteriologist then has a good pointer to the nature of the organism and its ultimate identification. But pigments may mislead, as in the case of bleeding polenta which is no longer considered to be a miracle but a phenomenon that can be produced experimentally by a bacterium and in nature is commonly produced by a yeast (Merlino, 1924; Gaughran, 1969; Cowan, 1956a, 1970). Bacteria present few gross diagnostic features and the bacteriologist must look closely at his organism; the characters he looks for and the tests he applies will depend on the field in which he practises and on his earlier experience of similar organisms; his approach to the identification will be conditioned by his professional training and his intuitive skill. The observations made and the tests applied are aimed at characterizing the organism so that it can be described (the technical term for the list of characters is a description) and compared with descriptions of other, previously identified and classified organisms.

4.1   Characterization
The difference between characterization for classification and for identification lies not so much in the tests as in the emphasis placed on the results of the tests. Although it is not universally accepted, most taxonomists now support the Adansonian concept that, in classification, equal weight should be given to each character or feature. The relations between strains can be calculated and expressed either as similarity of positive characters (Sneath, 1957b) or by taking into account both positive and negative features (Hill et al. 1961; Floodgate, 1962; Lockhart & Hartman, 1963); the results of such comparisons can be analysed laboriously by making

a large number of calculations, or more easily by letting a computer do the hard work (Sneath & Cowan, 1958).

Although we accept the Adansonian concept for classification, for identification we attach much weight to some characters, regarding them as having great distinguishing value, give less weight to others, and no weight at all to some features. Excessive weighting is given to coagulase production by the staphylococci; heavy weighting is placed on the urease and phenylalanine deaminase systems in identifying *Proteus* species, and on urease in distinguishing between *Alcaligenes faecalis* and *Alcaligenes bronchisepticus*. Little emphasis is placed on gelatin hydrolysis or liquefaction by staphylococci or micrococci but more weight is given to the same test among the enteric bacteria or the pseudomonads. The variable weighting attached to these characters is largely based on experience but it is always hoped that the assimilation of data from a wide range of bacteria will, in the future, enable us to express the value of a feature in a quantitative manner; this has been done for the Enterobacteriaceae by Edwards & Ewing (1972).

If everyone had ready access to a computer we should be able to use an almost unlimited number of characters or features, but with tables we are restricted by our memory or limited by our ability to recognize similarities and differences when making multiple comparisons simultaneously. These limitations led us to develop the mechanical aid we named the Determinator (Cowan & Steel, 1960, 1961) and to construct tables suitable for it. In the original Determinator we were restricted by its size to about twenty-five features, but in the simplified form this limitation was removed and, in theory at least, we could use fifty or more features in the

22

tables. We do not think that anyone (including ourselves) used this device, but the tables, which can be used by simple inspection, led to the development of this *Manual* and indirectly to a more elaborate mechanical device for the identification of the enterobacteria by Olds (1966, 1970). By selection – and weighting – we kept down the number of features used in the individual tables, and made the identification in stages. At one time we intended to make tables with the smallest number of tests essential for identification. In the event we included in each second-stage table sufficient detail to provide an adequate, but not exhaustive, characterization.

4.2 Choice of characters

In choosing characters for the tables we lean towards those that seem to be most constant and to tests that give most reproducible results. Unfortunately, nearly all tests are influenced by factors that are difficult to control, and we are not yet in a position to specify any standard methods. All we can do is to recommend that the materials used (media and reagents) should be controlled as far as it is possible to control them (see Appendix A), and that environmental factors such as temperature, and the time at which a test is done should be standardized. Various workers have discussed the choice of characterizing tests and methods, and each has his own preferences. Sneath & Johnson (1972) suggest statistical methods by which the influence of test error on the correctness of identification can be measured; they estimate that within one laboratory (where the error is likely to be least) test error will be about 5% and they consider that a test with a laboratory error greater than 10% will not be suitable for taxonomic work. We would emphasize the desirability of keeping to the same method of doing a test so that its idiosyncrasies and difficulties become known, and, within the one laboratory, the results become reasonably comparable. We have made innumerable comparative tests but seldom could we say unequivocally that one method was better than all the others. To keep our results reasonably comparable we chose certain methods and these became our laboratory standards. Often the choice of method was a compromise between two, sometimes conflicting demands: firstly to know

the truth, and secondly to be able to distinguish between two otherwise similar organisms. It is essentially a compromise to express qualitatively (as positive or negative) what is really a quantitative reaction. An example is the production of hydrogen sulphide; when an organism is grown in a medium with an adequate sulphydryl content, and a sensitive indicator (lead acetate paper) is used, the ability to produce even small amounts of H_2S can be detected, but the method is not discriminatory and the results are useless for distinguishing between those salmonellas that produce much and those that produce only a little H_2S. However, with a medium deficient in $-SH$ compounds and a poor indicator (ferrous chloride), only an organism with great ability to produce H_2S is positive in the test.

Sometimes a test is carried out by different methods when dealing with different groups of organism. Again taking H_2S production as the example; in the genus *Brucella* the organisms are grown on a medium rich in $-SH$ compounds and lead acetate papers are changed each day so that the result of the test can be expressed as 'H_2S produced on the first two days' or 'from the 1st to the 5th day'. We do not know of any other group of organisms in which this technique is used, and its application to other groups might give us information of value. On occasion we shall find it necessary to indicate the method to be used to obtain the results given in a table.

4.3 Characters not used in the tables

Before describing the characters chosen for use in our tables, we think we should state our reasons for omitting some time-honoured characters and tests. Certain features are not used in our diagnostic tables because they are subjective; for example, the smell of staphylococci growing on agar is unmistakable but also indescribable. The recognition of the finer shades of pigments is a subjective observation; we try to keep to the primary colours and eschew such indefinite subdivisions as baby-wool pink, coral red, and sky blue used by the female members of our staff.

Normally we do not describe colony morphology as this will vary with the medium on which the organism is grown and, except in bacteria such as *Corynebacterium diphtheriae* var. *gravis*, is seldom sufficiently characteristic to have diagnostic value. We do not consider that the descriptions of stroke cultures on agar slopes are worth the paper they are written on, and we rarely pay any attention to the type of growth in broth except to note the presence or absence of a pellicle. In a few cases (e.g. *Clostridium tetani* and *Bacillus anthracis*) the type of growth in gelatin stab cultures is characteristic, but the fir-tree and inverted fir-tree growths can only be seen when the gelatin columns are deep and the cultures are incubated at about 22 °C. On the whole we pay little attention to the type of lique-faction of gelatin and are content to record the test as 'gelatin liquefied' or 'not liquefied'.

Thus the reader will not find in this *Manual* diagrams of the different shapes, edges, surfaces, and elevations of colonies, and of the shapes of liquefaction seen in gelatin stab cultures; the elimination of these relics of nineteenth-century bacteriology makes unnecessary a glossary of descriptive terms that now have but limited use. However, lest we should be accused of too biochemi-cal an approach to classification and identification, we must state our belief that cell morphology has an important place in characterization and we depre-cate the tendency to abandon the microscope for the spectrophotometer and other instrumental aids.

We do not describe serological techniques since serology plays its part in classification and identifica-tion chiefly in the finer subdivisions made for epidemiological purposes. For those who wish to pursue serological analysis we recommend the monographs by Kauffmann (1954) and by Edwards & Ewing (1962; 1972); the latter is essentially a practical treatise and contains such relevant and important details as the identity of the best strains to use for immunization and absorption. One of the primary subdivisions of the streptococci is by the method of grouping introduced by Lance-field (1933) and this finds a place in Table 6.3*b*, *c*. The method of preparing extracts of streptococci is described in Appendix C.

We have not described fluorescence microscopy or fluorescent antibody (FA) methods for reasons that seem adequate to us. We do not think that laboratories that have the necessary equipment and skill to use it will need guidance from us, especially as (and this is our most compelling reason for omitting it) we have not used the method ourselves and do not think we should write on methods of which we have not had practical experience. The uninitiated who are looking for guidance should consult reviews by Cherry & Moody (1965) and Georgala & Boothroyd (1968).

4.3.1   Antibiotic sensitivity. To the clinician the only important character or set of characters of an infecting organism is its sensitivity to antibiotics that can be used therapeutically. Hence, anti-biotic sensitivity tests have become an important part of the clinical bacteriologist's routine and there is a tendency to regard the results of these tests, expressed in an antibiogram, as valuable characteristics in arriving at the identification of an organism. It is possible to say in general terms that certain species are sensitive or resistant to a par-ticular antibiotic but because so many strains come from patients who have been treated with antibio-tics it is likely that those strains isolated during treatment represent the antibiotic-resistant sur-vivors. Sensitivity to antibiotics, therefore, is not a character that has much diagnostic value among the bacteria of medical interest, and contrary to popu-lar belief, the antibiogram has only a minor part to play in identification work. While an unusual antibiogram can point to a misidentification (Abrams, Zierdt & Brown, 1971), the list of sensitivities and resistances of a strain from a treated patient merely reflects the effectiveness or failure of treatment. And, since strains made resistant *in vivo* do not change their other characters (Brown & Evans, 1963), the deletion of the anti-biogram removes only a highly variable character from consideration when the identification is made.

Non-fermenting and non-saccharolytic Gram-negative rods belong to groups of bacteria that have so many negative and so few positive characters that the identifier will clutch at the flimsiest straw and is tempted to accept the antibiogram as a useful tool, even if only as an auxiliary one (Pedersen, Marso & Pickett, 1970; Gilardi, 1971*c*). We think that this is unwise when trying to identify strains from patients, for it overlooks the possibility of resistance developing as a result of treatment, or from the influence of transfer and resistance factors (Anderson & Lewis, 1965*a*, *b*; Anderson, 1966). So, although the antibiogram is important to the clinician and should be reported to him, it is our view that it should have only a small part in the bacteriologist's armamentarium, and play no part whatever in the characterization and description necessary for accurate identification of organisms isolated from man and other animals that have been treated with or fed antibiotics. These objections are not made against bacteriostatic agents (such as lysozyme or the O/129 pteridine derivative) that are not used therapeutically or included in animal feeding stuff, and in fields other than medicine antibiotic sensitivity and sensitivity to antibacterial agents have been found helpful in identifying various pseudomonads and vibrios (Shewan, Hobbs & Hodgkiss, 1960).

4.4   Primary tests used in the tables

When we prepared our tables we started with the Gram reaction and for the next subdivisions used cytology and fundamental reactions such as ability to grow in air, catalase, oxidase production, and the method of carbohydrate breakdown. One of the advantages of a table is that several characters of different groups can be seen simultaneously and compared, a feat that is impossible with the genealogical type of chart or dichotomous key. We were surprised to find that on the results of a limited number of selected tests we could place most bacteria into a genus or a small group of genera.

4.4.1   Gram reaction.

Gram did not describe a stain but a method in which he used stains and solutions devised by others; to this day we do not fully understand its mechanism, but we do know that the reaction to Gram's method is a stable characteristic of a bacterium. Gram positivity (the ability to resist decolorization with ethanol or acetone) is a feature of relatively young bacterial cells of some species; as they age, the cells lose this characteristic and apparently become Gram negative. It is important, therefore, to examine young cultures, preferably before the end of the logarithmic growth phase. Genuinely Gram-negative bacteria do not retain the first stain which is easily removed by the decolorizing agent. Thus, as in many other tests, a positive finding (in this case retention of the purple stain) has much more

significance than a negative which may, in fact, be false due to (i) the age of the culture, or (ii) excessive decolorization with powerful solvents such as acetone. There are many variations of Gram's method (and each works well in the hands of those who practise it); the one we use under the name of Lillie's modification is simple and students obtain good results with it but, as acetone is used, the decolorization can be overdone. A modification by Preston & Morrell (1962) is claimed to be foolproof.

4.4.2   Morphology

is affected by the medium on which the organism is grown and the temperature of incubation. Organisms are in their most typical and natural state in young cultures and in wet, unstained preparations, and are best observed by phase-contrast or dark-ground microscopy. Such examination will show not only the shape(s) of organisms but, when preparations are made from suitable material (see Section 4.5.5), will show motility if it is present, and whether the cell remains rigid (as in most bacteria), flexes (spirochaetes), or glides (cytophagas). The distinction between spheres (cocci) and rods (bacilli) is not always clear-cut, and genera such as *Acinetobacter* and *Moraxella* cannot be categorically placed in one morphological group. Although it is usual to describe organisms of both these genera as either coccobacilli or short rods, electron micrographs clearly show the coccal nature of some acinetobacter strains (Thornley, 1967). Baumann, Doudoroff & Stanier (1968b) found that the differences in morphology of these genera corresponded with the growth phase: plump rods in the logarithmic, coccoid forms in the stationary phase. Brzin (1965) described what he called a sphaeroplasting effect, in that prolonged incubation of *Acinetobacter anitratus* strains at 37 °C produced polymorphism.

Bizarre-shaped cells may suggest particular genera to the microscopist, and the presence of clubs or dumb-bell shapes will call for staining methods such as Neisser's, Albert's, or Loeffler's methylene blue, capable of showing metachromatic granules.

Electron microscopy is not yet available in all diagnostic aboratories and one cannot determin accurately the site of insertion of bacterial flagella.

Fortunately such information is not essential for the identification of motile bacteria, and we do not mention it in the minidefinitions of genera given in Chapters 6 and 7. Scanning electron microscopy seems to have special advantages in the identification of the actinomycetes (Williams & Davies, 1967).

4.4.3 Acid fastness is shown when an organism resists decolorization by strong acids or mixtures of ethanol and mineral acid; this is a characteristic shown by few bacteria and when positive is diagnostic of mycobacteria, though one possible species, '*Mycobacterium*' *rhodochrous*, is only feebly acid fast. Nocardias are sometimes acid fast but seldom resist the vigorous decolorization which mycobacteria successfully endure. Ziehl-Neelsen's method is used to demonstrate acid fastness but methods using a cold stain have been described.

4.4.4 Spores are stained by a modification of Moeller's method (itself a modified Ziehl-Neelsen method) in which decolorization is by ethanol. The staining method is simple and seldom causes difficulty but the young spore does not resist decolorization and it may or may not take up the counterstain. In older cultures some bacilli may shed their spores so that in the rod-shaped bacterium an unstained area is seen, and stained spores may lie free of the cells from which they developed. An indirect method of showing the presence of spores is to show that a culture can survive heating at 80 °C for 10 minutes.

A problem that faces the diagnostician is the tendency for sporing organisms to lose the ability to produce spores. The asporogenous state may be permanent, or it may be a temporary reaction to an environment, when a change of medium or temperature of incubation could suffice to restore the strain's ability (or need) to form spores. Subculture to a starch-containing medium such as potato agar, is often successful in restoring the ability of an aerobe to form spores; in other instances a deficiency of manganese in the medium is the cause of the asporogenous state and the remedy is the addition of a 'trace elements' supplement. Often the cause is unknown and the best general advice we can give, based on the

restoration of many asporogenous strains of *Bacillus* in the National Collection of Type Cultures to the sporing state, is to grow the cultures on a medium containing soil extract (Section A2.7.28).

A frequent subject for discussion with R. E. Buchanan was the meaning of the word spore in bacteriology; as a purist (see also Cross, 1970) he insisted that bacterial spores were endospores, a term derived from endogenous spore; it was to be distinguished from the fragmentation spore of *Nocardia* species. But most bacteriologists do not consider that Nocardia is a sporing organism, and we think that the simple word spore tells us all we need to know about it. As we understand the spore, it is a resistant (to heat and disinfectants) body that is formed by few bacteria; of the animal pathogens the only sporing bacteria are members of the genera *Clostridium* and *Bacillus*, and of the last, only *B. anthracis* is certainly pathogenic. The importance of spore-forming bacteria in medicine is their association with war wounds, though they are not unknown as contaminants of other open wounds.

Sterilization techniques are checked by including spore suspensions in drums containing dressings and gloves; some spores are more heat labile than others, and spores of a resistant strain (usually of *Bacillus stearothermophilus*) are used. After sterilizer tests the spore suspensions returned to the laboratory should be incubated at about 50 °C and cultures observed for at least a week. It is important to identify any strain that appears to survive sterilization; a mesophilic spore-former suggests post-sterilization contamination.

In connexion with the acid-fast and spore-forming characters of organisms, certain other problems need to be discussed. Should we stain every culture by Ziehl-Neelsen's and Moeller's methods or apply heat-resistance tests, or do we restrict these tests to Gram-positive organisms or to those cultures which, by morphology, colony form, rate of growth, and other characters, we suspect may be acid fast or able to produce spores? We do not know of any Gram-negative bacteria that are genuinely acid fast and we think that it is reasonable to omit the Ziehl-Neelsen staining of Gram-negative organisms. Should we stain all cultures for spores and, failing to find them, try again after growing the cultures on soil extract agar or other spore-encouraging medium? We know that these tests are not done as a routine and, as the majority of cultures will show negative results we do not suggest that the search for sporing forms be made in all cases. All we would stress is that when spores are not looked for a mental note should be made that they have not been excluded, and their possible presence borne in mind.

4.4.5 **Motility** may be studied in a hanging-drop or other wet preparation. Some strains are only sluggishly motile when first isolated; motility may be speeded by using Craigie's technique (Craigie, 1931; Tulloch, 1939) in which the inoculation is made into a central tube of sloppy agar and, after incubation, a subculture is made from those organisms that, by their motility, have migrated outside the central tube. Motility may be inferred by observing the spreading growth in a semisolid agar (Tittsler & Sandholzer, 1936) which may be seen better when a tetrazolium dye is incorporated in the medium; as the organisms grow the dye is reduced, and the medium changes colour (Kelly & Fulton, 1953). The temperature of incubation is important: most motile organisms are motile at lower temperatures (e.g. 15–25 °C) and may not be motile at the temperature (e.g. 37 °C) optimal for growth.

The problem pertaining to motility is: do we test all strains or only rods? If we only examine the rods we shall overlook the motility of many strains of *Streptococcus faecium*, of *Micrococcus agilis*, and other cocci. When these tests become part of the daily routine they do not take up much extra time; they are only time consuming and upsetting of routine when they are 'special tests'. Our remarks refer to the motility shown by aerobic organisms; anaerobes present special problems in that motility will be inhibited by the air in hanging-drop preparations. Capillary tube preparations, sealed at each end, from cooked meat cultures, are more likely to show motility in clostridia.

Some bacteria (cytophagas) are motile by a gliding movement and to observe this special media and techniques are necessary. This type of movement is not only affected by the concentration of agar in the medium, but also by the concentration of peptone. Such organisms are not likely to be found

in pathological specimens because the methods used by medical bacteriologists are not suitable for showing this gliding motility. Lautrop (1961), Halvorsen (1963) and Piéchaud (1963) thought that they found a similar movement in *Bacterium anitratum* (*Acinetobacter anitratus*) and *Moraxella lwoffi* (*Acinetobacter lwoffii*), but this was not true gliding motility and the organism should be regarded as non-motile (Lautrop, 1965).

4.4.6 The **ability to grow in air** is a character shared by all bacteria except the strict anaerobes; it is a feature needed in Table 7.1 for the identification of certain anaerobes (especially *Clostridium welchii*) in which spore formation may be difficult to show, and which, without this line, would appear to be placed among the lactobacilli, corynebacteria, or other Gram-positive rods.

Failure to grow in air may be due to a deficiency in carbon dioxide, and growth in an atmosphere of air + CO_2 or in a candle jar should be attempted.

4.4.7 **Ability to grow under anaerobic conditions** is fairly widespread among bacteria but as it is not universal the knowledge that an organism cannot grow under these conditions can be diagnostically important. Some of these organisms are strict aerobes, others may need carbon dioxide.

4.4.8 The **catalase** test is simple and seldom causes difficulty, but because some strains of lactobacilli, pediococci, and a few strains of *Streptococcus faecalis* appear to form catalase, Gutekunst, Delwiche & Seeley (1957) questioned the validity of the test 'as an overriding classification feature'. False catalase reactions by some lactobacilli grown in low (0.05 %) concentrations of glucose (Dacre & Sharpe, 1956) are due to an azide-insensitive, non-haem catalase (pseudocatalase) and can be avoided by using media with 1 % glucose without added haematin (Whittenbury, 1964).

A few species (e.g. *Aerococcus viridans*) produce a weakly positive reaction which may easily be missed by those looking only for strong reactions. Gagnon, Hunting & Esselen (1959) devised a method that might be applied to bacteriology; the material under test was spread on disks of filter paper which were dropped into 3 % H_2O_2; when catalase was present the evolution of gas quickly brought the disks to the surface.

Those who work with mycobacteria have different standards for the catalase test; the methods are semiquantitative and positives are graded by the height of the column of froth in a standard test (see Section C3.9, method 3).

When aerosols might be dangerous, as with cultures of *Yersinia pestis*, Burrows *et al.* (1964) stab inoculate agar containing 0.5% H_2O_2 and using low power magnification, look for effervescence; the oxygen bubbles persist longer and reduce the danger from aerosols if a surface-tension lowering disinfectant (cetrimide, 0.5%) is added to the agar.

4.4.9 The **oxidase** test has been used to pick out colonies of *Neisseria* species in mixed cultures (Gordon & McLeod, 1928; McLeod *et al.* 1934; McLeod, 1947), but its wider use originated with the test devised by Kovács (1956) to distinguish pseudomonads from the enteric bacteria. When precautions are taken to avoid oxidation of the reagent, the test is sensitive and useful in classification and identification (Steel, 1961). Leclerc & Beerens (1962) use a similar technique to Kovács' but substitute the more stable dimethyl for the tetramethyl compound. Brisou *et al.* (1962) suggested a modification of Kovács' method that is said to make the result of the test more clear-cut and easier to read. In the USA the term cytochrome oxidase is used for the reaction, and the methods used are those of Gaby & Hadley (1957) and Ewing & Johnson (1960), which are less sensitive than Kovács' method.

Tests for oxidase resemble those for H_2S in that one can generally find a method of the sensitivity that one wants; and, as in the H_2S test, greater differentiation can be obtained by using a method with a low sensitivity. Steel (1962b) found Kovács' method too sensitive for staphylococci, some of which gave weak or delayed reactions; he obtained taxonomically more helpful results by using Gaby & Hadley's method, by which all staphylococci were oxidase negative.

4.4.10 **The Oxidation–Fermentation (OF) test.** To find out whether the attack on carbohydrate is by

oxidation or fermentation, the OF test is made by growing the bacterium in two tubes of Hugh & Leifson's (1953) medium; the medium in one tube is covered with a layer of soft paraffin (petrolatum). Oxidizers show acid production in the open tube only, fermenters show acid in the paraffin-covered tube and, starting from the bottom, in the open tube. The usual sugar included in the Hugh & Leifson medium is glucose but, because of the occurrence of organisms which do not seem to attack glucose but break down other sugars (Hugh & Ryschenkow, 1961; Koontz & Faber, 1963) the need for a test using the basal medium+maltose or pentoses should be considered. Park (1967), who had some indefinite results in a modified Hugh & Leifson medium, developed a simple test to show that the glucose had been utilized and was no longer present in the medium.

The OF base may be used for all the 'sugar reactions' used to characterize bacteria (Gilardi, 1971a). Various modifications to the medium have been suggested, including a useful peptoneless medium by Board & Holding (1960); to avoid confusion we do not use the term 'Hugh & Leifson test', but prefer the more descriptive term Oxidation–Fermentation (OF) test.

In connexion with the OF test three points deserve mention: (i) the organism may not be able to grow in the Hugh & Leifson type medium, in which case the test must be repeated using a basal medium enriched with 2% serum or 0.1% yeast extract; (ii) the organism may grow but not produce acid in either tube. This result should be confirmed by inoculation of Park's (1967) MHL medium+glucose; (iii) Leifson (1963) found that bromthymol blue was toxic to some bacteria, and modified the OF medium for marine organisms.

The OF test is one of the most important tests carried out in the early stages in the identification of aerobic bacteria. Most genera are composed of bacteria that either oxidize or ferment glucose; when a genus contains some species that attack glucose by oxidation and other species by fermentation, there would seem to be reason to reconsider the taxonomy of the genus and the desirability of dividing it.

Some organisms do not appear to be able to attack a sugar readily, and often show acid produc-

tion only after several days of incubation. Lederberg (1950) found that this delay was due to failure
of the sugar to reach the inside of the bacterial cell,
and a test (the ONPG, q.v. Section 4.5.34) was
devised to reveal quickly the potential fermentative
power of the 'late lactose fermenters'.

4.5   Secondary tests used in the tables
These notes give some background to the tests.
Details of special media used in the biochemical
tests will be found in Appendix A; reagents and
methods are described in Appendix C.

4.5.1   Acetylmethylcarbinol   production.   The
Voges–Proskauer or **VP test** can be carried out in
many ways and almost any desired degree of sensitivity can be obtained. It is now generally thought
that the older methods (Harden & Norris, 1912) are
too slow and insensitive, but there is less agreement
about the method to be recommended or the sensitivity that gives the best differentiation between
taxa. Although Clark & Lubs (1915) specified 30 °C
for the test, the MR and VP tests were often carried
out on cultures that had been incubated at 37 °C.
For many years water bacteriologists have recommended 30 °C (Report, 1956b) and we now know
that some enterobacteria such as the Hafnia group
·are often VP negative at 37 °C but positive at 30 °C
or lower. In a comparative trial we found that
incubation for 5 days (at 30 °C) was the minimum
time needed to detect by Barritt's method (1936) all
the positives among the enterobacteria; for other
organisms (e.g. staphylococci) longer incubation
up to 10 days gave more positive results. Others
have reported that acetylmethylcarbinol may be
broken down and used as a carbon source by various
coliforms (Linton, 1925; Paine, 1927; Ruchhoft
et al. 1931; Tittsler, 1938), Bacillus species (Williams
& Morrow, 1928) and staphylococci (Segal, 1940).
Taylor (1951) found that O'Meara's (1931) fumarate
medium prevented the breakdown of acetylmethylcarbinol by soft-rot bacteria and allowed it to
accumulate.

Outside the field of enteric bacteria it has been
found that phosphate may interfere with the
production of acetoin; Smith, Gordon & Clark
(1946) recommend a medium in which the phosphate
is replaced by NaCl, and Abd-el-Malek & Gibson

(1948b) use a simple glucose peptone broth without
salt or phosphate. For several years we compared
glucose phosphate broth with the media recommended by Smith et al. and by Abd-el-Malek & Gibson,
and we came to the conclusion that glucose peptone
was the most suitable for Bacillus and Staphylococcus and glucose phosphate broth was best for the
enterobacteria and most other organisms.

After comparing methods for the VP test over
several years we chose Barritt's (1936) method as
our standard; the sensitivity was found to be mid-
way between O'Meara's (1931) and Batty-Smith's
(1941) methods. For a useful review of the VP test
see Eddy (1961).

4.5.2   Aesculin hydrolysis is a test of value for
streptococci and some other groups, and may be
demonstrated in one of two ways. The usual
method is to incorporate the glycoside in a nutrient
base together with a ferric salt; hydrolysis is indicated by a brown coloration due to reaction of
the aglycone (6:7-dihydroxycoumarin) with the
iron. Alternatively, use of the glucose portion of
the molecule can be detected by acid or acid and
gas production.

4.5.3   Bile solubility is used to distinguish pneu-
mococci from the viridans types of streptococci;
however, the test is not specific for Streptococcus
pneumoniae. The pneumococcus differs from other
streptococci in having an autolytic enzyme which
can be demonstrated by allowing a digest broth
culture to age in the incubator; at 24 hours the
broth is turbid; after a few days the medium will
become clear. Bile and bile salts activate the autolytic enzyme, and so will not produce clearing of a
heat-killed culture or one that is too acid; the
suspension to be tested should be about pH 7.2.
At one time crude bile was used for the test but the
isolation of various bile salts in a pure state showed
that certain of them were more active than others
(Downie et al. 1931). Sodium deoxycholate is used
as it can be obtained in a reasonable state of
purity.

4.5.4   Buffered single substrate (BSS) tests are,
as their name implies, attempts to get away from
the usual biochemical tests made in complex

media with the concomitant risk that metabolic products will interfere with the specific reaction under test. The risk is a real one and is most obvious in sugar reactions made in peptone-containing media on organisms that oxidize carbohydrates, and as long ago as 1955 Pickett showed that brucellas were able to produce acid from several sugars in an otherwise inert milieu.

Various methods have been used to exploit the BSS principle; tablets containing substrate and buffer (Hoyt, 1951; Pickett & Scott, 1955; Hoyt & Pickett, 1957) were dissolved in small volumes of water, steamed, and the solutions were heavily inoculated with the test organism. Biochemical tests were carried out within a few hours, and the results probably depended on the presence of preformed enzymes. Our micromethods (Clarke & Cowan, 1952), which largely depended on preformed enzymes, had the disadvantage that the preparation of the heavy suspensions of test organisms involved too many manipulations for use in a routine laboratory.

Pickett (1970) and Pickett & Pedersen (1970b) have developed a series of tests (or rather of test surroundings) in which the organism can act on one substrate at a time; the principle is applied to sugar reactions, decarboxylases, deamidases, and hydrolases. The tests are particularly useful for characterizing non-saccharolytic bacteria and those that oxidize carbohydrates, the non-fermenters. We should point out that characterizations based on BSS tests will not always be the same as those made by conventional methods, neither will they match the characters shown in most of our tables; if these tests come into regular use new tables will be necessary (cf. Table 7.6a and b).

4.5.5 A positive **CAMP test** is the production of a clear zone around a colony in an area of a blood plate that has been affected by staphylococcal β-toxin; this bald statement needs amplification, for the clearing takes place only on blood agar made with sheep or ox blood, and not on media made with human, rabbit, horse, or guinea-pig blood. The important point in carrying out the test is that the agent produced by the bacterial cells must come in contact with the sheep (or ox) red cells before the staphylococcal β-haemolysin. The

test is almost specific for strains of *Streptococcus agalactiae* from man or animals; Christie, Atkins & Munch-Petersen (1944) did not find any other species to produce the clear zone, but some haemolytic strains of groups E, P, and U give positive CAMP reactions (Shuman *et al.* 1972); *Pasteurella haemolytica* also gives positive reactions (Bouley, 1965).

Fraser (1961) described a somewhat similar synergic haemolytic effect that may occur when *Corynebacterium ovis* and *C. equi* are grown together on blood agar made with washed blood cells from sheep but not from the horse. Unlike the phenomenon described by Christie *et al.*, this observation does not seem to have led to the development of a useful specific diagnostic test.

4.5.6 **Carbohydrate breakdown.** The division of bacteria into fermenters, oxidizers, and non-utilizers by the OF test is one of the most heavily weighted of the primary tests used in our progressive system of identification, and carbohydrate utilization also features in our secondary tests. The so-called 'fermentation tests' were used by the early bacteriologists to distinguish one organism from another and elaborate diagnostic tables were based on them (see for example Castellani & Chalmers, 1919). The introduction of the simple gas tube (Durham, 1898) and indicators enabled the production of gas and acid to be detected by inspection. Screw-capped bottles and tubes are not satisfactory for sugar tests since the CO_2 evolved by the bacteria is trapped and, by lowering the pH value of the medium, may change the colour of the indicator and suggest a (false) positive test. If screw-capped containers are used the caps should be loosened an hour before the indicator colour is observed.

Possibly we put too much emphasis on differentiation by the reactions of individual sugars (apart from glucose, Section 4.4.10); in classification by numerical methods the composition of taxa is essentially the same whether or not the sugar reactions are included in the characters analysed (Focht & Lockhart, 1965). In the genus *Acinetobacter* acid production from several sugars is mediated by a non-specific aldolase (Baumann *et al.* 1968b).

The failure to standardize methods has led to

30

discrepant results in the hands of different workers, and it is only within recent years that taxonomists have given adequate thought to the significance of acid production by a bacterium growing in a medium containing a carbohydrate. In such a medium we provide peptones which, during growth of the organism, are broken down to substances that are alkaline in reaction; if, in the medium, there is a carbohydrate, alcohol, or other substance commonly called a 'sugar' that can be broken down by the bacteria either by oxidation or by fermentation, acid will be produced, but it will be detected by an indicator in the medium only when the acid produced from sugar exceeds the alkali from peptone. The visibility of the reaction is also influenced by (i) the buffering properties of the medium, and (ii) the indicator used, e.g. bromthymol blue shows acid production when the pH value falls to 6.0 or less, whereas bromcresol purple does not change colour until the pH has fallen to about 5. Peptone water sugars, which are commonly used in this country and continental Europe, have less buffering power and yield less alkali than the broth-based sugars used extensively in the USA and elsewhere. With peptone water sugars we normally use Andrade's indicator (which becomes pink at about pH 5.5) or bromcresol purple (yellow at about pH5), and it is fortunate that in these media the enterobacteria give similar results to those given in broth-based sugars with bromthymol blue (yellow at about pH 6.0).

With apparently non-saccharolytic bacteria the results obtained in peptone-containing sugar media may be misleading in assessing the carbohydrate-attacking ability of a bacterium, because a small amount of acid produced will be masked by the breakdown products from peptone. Pickett (1955) and Pickett & Nelson (1955) overcame this difficulty by using peptoneless media and, with cresol red as indicator showed that acid was produced from several sugars by the apparently 'non-fermenting' Brucella species. For the development of these methods see Section 4.5.4 and Pickett (1970). Another method to reveal the acid-producing potential of Acinetobacter anitratus (Stuart, Formal & McGann, 1949) and of slow-lactose-fermenting coliforms (Lowe & Evans, 1957) is to increase the carbohydrate concentration to five or even ten per cent. A peptoneless modification of the Hugh & Leifson (1953) OF medium has been suggested (Board & Holding, 1960; Holding & Collee, 1971) in which acid production correlates well with utilization of glucose; it can be used for aerobic, oxidizing bacteria, and also for bacteria that require additional growth factors.

Some bacteria will not grow on simple media and need an enriched sugar medium. Many streptococci and corynebacteria are grown in media containing serum; neisserias in media enriched by serum or ascitic fluid; haemophilic bacteria in sugar media to which X and V factors have been added.

Organisms that oxidize sugars do not readily show acid production when they are grown in tubes of liquid media, and more reliable results are obtained when they are grown on the surfaces of solid media, which expose the organism to an adequate supply of air. Oxidizers such as Pseudomonas species do not give reliable 'sugar reactions' on peptone-containing media and should be grown on media with an ammonium salt as the main nitrogen source. Smith, Gordon & Clark (1952) used ammonium salt sugars (ASS) for their work on Bacillus species, some of which ferment and others oxidize carbohydrates. Bacteria may be grown on peptone-containing medium and then spun out and resuspended in water or saline so that, when added to a buffered solution of carbohydrate, the bacterial enzymes act on a single substrate (see, for example, Davis, 1939; Clarke & Cowan, 1952; Le Minor & Ben Hamida, 1962).

Snell & Lapage (1971) compared four methods of detecting glucose breakdown, one of which was positive only when all the glucose had been utilized. Peptone water sugars gave the fewest positives and the ammonium salt sugars the most; a modified OF medium (Park, 1967), tested for residual glucose, gave results almost as good as those with ASS. Snell & Lapage confirmed that Pseudomonas maltophilia could attack glucose when methionine, an essential growth factor, was added to the ASS medium, showing that it was suitable, when supplemented, for testing fastidious bacteria.

Carbohydrate utilization by anaerobes can be shown in liquid media in an anaerobic jar or, without using a jar, in deep columns of agar medium under a seal; beware, for the gas produced may

31

blow the seals out of the tube and your incubator becomes contaminated with plugs, seals and perhaps agar. Gas production may be from protein and is not, in itself, evidence of carbohydrate utilization. So many anaerobes decolorize indicators that it is usual to add the indicator after completion of incubation.

4.5.7   Carbon source utilization (CSU) tests are used extensively in classificatory work and their application to identification is limited mainly to tests for the utilization of citrate, but an extension to other substrates is anticipated (Snell & Lapage, 1973). The mineral basal medium used by Owens & Keddie (1969) for studies on nitrogen nutrition can be used for the CSU tests; it may be supplemented when necessary with an amino acid mixture or with yeast extract (0.02%) and vitamin B_{12}, 2 µg/l (R. M. Keddie, personal communication).

Gordon & Mihm (1957) used organic acids as carbon sources in the basal medium described in Section A2.7.5. But few CSU tests are yet ready for use in routine diagnostic laboratories, since nitrogenous supplements to make growth possible may provide enough carbon to eliminate the need for more.

Citrate utilization is tested in Koser's (1923) citrate medium or in a similar medium solidified by agar (Simmons, 1926). Vaughn *et al.* (1950) believe that the addition of agar invalidates the test. The medium must be in chemically clean tubes (see Section A1.1). In tests of this kind the inoculum should be small and free from medium on which the organism has grown. To avoid carry-over, use a straight wire instead of a loop, and inoculate from a light suspension in water, saline or buffer. All growth should be confirmed by subculture (again using a wire) to another tube of the same citrate medium.

Other citrate media, such as Christensen's, contain additional nutrients and do not test the ability of the organism to use the citrate radical as a sole carbon source. An organism growing in Koser's or Simmons' medium will grow on Christensen's medium, but one growing on Christensen's medium may not grow on the other two media (but see Piéchaud & Szturm-Rubinsten, 1963).

4.5.8   Chitinolytic activity can be shown as a clear halo around growth on chitin agar. As chitin is insoluble in water a purified preparation is suspended in salt (for halophils) or water agar and layered on a base of nutrient agar (Section C3.10).

4.5.9   The coagulase test was developed from observations that certain staphylococci clotted plasma from the goose (Loeb, 1903), man, horse, and sheep (Much, 1908), and Gratia (1920) introduced the name staphylocoagulase for the active agent. At least two substances go to make up staphylocoagulase, bound and free coagulases, but the tube methods of carrying out the coagulase test do not distinguish between them; the slide test (Cadness-Graves *et al.* 1943) detects bound coagulase.

The type of plasma used in the test may affect the result; the anticoagulant should not be citrate alone for this will be removed by citrate-using bacteria such as *Klebsiella aerogenes* (Harper & Conway, 1948) or certain streptococci (Evans, Buettner & Niven, 1952), with the result that a clot will form after prolonged incubation and give the (false) appearance of a delayed positive coagulase test. Harper & Conway recommend that heparin be added to citrated plasma to prevent clotting of fibrin when the citrate is withdrawn. A filterable coagulase-like factor produced by some streptococci will not clot heparinized plasma (Wood, 1959). The species of animal from which the plasma is derived is important; for staphylococci of human origin plasma from man or rabbit should be used, sheep or bovine plasma gives fewer positives and guinea-pig plasma gives even fewer. When strains from animals other than man are under test, it is advisable to run the test with plasmas of several animal species, including the one from which the strains were isolated.

The coagulase test is simple, so simple that there are almost as many ways of doing it as there are bacteriologists. There is now an internationally agreed (or recommended) method of testing for free coagulase (Subcommittee, 1965), see Section C3.11. Williams & Harper (1946) compared many of the methods, and those given in Appendix C are based on their recommendations and our own experience and preference. We draw attention to points that we regard as important. Occasionally a strain will be isolated that produces so much fibrinolysin early in its growth that a clot from coagulase action never becomes visible. Sometimes a small clot forms early but lyses quickly; for this reason a reading should be made an hour after the test has been put up. Some strains produce only small amounts of coagulase and the clot may only be seen after overnight incubation. Each batch of plasma should be tested to show that it is suitable for the coagulase test; filtered plasma is generally unsuitable. Positive and negative controls should be included in the tests put up each day. The use of fibrinogen was investigated by Cadness-Graves *et al.* (1943) and was found to be a suitable substitute for plasma. Dried plasma can also be used (Colbeck & Proom, 1944).

4.5.10   Decarboxylases for amino acids are characteristic for different bacteria within the Enterobacteriaceae (Møller, 1954a, c). Initially the determination of the decarboxylases was a research problem but Møller (1955) developed simpler technical methods so that the decarboxylase pattern became a useful taxonomic tool at a higher level than antigenic structure. The method is not specific for decarboxylation and may indicate other metabolic processes such as deamination, deamidation, and transamination (Cheeseman & Fuller, 1966); we do not make these distinctions in this *Manual*. Glutamic acid decarboxylase, which is characteristic of *Escherichia*, *Shigella*, and *Proteus* (including Providence), cannot yet be determined simply, but arginine dihydrolase, and lysine and ornithine decarboxylases can now be detected simply by observing the colour change of an indicator. Falkow (1958) introduced even simpler tests but we found that they were not satisfactory with klebsiellas; they cannot, therefore, be used with organisms of unknown identity. Arginine is hydrolysed by some but not all streptococci and corynebacteria (Niven, Smiley & Sherman, 1942); methods of detecting arginine hydrolysis by pseudomonads are described by Sherris *et al.* (1959) and Thornley (1960). Steel & Midgley (1962) found the decarboxylase pattern of different genera and species taxonomically useful. Møller's methods are not always satisfactory with the non-fermentative bacteria, and

BSS decarboxylase tests (Pickett & Pedersen, 1970b) may give more positive results.

4.5.11   Denitrification. Many bacteria isolated in medical laboratories are denitrifiers, that is, they not only reduce nitrate to nitrite but also reduce nitrite to nitrogen gas. And this in itself upsets the reading of the nitrate reduction test (see Section 4.5.30 and Table 4.1). The gas may be detected in a Durham tube in nitrate broth or in the butt of FN medium of Pickett & Pedersen (1968).

4.5.12   Deoxyribonuclease (DNase) can be shown by growing the test organisms as streaks on a medium (either defined or complex) containing DNA, and after incubation for 36 hours, flooding the plate with N-HCl. A clear zone around a streak indicates DNase production. The temperature of incubation may be important and Jeffries *et al.* (1957) advise incubating at several temperatures as the enzyme may act at a temperature other than the growth optimal; with *Bacillus megaterium* they obtained zone sizes of 0.2 cm at 37 °C, 0.5 cm at 30 °C, and 0.9 cm at 25 °C.

4.5.13   Digestion of meat, inspissated serum, Dorset egg or casein are used as indicators of proteolytic activity. At one time gelatin liquefaction was used to detect proteolysis, but gelatinase is not a true proteolytic enzyme.

4.5.14   Ethylhydrocuprein or **optochin inhibition** of the pneumococcus was described by Moore in 1915, but as a diagnostic test it has had a chequered career. Soon after its introduction it fell into disrepute and, as a means of distinguishing pneumococci from viridans streptococci, it was superseded by the bile solubility test, especially when the more highly purified bile salts became available (Downie *et al.* 1931). The optochin test has now come into its own again; ethylhydrocuprein is applied to localized areas of a plate by impregnated paper disks (Bowers & Jeffries, 1955; Bowen *et al.* 1957). In the concentration recommended by Bowers & Jeffries a small zone (1–2 mm beyond the disk) of inhibition may occur with a few viridans streptococci but pneumococci are inhibited more obviously and the zone extends 5 mm or more. The advantage of the optochin test over bile solubility is that the disk can be applied to any plate culture of the organism under test, whereas for bile solubility the suspension or broth culture must be of about neutral pH value. When small zones of inhibition are ignored and 5 mm is the minimum to be recorded as positive, the specificity of the optochin test for the pneumococcus is claimed to be high. Bowers & Jeffries (1955) found that only one of 243 pneumococci failed to be inhibited; the exception was found to be avirulent for mice and was thought to be in the R form (however, the R pneumococci are bile soluble).

4.5.15 Biochemical tests in enriched media. Delicate or fastidious organisms are often grown in media enriched with serum, ascitic or hydrocele fluid, and these supplements can introduce uncontrolled and uncontrollable side-effects. Whenever such enrichments are used the supplemented medium (without the test substrate) should be used as a control. For example, Cobb (1966) reported that *Corynebacterium bovis* produced ammonia from Christensen's urea medium supplemented by 3% serum. In a control experiment he found that the organism produced acid from the basal medium without urea (the basal medium contained glucose); when urea was present the test culture produced an alkaline reaction, confirming that alkalinity (the positive urease indicator) of the test was due to urea breakdown (Cobb, personal communication).

An alternative method of dealing with fastidious organisms is to grow them on a suitable medium, wash off with water or saline, spin, resuspend in water and use the suspension in a BSS test (Section 4.5.4). In this way we once showed that *Haemophilus influenzae* produced a powerful urease, a characteristic confirmed by Joyce Frazer (personal communication) and by Sneath & Johnson (1973).

4.5.16 Gelatin hydrolysis or liquefaction is shown by a test in which the organism grows in a nutrient medium solidified by gelatin; the disadvantages of the liquefaction test are (i) different samples of gelatin vary in gelling power; (ii) the cultures are incubated at a temperature (22 °C) below the melting point of the medium (about 25 °C) and mesophilic organisms may grow very slowly or not at all; (iii) some bacteria will not grow in the medium. To overcome the second of these difficulties the cultures may be incubated at the

optimal temperature for growth and later refrigerated to see whether the gelatin has retained its gelling property; a suitable control is uninoculated medium exposed for the same length of time to the same temperature.

Gelatin stab cultures may need weeks of incubation before showing liquefaction. Hucker (1924*a*), working with micrococci, found a curious relation between length of incubation and the first appearance of liquefaction; when the number of liquefying strains was plotted against duration of incubation there were two peaks, one after about 1–2 weeks, the second after about 3 months incubation. The significance of tests of such long duration is doubtful (the gelatin may be denatured) and they are quite useless in identification work. However, the gelatin stab test should not be discarded; some species will liquefy it overnight, others will take longer, and these differences may be helpful in distinguishing between species (e.g. *Enterobacter cloacae*, which takes a week or more, and *Serratia marcescens*, which liquefies gelatin in 1–2 days). For identification work the duration of incubation must be limited to a reasonable period, and we suggest that one of the rapid methods should be run in parallel. Frazier's (1926) test has the advantage that the gelatin is in agar and the medium does not melt at 37 °C. After growth of the organism, the plate is flooded with an acid mercuric chloride solution which reacts with the gelatin in the medium to produce an opacity; where gelatin has been hydrolysed the medium remains clear.

A rapid method devised by Kohn (1953) uses gelatin–charcoal disks hardened by formaldehyde; these do not melt at 37 °C and can be added to peptone water cultures which are then returned to the incubator; preformed or induced enzyme will hydrolyse the gelatin and liberate the charcoal particles. Our experience with these disks is limited but there seem to be uncontrolled factors that produce considerable variations between different batches of disks. However, Lautrop (1956*a*) found that the action of gelatinases was influenced by the presence of Ca ions and recommended that test organisms should be suspended in physiological saline + 0.01 M-CaCl$_2$. Using Difco gelatin, he reported favourably on the modified method. Green & Larks (1955) devised an even quicker micromethod in which Kohn's disks were used (see Section C3.21). Thirst (1957b) and Hoyt & Pickett (1957) developed microscope-slide techniques which were similar to one described by Pickford & Dorris (1934), who found that the gelatin of photographic plates and film could be removed by proteolytic enzymes and bacteria. LeMinor & Piéchaud (1963) describe a method in which the silver sulphide of exposed and developed film can be seen to be released when the gelatin is liquefied.

4.5.17 Gluconate is converted by some bacteria to 2-ketogluconate which can be detected by the appearance of a reducing substance in the medium. Haynes (1951) found this test helpful in identifying *Pseudomonas aeruginosa*. Shaw & Clarke (1955) simplified the test and reported that it was useful for klebsiellas. When *Klebsiella* species were compared with *Enterobacter*, Cowan et al. (1960) found that klebsiellas with IMViC reactions − − + + and *Enterobacter* species were gluconate positive, but that klebsiellas with other IMViC reactions were often gluconate negative.

4.5.18 Growth or failure to grow on specified media can, depending on the media themselves, indicate (i) nutritional needs; (ii) sensitivity or insensitivity to substance(s) in the medium; (iii) ability to use a specified compound as source of a particular element. Examples of the characters revealed are: (i) growth on blood agar but not on the basal medium indicates a need for enrichment with blood; (ii) (a) failure to grow on MacConkey accompanied by growth on nutrient agar, shows sensitivity to bile salt; (b) growth on media containing 6.5% NaCl shows an unusual degree of salt tolerance; (iii) failure to grow on Koser's citrate medium shows that the organism cannot use citrate as carbon source under the conditions tested. These utilization tests must be adequately controlled to prevent carry-over from the medium on which the inoculum was grown (see citrate utilization, Section 4.5.7).

4.5.19 Haemolysin production and **haemolysis** are not always cause and effect, and the ability to produce a soluble haemolysin is not necessarily associated with zones of haemolysis on blood agar

plates (Elek & Levy, 1954). Streptococci produce haemolytic zones on the surface of blood agar made from the blood of most animal species and these organisms are rightly named haemolytic streptococci. The haemolysins produced by streptococci may be oxygen labile (streptolysin O) or oxygen stable (streptolysin S) and they need different conditions for their production; on blood agar plates, however, similar zones of haemolysis are produced. Brown (1919) studied the haemolytic zones around streptococcus colonies in poured plates and labelled the types of haemolysis α (green zone, cell envelopes intact), β (clear, colourless zone, cell envelopes dissolved) and γ (no action on red cells). The term γ-haemolysis is an anachronism and describes a negative result. The application of the first two terms, α and β, has been extended to the haemolytic zones seen around colonies on the surface of blood agar, and although this is not in accordance with Brown's usage, it is a convention that is well understood.

Streptococci that produce α-haemolysis or green zones on blood agar are often described as the 'greening streptococci'. The species name *Streptococcus viridans* has been attached to several different kinds of greening streptococci, but as the species has never been adequately characterized, the name is now seldom used; *Streptococcus mitior* is probably most representative of organisms that were named *S. viridans*.

Staphylococci behave differently on plates made with the blood of different species and it is misleading to speak of haemolytic staphylococci because the haemolysis may be due to a haemolysin or to a lipolytic enzyme (Orcutt & Howe, 1922). The soluble haemolysins can be used to detect the toxins produced by some strains of staphylococci; thus rabbit cell haemolysin is one manifestation of α-toxin, and sheep cell 'hot–cold' lysin is a characteristic of β-toxin. These toxins are not used in characterizing different species of *Staphylococcus* and so do not appear in our diagnostic tables.

Among strains of *Clostridium*, however, the different kinds of toxin produced may determine the species, and as some of the toxins are haemolytic, these could appear in tables showing the finer subdivision of the genus. The haemolytic activity of certain vibrios is said to have distinguishing value; with these organisms not only is the species of red cell attacked important, but also we should know whether calcium is needed for or inhibits haemolysis (De *et al.* 1954).

4.5.20   Hippurate may be hydrolysed to benzoate by bacterial action, and the ability to do this is limited to certain bacteria, of which it is an important characteristic. The end product is tested for by the addition of ferric chloride which precipitates both hippurate and benzoate but the hippurate is more readily soluble in excess. The final concentration of iron is critical and to find the optimal amount of $FeCl_3$ to add, uninoculated tubes of medium, on which a titration can be made, are incubated with the test cultures.

The methods of Ayers & Rupp (1922) and Hare & Colebrook (1934) for streptococci use a relatively rich basal medium in which the organism will grow without hippurate. The Hajna & Damon (1934) method for coliforms uses Koser's medium (without citrate) as a base and so becomes a test of the organism's ability to use hippurate as a source of carbon as well as its ability to hydrolyse it. Thirst (1957a) added an indicator so that the growth may be seen more readily.

4.5.21   Hydrogen sulphide production by bacteria is such a common feature that, of itself, it has little differential value. The H_2S test is one that can be made as sensitive as a worker wishes (for a review see Clarke, 1953a); with an adequate sulphur source (cysteine) and a delicate indicator (lead acetate papers) almost all the enteric bacteria can be shown to have the ability to produce H_2S. Tested in this way we obtain an accurate estimate of an organism's katabolic power in relation to sulphur compounds but we cannot distinguish readily between those organisms that have much and those that have little ability to produce H_2S. With a poor medium or a less sensitive indicator (ferrous chloride or lead acetate in the medium) we detect only the strong H_2S-producers. This is the kind of test used by the enterobacteriologists who have developed tests of low sensitivity that make possible clear distinctions between *Escherichia* and *Salmonella* and even between different salmonellas. Two media yield results of this kind, ferrous chloride gelatin

and triple sugar iron agar (TSI); both are recommended by the international Enterobacteriaceae Sub-Committee (Report, 1958), and their formulae are given in Appendix A. Lead acetate papers are not only ten times more sensitive than lead acetate in the medium, but they eliminate the toxicity of lead for the growing bacteria (ZoBell & Feltham, 1934). In the Brucella group the time of H_2S production may be significant; this is found by changing the lead acetate papers each day.

4.5.22   Indole is volatile and can be detected either by testing the medium with *p*-dimethylamino-benzaldehyde or by a paper strip impregnated with oxalic acid held near the mouth of the test tube by the cotton plug. Both methods are sensitive and usually give the same result; occasionally all the indole volatilizes and only the paper strip is positive. Extraction of the indole from the liquid culture increases the sensitivity of the test; ether, xylol and petroleum have been used, but all are potentially dangerous if, following the usual bacteriological techniques, the mouth of the tube is flamed. Kovács' (1928) reagent has the advantage that the solvent (amyl alcohol) is present in the test solution. Oxalic acid papers (Gnezda, 1899; Holman & Gonzales, 1923) and papers soaked in *p*-dimethyl-aminobenzaldehyde (Kohn, 1954) are sensitive indicators of indole.

Temperature of incubation may affect the result; Taylor (1945–6) found three strains of *Escherichia coli* that were indole negative at 37 °C but positive at 30 °C. Some organisms (e.g. *Clostridium* species) may break down indole; Reed (1942) found that with some species this happened so slowly that indole could always be detected in cultures 1–10 days old, but *C. sporogenes* used it so quickly that they gave negative results when cultures were grown for only one day in a medium containing 1 mg indole per 100 ml broth.

Unless indole has previously been extracted with xylol, sodium nitrite present in broth may interfere with its detection by Ehrlich's or Kovács' reagents (Smith, Rogers & Bettge, 1972).

4.5.23   Inhibition of growth by a defined or a biological agent may be a useful identifying characteristic and is used in several of our tables; it occurs in rather different forms, ranging from inhibition by chemicals such as KCN or dyes to inhibition by antibiotics. Inhibition by KCN (C3.29), optochin (C3.20), and the pteridine derivative O/129 (C3.38) are described in the sections indicated; here we mention inhibition by antibiotics (or antibiotic sensitivities) which are not discussed at length in this *Manual* (see Section 4.3.1).

Commercially available antibiotic disks keep pace with prevailing fashion; there are single disks containing different amounts of antibiotic and also rings with several antibiotics. While all the requirements of the inveterate antibiotic sensitivity tester are readily available, the enthusiast should not imagine that antibiotic sensitivities will help him to identify an organism he has isolated. If readers think that this is a cynical or prejudiced view they are probably correct.

4.5.24 The **KCN** test distinguishes those bacteria that can grow in the presence of cyanide and those that cannot grow in the stated concentration. When we report a strain as KCN positive we mean that it is resistant and that it grows in Møller's (1954b) KCN medium. KCN-negative strains, i.e. those that do not grow, should be subcultured to the basal medium without KCN; if they cannot grow in the basal medium the test is without significance. Møller (1954b) used waxed corks to prevent loss of cyanide from the tubes; these are unpleasant to handle and we prefer to use small screw-capped bottles (Rogers & Taylor, 1961).

Those who use the test assume certain responsibilities; KCN and HCN are extremely toxic and the KCN solution should be kept in a locked cupboard. After use the cyanide in the medium should be destroyed by adding ferrous sulphate and alkali before the tubes or bottles are put in the autoclave.

4.5.25 Lecitho-vitellin (LV) is the lipoprotein component of egg-yolk and can be obtained as a clear yellow liquid by mixing egg-yolk with saline. This liquid becomes opalescent when mixed with certain bacterial toxins or lecithinases; flocculation and separation of a thick curd of fat may follow. When lecithinase-forming organisms are grown on a solid medium containing LV, the lecithinase diffuses into the agar and produces zones of opalescence around individual colonies. This reaction can be inhibited by adding certain antitoxic or antilecithinase sera to the surface of the medium before inoculation. Lipolytic organisms also produce an opalescence on LV agar and it is often accompanied by a distinctive 'pearly layer' or iridescent film; the presence of free fatty acid can be demonstrated by treating the medium, after incubation, with copper sulphate solution (Willis, 1960). The ability to produce an opacity on LV agar is useful in the division of the genera *Bacillus* and *Clostridium*, but other organisms, such as *Staphylococcus aureus*, may give positive reactions.

The LV reaction is not due solely to a lecithinase, and Willis & Gowland (1962) consider that separation of insoluble protein, splitting of fats from lipoprotein complexes, and coalescence of particles of free fat are all involved. In many laboratories medium containing human serum (Nagler, 1939) has been replaced by egg-yolk medium.

Although *Pseudomonas aeruginosa* is known to produce a lecithinase, the egg-yolk reaction is usually negative; from this Stanier *et al.* (1966) argue that the egg-yolk reaction is specific for only one kind of lecithinase and that other types do not produce an opacity of egg-yolk. The actions of four types of lecithinase are discussed by Willis (1969); lecithinase C (but the terminology is confused) is the one usually produced by bacteria.

4.5.26 The **malonate** test was introduced by Leifson (1933) to help distinguish *Escherichia coli* from *Klebsiella aerogenes*, and with these organisms he found a perfect correlation with the VP test. Shaw (1956) showed that most strains of the Arizona group were malonate positive and most other kinds of salmonella were malonate negative. Both these groups are VP negative and there is clearly no correlation between the malonate and VP tests. The test was described as a fermentation by Leifson and as a utilization by Shaw in spite of the fact that she added yeast extract to stimulate growth.

4.5.27 The **methyl red (MR)** test and Voges–Proskauer (VP) test for acetylmethylcarbinol or acetoin may be carried out on the same tube of culture. The tests are mainly used to distinguish various coliform organisms from each other; all these ferment glucose vigorously and the pH value of the glucose medium falls quickly. When methyl red is added after overnight incubation the cultures of all these organisms will be found to be acid to the dye, i.e. MR positive. After further incubation *Escherichia coli* cultures produce even more acid and in spite of phosphate buffer in the medium may be self-sterilizing; the MR test remains positive. *Klebsiella aerogenes* cultures, on the other hand, decarboxylate and condense the pyruvic acid to form acetylmethylcarbinol, the pH value rises and, when methyl red is added, the colour is yellow, i.e. MR negative. Nowadays there is a tendency to do biochemical tests earlier but the temptation to speed up the MR test must be resisted; the MR should never be read until the cultures have been incubated for at least 2 days at 37 °C or 3 days at 30 °C. The reaction cannot be accelerated by increasing the glucose content of the medium; Clark & Lubs (1915) found that, in media with much above 1% glucose, cultures of *K. aerogenes* did not revert to become MR negative.

4.5.28 Milk (usually as litmus milk or bromcresol purple milk) is a good nutrient medium in which most organisms will grow and it has a fairly constant composition since man only interferes by removing the cream and adding an indicator. Although highly esteemed elsewhere, in the medical laboratory litmus (or bromcresol purple) milk occupies a secondary position and most bacteriologists believe that the information it gives can be obtained more certainly in other media. An objection to milk is that unless a change takes place in the appearance of the medium (e.g. acid or clot formation) one cannot be sure that growth has occurred.

Milk contains lactose, galactose, a trace of glucose, casein, and mineral salts. Acid production from the fermentation of lactose is shown by a change in colour of the indicator, and, when much acid is produced, by the formation of a clot. But another form of clot may be produced by rennet; in this case the clot forms and later, like the fibrin clot in blood, contracts and expresses a clear whey. By contrast the acid clot does not contract. When the bacterium also produces proteolytic enzymes the clot may be peptonized. Apart from the rennet clot (for which milk is a unique medium) all the

other reactions can be detected more easily by using media appropriate for each reaction.

4.5.29 Niacin (nicotinic acid) production is a characteristic feature of human tubercle bacilli and distinguishes them from bovine tubercle bacilli and other mycobacteria (Pope & Smith, 1946). Several modifications of the test method have been devised; all are based on the extraction of niacin from the bacterial growth and subsequent detection by a colorimetric reaction. Users of the test must exercise caution as one of the reagents (cyanogen bromide) is lachrymatory and toxic.

4.5.30 Nitrate reduction may be shown either by detecting the presence of one of the breakdown products, or by showing the disappearance of nitrate from the medium. The products of reduction may include nitrite, hyponitrite, hydroxylamine, ammonia, nitrous oxide, or gaseous nitrogen. The first test to be applied aims at showing the presence of nitrite. When this test is negative (i.e. nitrite is not detected) we test the medium to see whether there is residual nitrate; if this test also is negative we know that the first stage of the breakdown has been completed and the nitrite further broken down.

In uninoculated nitrate broth or cultures of organisms that do not reduce nitrate the test for nitrite is negative until zinc dust (ZoBell, 1932) or other reducing agent is added to the culture medium to reduce the nitrate contained in it. To detect small amounts of residual nitrate the amount of zinc added may be critical (Steel & Fisher, 1961). The tests are very sensitive and it is important to check the uninoculated medium for nitrite, which should not be present.

Some workers prefer to carry out the test in a semisolid medium (ZoBell, 1932); others insist that free access to oxygen is necessary for nitrate reduction by aerobes.

Conn (1936) discussed the difficulty of recording the results of the nitrate reduction test, and advised that the terms positive and negative be avoided. Instead the actual finding(s) should be recorded; the possibilities are shown in Table 4.1.

An entirely different method was described by Cook (1950) who found that when nitrate was included in blood agar base, nitrate-reducing

Table 4.1 *Interpretation of tests for reduction of nitrate and nitrite*

Culture grown in	Test Applied	Result	Interpretation
Nitrate broth	1 For nitrite	Colour not changed (negative)	Nitrite not present (see 3 below)
	2 For nitrite	Red colour (positive)	Nitrate reduced to nitrite
	3 Zinc dust added to 1	A Colour not changed	Nitrite not present: therefore $-NO_3$ in original medium has been reduced by the bacteria
		B Red colour	$-NO_3$ in medium reduced to $-NO_2$ by zinc but not by bacteria
Nitrite broth	4 For nitrite	C Red colour	Nitrite present; not (all) reduced
		D Colour not changed	Nitrite reduced by bacteria and has disappeared from the medium

bacteria growing on the blood agar reduced the haemoglobin to methaemoglobin; this method has the advantage that the change seen is apparent even when the organism can reduce nitrite.

4.5.31 Nitrite reduction can be brought about by certain bacteria incapable of reducing nitrate (ZoBell, 1932). It can be shown by growing the organism in a broth containing 0.01 % $NaNO_2$ and, after sufficient time for the reduction to take place, testing for residual nitrite (Table 4.1).

4.5.32 The **nitrogen nutrition** of bacteria can be studied in a mineral base plus a chelating agent (Owens & Keddie, 1969). The method has considerable interest in classification work but the standards of chemical cleanliness required are higher than some bacteriological laboratories can meet. But this should not deter anyone from trying the method.

4.5.33 O/129 sensitivity. The pteridine derivative O/129 is almost specific in its inhibition of vibrios, and it is useful to apply to any non-fluorescent, oxidase-positive, Gram-negative rod. Simple methods, dropping one or two crystals (Davis & Park, 1962) or drops of 10% suspension (Barrow, personal communication) on to an inoculated plate, seem to be satisfactory.

4.5.34 The **ONPG** (*o*-nitrophenyl-β-D-galactopyranoside) test is used to detect potential lactose fermenters which, in ordinary media, either take several days to produce acid or do not produce any acid. Lactose fermentation depends on two enzymes, (i) an induced intracellular enzyme, β-galactosidase, which attacks lactose, and (ii) a permease which regulates penetration of the cell wall. Kriebel (1934) found that late lactose-fermenters produced acid more quickly when the concentration of lactose was increased to 5%; Chilton & Fulton (1946) recommended 10% lactose in agar. However, the results of the 5 and 10% lactose tests and the ONPG test for β-galactosidase do not always agree (Lapage, Efstratiou & Hill, 1973). Lederberg (1950) used ONPG for the study of β-galactosidase, and Le Minor & Ben Hamida (1962) developed a rapid ONPG test on toluene-treated bacterial cultures. Lowe (1962) found that toluene treatment was not essential to liberate the β-galactosidase and that overnight incubation of cultures in peptone water containing ONPG hydrolysed the colourless substrate to the yellow *o*-nitrophenol.

4.5.35 Phenylalanine can be converted by oxidative deamination to phenylpyruvic acid (PPA) which, like many other keto acids, can be identified by adding ferric chloride (Singer & Volcani, 1955). The phenylalanine test was used by Henriksen & Closs (1938) who found that *Proteus* species gave the strongest reactions but *Klebsiella aerogenes* also gave some positives. Since then Henriksen (1950) and other users of the test (Buttiaux *et al.* 1954; Singer & Bar-Chey, 1954; Shaw & Clarke, 1955) have found it to be almost specific for *Proteus* and Providence. This specificity prompted Singer & Bar-Chey to put the Providence organisms into the genus *Proteus*.

The phenylalanine deaminase of *Moraxella phenylpyruvica* seems to be weaker than that of *Proteus* species and the usual methods do not work well. Snell & Davey (1971) describe a method in which the tubes are agitated at 37 °C and give positive results in about an hour.

Most strains of *Erwinia herbicola* are PPA positive.

4.5.36 Phosphatase activity was used by Barber & Kuper (1951) to aid the identification of pathogenic staphylococci; they found a high degree of correlation between phosphatase and coagulase production. By prolonging the incubation period, Baird-Parker (1963) demonstrated phosphatase production in 378 of 546 strains of staphylococci and 10 of 677 strains of micrococci. Some workers prefer a liquid medium and Lewis (1961) compared the plate and tube methods; he found that essentially similar results were obtainable in a liquid medium incubated for 6 hours and on a solid medium incubated for 18 hours with coagulase-positive staphylococci, but the tube method showed far fewer phosphatase-positive coagulase-negative strains. Among enteric bacteria, Vörös *et al.* (1961) found phosphatase to be produced only by strains of *Proteus* and Providence; using the same technique we were unable to confirm this specificity and found positives also in the *Salmonella, Shigella, Klebsiella,* and *Escherichia* groups.

4.5.37 Pigment formation often has considerable diagnostic value and it is an advantage to know how to encourage it. Although the pigments produced are seldom photosynthetic, most bacteria dealt with in this *Manual* form pigment better in the light; this is most noticeable in the staphylococci

and serratias, but also occurs in the pseudomonads and in chromobacteria. The effect of light on pigment production by mycobacteria has become a means of distinguishing species. Temperature and medium also influence the intensity of pigmentation; most bacteria produce pigments better at temperatures below the optimum for growth. In England room temperature is usually so low that the organism may fail to grow; in such cases a 22 °C incubator will be useful.

Medium probably has the biggest effect on the development of pigment. In some cases the simple addition of glucose will enhance pigmentation, in other cases this will inhibit it. The old adage that 'one man's meat is another man's poison' applies to bacterial pigment production and different formulae are needed for different organisms. The elimination of all meat extracts and the addition of mannitol are beneficial for *Chromobacterium* species and may improve pigmentation of *Serratia* (Goldsworthy & Still, 1936, 1938); quite different media are needed to encourage pigmentation by pseudomonads (see Section A2.5). In a personal communication, Dr M. J. Pickett tells us that all strains of *Pseudomonas cepacia* produce pigment on Kligler's iron agar (KIA) and on TSI, but not on any other medium (used in American clinical laboratories). This observation could not have been made in England, where KIA and TSI are less often used, and probably never for observing pigment production.

4.5.38 Poly-β-hydroxybutyric acid (PHB) may accumulate as a cellular reserve material, and was used by Stanier *et al.* (1966) in their characterizations of *Pseudomonas* species. The chemical method of extracting and identifying the polymer (Williamson & Wilkinson, 1958) is not suitable for routine use, but examination of wet preparations of the organism by phase-contrast microscopy or of films stained by weak carbol fuchsin will reveal the intracellular deposits. PHB is produced most abundantly when the organism is grown in a medium containing DL-β-hydroxybutyrate.

4.5.39 Survival under certain adverse conditions (usually heat) may have diagnostic significance; e.g. a streptococcus that survives heating at 60 °C for 30 minutes is likely to be a group D streptococcus. The tests themselves are not easy to standardize and the methods used by different authors vary greatly. For example, after the heating test for *Streptococcus faecalis* an immediate subculture may fail to show growth, whereas if the heated broth is incubated overnight before a subculture is made, this later subculture is more likely to grow. Other factors that may affect the result are the medium or suspending fluid in which the heating is carried out, its pH value, the time allowed for the medium to heat up to the desired temperature, and the type of container, particularly the thickness of the glass, in which the sample is heated. Some authors (Abd-el-Malek & Gibson, 1948a) always use milk which they regard as a medium of more constant composition than man-made infusions and enzymic digests.

While the testing of vegetative bacteria for survival has its difficulties, the testing of spore suspensions is even more full of pitfalls. The heat stability of spores varies from one species to another, but even in the same species it will vary from strain to strain, and spores of the same strain grown on different occasions do not necessarily have the same resistance to heat. For a discussion of this subject the reader is referred to papers by Kelsey (1958, 1961).

4.5.40 Temperature range for growth and optimal temperature are characteristic of different groups of bacteria; of those in the medical and veterinary fields the optimal temperature is usually between 35 and 40 °C but the range for growth varies considerably. Some species (e.g. *Neisseria gonorrhoeae*) have only a narrow range and rapidly die at temperatures outside the range; other organisms have a wide growth and an even wider survival range. In all cases the optimal temperature is near the maximum for growth.

Biochemical tests are usually made on cultures grown at the temperature optimal for growth; that this may not be optimal for the development of the product which is being tested is shown in acetoin production by hafnias which occurs at a lower temperature than the growth optimum. We have found that some salmonellas are able to grow on a medium containing an ammonium salt as nitrogen source at 30 °C but will not grow on this medium at 37 °C, the optimal temperature for growth on media providing organic nitrogen.

The ability of an organism to grow at 20–22, 30, and 37 °C are tested in many laboratories and our diagnostic tables show, in general, the more specialized tests used by experts in different groups of bacteria; for these, easily adjusted water baths or incubators are needed. In the differentiation of species of *Mycobacterium* (Table 6.10b) growth or survival is shown at several different temperatures.

4.5.41 Temperature tolerance. Most mesophilic bacteria in the vegetative state are killed at 56 °C for 30 minutes, but a few species such as *Staphylococcus aureus*, *Aerococcus viridans*, and some species of *Streptococcus* survive such heating. Indeed, most group D strains survive heating at 60 °C for 30 minutes, and a test for this degree of heat tolerance is useful for making a quick identification of these species (see Table 6.3c).

4.5.42 Tween 80 test for lipolytic activity (Sierra, 1957). Tween 80 is the oleic acid ester of a polyoxyalkylene derivative of sorbitan. It can be included in a suitable nutrient medium and the test culture(s) streaked on the surface; after incubation at the optimal temperature for the organism(s) under test, the plate is examined for opaque haloes around the growth. The opacity, which indicates lipolytic activity, is due to crystal formation.

Tween 80 can also be incorporated in a liquid medium, which is used for the much longer period of incubation (up to 21 days) needed by mycobacteria (Kubica & Dye, 1967).

4.5.43 Urease activity is tested in Christensen's (1946) urea medium which supports the growth of many bacteria. The urease activity of *Proteus* species can be shown in a highly buffered urea medium (Stuart, van Stratum & Rustigian, 1945) in which other enterobacteria appear to be urease negative; *Proteus* species can use urea nitrogen but most other urease-producing organisms need an additional nitrogen source. Urease activity is shown by alkali production from urea solutions, but, in at least two methods (Elek, 1948; Ortali & Samarani, 1955), Nessler's reagent is added to show the presence of ammonia.

5
Theory and practice of bacterial identification

Unlike authors of texts with chapters headed 'Xococcal infections' and the like, we do not think that clinicians are able or skilled enough to make a bacteriological diagnosis or to guide the laboratory worker to the appropriate chapter; on the other hand, we think that his notes and the information he passes to us should be sufficiently full to help us to choose the appropriate media for the primary isolation.

We believe that we should approach a bacteriological investigation without preconceived ideas, consider our organism as quite unknown, and start the identification from the basic (primary) characters.

5.1   Theory of identification

In theory the identification of a bacterium consists of a comparison of the unknown with the known, the object being the ability to say that the unknown is like A (one of the knowns) and unlike B–Z (all other knowns); a subsidiary (some would say a more important) objective is to say that the unknown is A, i.e. to give it a name or identification tag. When we say that it is A we imply that it is different from the other knowns, B–Z. All identification schemes depend on knowing a great deal about the already identified (or known) units, but the human memory can cope only with a small proportion of this knowledge and memory aids make up the treasure chest of the diagnostician. In practice there are at present two distinct methods of making the identification, but a third method using a computer suggested by Payne (1963), although a practical possibility (Lapage et al. 1970; Whitby & Blair, 1970) is not readily available and is not described here.

The first method is familiar to all biologists and uses the dichotomous key. Characters are taken in turn and the keys are most successful when the features can be expressed unequivocally as positive or negative. Although *Streptomyces* species are not described in this *Manual*, Küster's (1972) claim that dichotomous keys are the most workable for the classification and identification of that genus deserves notice. In choosing the sequence of characters he tried to take first those that were easiest to determine, and he followed the same sequence for all subdivisions of the genus. Küster's scheme used seven characters which he was able to determine from observations made on cultures grown on two media only. With this economy of effort he (i) made primary groupings on the colour of the aerial mycelium, and (ii) subdivided these groups by the presence or absence of a distinctive pigment on the reverse side of the vegetative mycelium. Other characters used were, in order (iii) melanin reaction, (iv) formation of a soluble pigment, (v) morphology of sporophores, (vi) morphology of spores, and (vii) further subdivisions made on the utilization of one or more carbohydrates. The only dichotomous key to deal comprehensively with bacteria is that developed by Skerman (1949, 1959, 1967) and the successive versions have been increasingly useful.

Another form of dichotomous key is named a flow chart, and the one worked out by Manclark & Pickett (1961) makes allowance for the variable reactions given by strains of some species. Thus, what we in this *Manual* call a 'd' character (different in different strains, positive in some, negative in others) is treated in the flow chart as both positive and negative, and the species appears in at least two places at the extremities.

Tables make up the second memory aid, and these are widely used in all laboratories. It is easier to see the essential characters in a table than in pages of descriptive matter, which is seldom precise

and often made unnecessarily vague by phrases such as 'most strains are . . .', 'some strains do not . . .', 'not infrequently strains . . .', and the impossible 'strains showing no . . .'.

The construction of tables would be simplified if all strains of one species behaved alike, and if the results of all tests could be expressed as clear-cut positives and negatives. Unfortunately neither of these desiderata is likely to happen, and we are forced to use various symbols to indicate the constancy or inconstancy of characters.

The symbols now in use were developed from those used by Kauffmann, Edwards & Ewing (1956), and later adopted in reports of the Entero-bacteriaceae Subcommittee of what has become the International Committee on Systematic Bacteriology of the International Association of Microbiological Societies (ICSB of IAMS). Neither Kauffmann nor the Subcommittee fixed any numerical values to the symbols and in the first edition of this *Manual* we gave a small table showing the values we had used in preparing tables for that edition. In Table 5.1 we show the assessment of these values and the gradings used in Chapters 6 and 7 of this edition; we also show the approximate equivalents of descriptive terms used for reactions or expressing the results of tests; these equivalents (which are subjective) are necessary because so few characterizations are expressed quantitatively. Few laboratories have examined a sufficient number of strains of the less common bacteria to make percentages meaningful; an exception to this statement is the Center for Disease Control, Atlanta, Georgia which, over a period of many years, has handled large numbers of cultures and turned out many publications in which the results are expressed quantitatively. The tables of King (1964, 1972) for a large range of bacteria, and those of Edwards & Ewing (1962, 1972) for a more limited range, are particularly valuable.

Some characters are almost invariably positive or negative; unfortunately characters of such constancy are usually shared by similar organisms, and although they are important in characterizing an organism (and may appear in the miniature definitions given in Chapters 6 and 7), they have little value in distinguishing it from its neighbours, and seldom appear in our second-stage tables.

The tables can form the basis of a set of diagnostic punched cards to be used with similar cards on which the characters of the unknowns are punched. Sorting the cards of the unknowns with those of the knowns can be one of the quickest, most accurate and least burdensome ways of arriving at an identification (cf. Riddle *et al.* 1956).

The use of our tables in a punched card system of identification will be described in Chapter 8 and Appendix D.

5.2 Practice of identification

So far in this *Manual* we have discussed principles and indicated how all identification is based on a comparison of the organism we wish to identify with organisms of known identity. The accuracy of the identification depends on the thoroughness of the preparatory work such as media making, preparing stains and reagents, and the degree of care taken in carrying out, observing and recording the results of the various tests.

In Chapter 3 we drew attention to the fact that bacteria isolated on inhibitory and selective media were likely to be mixed cultures, and we indicated some of the steps to be taken to purify a culture. It is not easy to be sure that the purified culture is incontrovertably pure, and when there is any doubt whatever, it saves time to repeat the purification process. To identify a culture takes a great deal of effort and to suspect at the end that the culture is impure is not only aggravating to the laboratory worker and the delay in receiving the report frustrating to the clinician, but indicates that the bacteriologist has wasted much of his time and material. Common organisms really are the commonest; when an organism cannot be identified or seems to be an exotic species, we should consider the possibility that either our culture material is impure, or that we have made some error in observation or recording. This happens to all of us and it reflects adversely on our ability and integrity when we fail to repeat observations, and go ahead believing that our results are infallible.

There are various routes by which an identification can be arrived at; the medical bacteriologist often has the advantage that he known what he is looking for, and at an early stage directs his investigation into certain special channels. This may turn out to be a disadvantage, and the selective media used may inhibit the growth of a pathogen whose presence is unsuspected. Steel (1962*a*) discussed the different techniques used in making identifications of pure cultures. Basically there are three approaches to the problem; in the first, which we call the *blunderbuss* method, every conceivable test is made, and when all the results are available, the characters of the organism are compared with those listed in standard texts and *Bergey's Manual*. If all tests appropriate to the organism have been included, it should be possible to make the identification, but quite often we find that other (possibly unheard of) characters are mentioned and additional tests are needed: this is such a common experience that few bacteriologists follow the blunderbuss method. However, such a comprehensive investigation is necessary when the organism has to be characterized for its description as a new species.

The second approach is based on *probabilities* and a judicious assessment of what sort of organism is causing the particular infective process. Thus, from a boil one would expect to isolate *Staphylococcus aureus*, or from the stools of a patient with an intestinal upset, one of the enterobacteria, and it would be reasonable to put up tests that are likely to lead to as rapid an identification as is consistent with accuracy. When the most probable causal organism seems to be excluded, the investigator should continue with an open mind and follow the third approach.

The third approach is the step-by-step or *progressive* method used in this *Manual*, in which the first step aims at determining a few fundamental characters such as those used in Tables 6.1 (p. 46) and 7.1 (p. 78). When these characters are known (usually in 24 hours but occasionally needing 48 hours) another set of media can be inoculated to enable the appropriate tests (to be found in a second-stage table) to be made; the number of these tests will always be less than that needed when the blunderbuss method is followed. Sometimes additional tests are needed for the better identification of a species, and these are shown in third-stage tables.

In deciding what media to inoculate we are guided

by the tests to be carried out, and we must decide for or against classical methods that are slow, e.g. gelatin stab cultures to show liquefaction or hydrolysis. Time can be saved by using multitest media in which several reactions can be observed at one time; such methods are used mainly in the preliminary screening of large numbers of cultures, and they are useful in that 'non-pathogens' or organisms thought to be of low-grade pathogenicity can be detected and discarded without more ado, and further tests restricted to those organisms that appear to fit into groups that contain potential pathogens.

Other rapid methods may be considered. Not only are the methods quicker than standard procedures but some, at least, give more clear-cut results. We should warn users of these methods that the Clarke (1953*a*) H₂S microtest is very sensitive and gives more positives than are shown in our tables.

When all the tests are completed the results are compared with the appropriate table(s); in this edition some species can be identified at the second stage, in others both the second- and third-stage tables should be consulted. For various reasons a species (or genus) may be shown in more than one table; we hope that these double entries will make identification easier for users of the *Manual*.

In using the progressive tables in Chapters 6 and 7 we should remember that occasionally an organism of undoubted identity will have an anomalous character (such as a positive oxidase reaction in a strain of *Salmonella typhi*) so misleading that it will be impossible to make the identification from the tables. We have not made provision for exceptions such as this; neither have we made double entries for motile and non-motile variants of the same species. Asporogenous variants of *Clostridium welchii* are so common that entries are justified in two tables, and the user of Table 6.1 is reminded of the possibility of asporogenous strains of *Bacillus* species. Not all *Bacillus* species are Gram positive but those likely to be isolated in medical laboratories are, and the genus is shown in Chapter 6. *Gemella*, because its staining character (usually Gram negative) is misleading, is shown in tables in both Chapters 6 and 7.

6
Characters of Gram-positive bacteria

In our characterization by stages, the first-stage table is combined with a figure and shows how, by a small number of selected characters, it is possible to divide Gram-positive bacteria into groups that correspond to those used in orthodox classifications. Not all of the theoretically possible combinations of characters are shown in Table 6.1 because many do not seem to occur in nature. Each shaded square indicates the genus or genera that have the characters shown in the same column in the table above it. Equivocal characters, characters difficult to determine, and characters markedly influenced by medium or method can make a genus span more than one column; generally we concentrate on the reactions given by most strains of a species in the kind of media likely to be used (majority reactions or characters); in doing this we may perhaps have introduced a tidiness that is unwarranted by the biological nature of the scheme. An example of generic spread is seen in *Aerococcus* which appears in the third and fourth columns of Table 6.1; in this case the reason for the spread is that the cata-lase reaction is not always easy to read and may be interpreted in contrary ways by different workers. Those who expect a large volume of gas to be pro-duced may record the feeble reaction of *A. viridans* as negative whereas others, who habitually work with streptococci and are conversant with truly negative results in this test, will take more notice of the small bubble of gas that may be produced and record it as positive. Conflicting readings of this kind were made in the NCTC and the (then) Streptococcus Reference Laboratory at Colindale when the two laboratories co-operated in the work which led us to describe the new species *Aero-coccus viridans* (Williams, Hirch & Cowan, 1953).

6.1   Division into major groups

In this edition we have divided the Gram-positive bacteria into several major groups, using the characters shown in the upper part of Table 6.1; they are shown as rectangles with broken lines and they are numbered to correspond to the tables in which further characterizing detail will be found. In making these major groups, most composed of several genera, we may be accused of reverting to a hierarchy, but that is not so and would misrepresent our thinking. Our major groups are not accretions of related (whatever that may mean) genera but are groups of convenience, groups of similarly shaped organisms, or groups of organisms that produce similar results in the limited number of tests applied in the first stage of our identification scheme. When we deal with the Gram-negative bacteria in Chapter 7, we shall see that one group consists of a collection of miscellaneous bacteria that cannot reasonably be attached to other groups; in this edition we do not have a chapter on miscellaneous bacteria or bacteria of uncertain taxonomic position (the 'odds and sods' of here-tical taxonomy). We do not wish to be either provocative or theoretical, our intention in using major groups is to be strictly practical; to some extent the size of a group is determined by the size of tables that will fit into the page without resorting to minute type; we think that the major groups help us to follow in a logical manner our aim of identify-ing bacteria in stages or by steps. The consequences of the grouping can be seen in Chapter 8, which uses information from Tables 6.1 and 7.1 in a scheme of identification to the level of genus by the use of punched cards. We do not name the groups but colloquial tags may be applicable to some (anaerobic cocci, enterobacteria). Some of our groups overlap (and to this we do not object) and

Table 6.1 *First-stage table for Gram-positive bacteria*

	1	2	3	4	5	6	7	8	9	10	11	12	13	14	15	16	17	18	19	20	21
Shape	S	S	S	S	S	S	S	R	R	R	R	R	R	R	R	R	R	R	R	R	R
Acid fast	−	−	−	−	−	−	−	−	−	−	−	−	−	−	−	−	−	−	−	w	+
Spores	−	−	−	−	−	−	−	−	−	−	−	−	−	−	−	−	+	+	−	−	−
Motility	−	−	−	−	+	−	−	+	−	−	+	−	−	−	−	−	D	D	−	−	−
Growth in air	+	+	+	+	+	+	−	+	+	+	+	+	+	−	−	−	−	+	+	+	+
Growth anaerobically	−	+	w	w	+	+	+	−	+	+	+	+	−	+	+	+	+	D	−	−	×
Catalase	+	+	w	−	−	−	−	+	+	+	+	−	+	+	−	−	−	+	+	+	+
Oxidase	−	−	−	−	−	−	−	−	−	−	−	−	×	×	×	×	×	d	−	−	−
Glucose (acid)	D	+	+	+	+	+	+/−	−	−	+	+	+	+	+	+	−	D	D	+	+	+
OF	O/−	F	F	F	F	F	F/−	−	−	F	F	F	F	F	F	−	F/−	F/O/−	O	O	O/NT

Genera (rows, with typical-form cells shaded and sub-table references indicated):
Micrococcus (6.2), Staphylococcus, Aerococcus, Streptococcus (6.3), Pediococcus, Gemella, Anaerobic cocci* (6.4), Kurthia, Corynebacterium (6.5), Listeria, Erysipelothrix (6.6), Lactobacillus, Arachnia†, Rothia, Propionibacterium, Actinomyces (6.7), Bifidobacterium, Eubacterium (6.8), Clostridium, Bacillus (6.9), Nocardia, Mycobacterium (6.10)

* *Peptococcus, Peptostreptococcus* (also *Leuconostoc*).
† Also *Actinomyces odontolyticus*.
D Different reactions in different species of the genus.
d Different reactions in different strains.
F Fermentation.
O Oxidation.
w Weak reaction.
× Not known.
[<>] Asporogenous variants.
▒ Typical form.

[ ] Cultural characters of these organisms can be found in tables with the number indicated.

S Sphere (coccus).
R Rod-shaped (bacillus).
NT Not testable.

Other symbols used in the table are explained in Tables 5.1 and 5.2 (facing p. 43).

this shows that our groups are not conventional taxa.

Some characters that need the help of biochemists and molecular biologists are very useful in bacterial classification but they cannot be used in day-to-day diagnostic work. The chemical composition of cell walls of Gram-positive bacteria is distinctive (Baird-Parker, 1965a, 1970; Colman & Williams, 1965; Cummins, 1962, 1970; Cummins & Harris, 1956, 1958; Kandler, 1970; Work, 1970) and helpful in classification, though Gooder (1970) has reservations and thinks that the listing of streptococcal cell wall sugar patterns is unrewarding. Group antigens of lactobacilli are located in the cell membranes or walls and are either teichoic acids or polysaccharides (Sharpe, 1970). These, and other complex analyses may be of great importance in classification but, like DNA-base ratios, they are not characters that can be determined by simple tests; they do, however, play an essential part in identification at the reference laboratory level.

6.2   The staphylococci
(*Staphylococcus*, *Micrococcus*, and *Aerococcus*)
Characters common to members of the group: **Gram-positive cocci; aerobic. Catalase positive; oxidase negative (some exceptions). Indole and H$_2$S not produced.**
The seemingly interminable arguments about *Staphylococcus* and *Micrococcus*, whether they should be separate or combined, and if combined what they should be named, were reviewed by Cowan (1962b); that survey will be taken as read and few of the 133 references quoted in it will be repeated here. In the early 1950s the general opinion among bacteriologists was that only one group of catalase-positive, Gram-positive cocci was justified, and while the name Micrococcus was popular among the non-medical bacteriologists, Staphylococcus reigned supreme in medical circles. By the late 1950s distinctions were being made between those cocci that fermented glucose anaerobically (the staphylococci) and those that oxidized the sugar or did not attack it (the micrococci). The distinction was made either in the complex medium of Evans, Bradford & Niven (1955) or in a modification of Hugh & Leifson's (1953) OF medium. As

with the oxidase test (Steel, 1962b) and tests for H$_2$S production (Clarke, 1953a), media and techniques have considerable influence on the results of tests for these characters, both in sensitivity and specificity. A satisfactory method for detecting the ability of cocci to ferment glucose uses an anaerobic jar (Cowan & Steel, 1964); paraffin seals do not exclude air sufficiently well to prevent oxidative organisms from attacking glucose. It is fortunate that in practice less stringent anaerobic conditions suffice. The standard method recommended by the Subcommittee on the taxonomy of staphylococci and micrococci (Subcommittee, 1965) uses a modification of Baird-Parker's (1963) medium; Evans & Kloos (1972) use a medium containing thioglycollate and dispense with an oily seal; the test is read by observing where growth occurs (in relation to the air/medium interface) and is independent of coloured indicator. Growth is observed by transmitted light, and readings are made after incubation for 1, 2, or 3 days. Staphylococci produce growth (and opacity) throughout the tube but *S. epidermidis* produces lighter growth in the depth of the agar. Micrococci grow near the air, immediately below the interface, and growth does not occur in the deeper parts of the medium.

Kocur & Martinec (1962) thought that the best character for separating the two genera was acetylmethylcarbinol production. To be useful, a test for this character should be well standardized, particularly in regard to temperature and duration of incubation, since 80% of *Staphylococcus albus* (probably *S. epidermidis*) strains can break down acetylmethylcarbinol (Segal, 1940), and if incubation is prolonged, false negative results will be recorded.

All staphylococci are oxidase negative but some micrococci are oxidase positive (Boswell, Batstone & Mitchell, 1972); a positive oxidase test, therefore, indicates that the organism is not a staphylococcus.

The sensitivity of strains of the two genera to two lytic substances may be of help in distinguishing them; lysozyme (Fleming, 1922) lyses micrococci but usually not staphylococci; lysostaphin (Schindler & Schuhardt, 1964) lyses staphylococci but not micrococci.

Other characters used by taxonomists to separate staphylococci from micrococci are convincing instruments for research in classification; they include the chemical nature of the cell wall components and the guanine and cytosine content of the DNA (Auletta & Kennedy, 1966). Because of technical difficulties involved in the determination of these characters they are not described in this *Manual*; for those seeking this information Baird-Parker (1970) summarizes the cell wall constituents and Kocur, Bergan & Mortensen (1971) give the DNA-base compositions of 343 strains of Gram-positive cocci.

Serology (slide agglutination) has been used successfully for distinguishing between micrococci and coagulase-negative staphylococci (Nakhla, 1973).

Table 6.2a shows the main distinguishing features of the three genera in this group. Aerococci have not been mentioned in the preceding paragraphs because they can be distinguished fairly readily from both staphylococci and micrococci; they are the α-group of Shaw *et al.* (1951), more closely resemble the streptococci and will be considered in Sections 6.2.3, 6.3, and 6.3.2.

The aerobic packet forming cocci (the sarcinas) are best considered as micrococci, and the genus *Sarcina* limited to anaerobic packet-forming cocci (Shaw *et al.* 1951; Hubálek, 1969).

6.2.1 Staphylococcus (Table 6.2b).

The cocci are rather smaller than the micrococci but variations due to media and age of the culture are too great to make size a reliable criterion for their differentiation. As they age, the cells become Gram negative but Gram-positive forms can usually be found without difficulty. Pigmentation has received much attention and been greatly stressed but in our view it is one of the least important characteristics of the genus; pigmented strains continually throw off non-pigmented (white) variants which retain the pathogenic (Downie, 1937) and other characters except clumping by plasma (Barber, 1955) of the parent. The presence of fermentable carbohydrate in the medium is said to enhance pigment production (Sevag & Green, 1944; Brown & Harris, 1963), but this is denied by Willis, O'Connor & Smith (1966) who think that fatty acids are more important and recommend a cream agar. Contrary to the usual experience, O'Connor, Willis & Smith (1966) did not find that exposure to daylight improved pigmentation.

Table 6.2a *Second-stage table for* Staphylococcus, Micrococcus *and* Aerococcus

	1	2	3
Growth under anaerobic conditions	+	−	w
Catalase	+	+	w
Oxidase	−	d	−
Carbohydrate attack	F	O/−	F
VP	+	−	−
Nitrate reduced	+	d	−
Arginine hydrolysis	+	−	−
Phosphatase	+	−	.
G+C mole per cent	30–40	66–75	38–43
Lysozyme	r	s	.
Lysostaphin	s	r	.

1 **Staphylococcus**
2 **Micrococcus**
3 **Aerococcus**

r resistant
s sensitive
w weak reaction/growth

Staphylococcus aureus produces several toxins; one, an enterotoxin is powerful in its effect on man and brings on vomiting within a few hours. Of the other known toxins the most important in human infections is probably the PV leucocidin (Panton & Valentine, 1932) which, unlike the NW leucocidin of the α-toxin, destroys human leucocytes. The haemolysins (α-, β-, and δ-toxins) do not seem to have much significance in the pathogenicity of staphylococci for man, or their antitoxins any effect in the prevention and treatment of staphylococcal infections.

The distribution of haemolytic activity among staphylococci may give useful information about the origin of strains; β-haemolysin-producing strains are more commonly isolated from animals than from man, but attempts to divide strains of *Staphylococcus aureus* by the haemolysins produced or by the usual biochemical characters have not been very successful (Cowan, 1938b) and better distinctions can be made by serology and phage typing. Although we do not agree with Meyer (1967b) that three varieties of *S. aureus* should be recognized, we think that some characters can be helpful in indicating the sources of strains; these are:

Table 6.2b *Third-stage table for* Staphylococcus, Micrococcus *and* Aerococcus

	1	2	3	4	5	6
Growth under anaerobic conditions	+	w	–	–	–	w
Oxidase	–	–	d	–[a]	–[a]	–
Carbohydrate breakdown [F/O/ –]	F	F	–/O[b]	O	O/–	F
Carbohydrates, acid from:						
glucose	+	+	–[b]	+	+	+
lactose	+	d	–	d	–	+
maltose	+	+	–	d	–	+
mannitol	+	d	–	d	–	d
mannitol (anaerobic)	+	–	–	–	–	.
sucrose	+	+	–	d	d	+
xylose	–	–	–	d	–	–
VP	+	d	–	–	–	–
Nitrate reduced	+	d	–	d	+	–
Gelatin liquefaction	+	d	d	d	–	–
Urease	+	d	d	+	d	–
Arginine hydrolysis	+	+	–	–	–	–
LV (egg-yolk reaction)	+	+	–	–	–	–
Pigment formation[e]	+/–	–/+	+	+	+	–
Phosphatase	+	d	–	–	–	.
Coagulase	+	–	–	–	–	–

1 **Staphylococcus aureus**; *S. pyogenes*; *Micrococcus pyogenes* var. *aureus*
2 **Staphylococcus epidermidis**; *S. saprophyticus*; *S. albus*; *Micrococcus pyogenes* var. *albus*
3 **Micrococcus luteus**; *M. afermentans*; *M. lysodeikticus*; *Staphylococcus afermentans*
4 **Micrococcus varians**; *M. lactis*; *Staphylococcus lactis*
5 **Micrococcus roseus**; *Staphylococcus roseus*
6 **Aerococcus viridans**

[a] Result may vary with the method; see Steel (1962b).
[b] May be positive on ammonium salt sugars; see Section 6.2.2.
[e] Pigments usually gold, cream or yellow; *M. roseus* pigment is pink. – on the pigment line = white or grey.

Other symbols used in the table are explained in Tables 5.1 and 5.2 (facing p. 43).

(i) *Fibrinolysin*: human fibrin is lysed only by human strains (Madison, 1935; Madison & Dart, 1936); in Hájek & Maršálek's (1971) view this is the most significant characteristic of human strains.

(ii) *Coagulases*: human, rabbit, and horse plasmas are coagulated regularly by human strains of *S. aureus*, bovine and ovine plasmas are less frequently clotted by them (Shaw *et al*. 1951). On the other hand, human plasma is coagulated less often by dog strains than are rabbit or ovine plasmas (J. E. Smith, 1962); Live's (1972) canine strains were more exacting for they only clotted canine plasmas. Coagulation of bovine plasma is characteristic of animal (other than human) strains (Hájek, Maršálek & Černá, 1968).

(iii) *Serology*: sera against human strains (the serotypes of Cowan (1939), Christie & Keogh (1940), Hobbs (1948), and of Oeding (1952, 1960)) seldom agglutinate animal strains, and an entirely different set of serotypes infect the bovine udder (White, Rattray & Davidson, 1962). The nucleases of human, bovine, and canine strains are serologically specific (Scharman & Blobel, 1968).

(iv) *Phage sensitivity*: phages used for the phage typing of human strains (Fisk, 1942; Wilson & Atkinson, 1945; Williams & Rippon, 1952; Blair & Carr, 1953) except the 42D group (recognized as an animal group) are not suitable for phage typing animal strains (Meyer, 1967a) and special sets of phages have been developed for typing them (Frost, 1967). In distinguishing animal from human strains Marandon & Oeding (1966) found that all 42D strains were β-toxin producers and were fibrinolysin negative, characteristics of bovine strains.

To the medical bacteriologist the potential pathogenicity of a strain is its most important characteristic. It has been assumed, certainly since Cruickshank published his paper in 1937, that coagulase positive staphylococci are potentially pathogenic, and this is probably correct for acute and severe infections such as osteomyelitis. In more chronic infections, secondary infections, and infections associated with anatomical or mechanical abnormalities such as urinary calculi, coagulase-negative strains may be incriminated (see, for example, Cunliffe, Gillam & Williams, 1943; Holt, 1969). DNase activity (Elston & Fitch, 1964) and lysozyme production (Grossgebauer *et al.* 1968) have been suggested as indicators of potential pathogenicity, but coagulase remains the most easily determinable and most reliable indicator of pathogenicity for man.

For the coagulase-negative staphylococci we think that only one species is justified, but our view is not shared by Jones, Deibel & Niven (1963a) who think that *Staphylococcus epidermidis* should be restricted to mannitol-negative strains. The description we give of this species in Table 6.2*b* is compiled from those given by Hugh & Ellis (1968) and Baird-Parker (1965*a*, *b*) for *S. epidermidis* and that of Shaw *et al.* (1951) for *S. saprophyticus*. This lumping contrasts with the splitting practised by Holt (1969) who subdivided Baird-Parker's subgroup II into 15 subdivisions.

With increasing recognition of the potential pathogenicity of *Staphylococcus epidermidis*, both serological and phage typing schemes have been developed (Williams & Corse, 1970; Verhoef, van Boven & Winkler, 1972).

For the selective isolation of staphylococci media containing egg-yolk and tellurite have been devised by Alder, Gillespie & Waller (1962), Baird-Parker (1962), and Alder, Brown & Mitchell (1966). For food-poisoning investigations, De Waart *et al.* (1968) commend Baird-Parker's ETGPA medium.

In spite of our long discussion on the characters, pathogenicity, and the possible subdivision of staphylococci by mammalian source, every medical bacteriologist knows that *Staphylococcus aureus* is one of the easiest organisms to isolate and to identify, and it does not need a wide range of tests to do it. Table 6.2*b* is informative, but such detail is not essential for identification.

> **Minidefinition:** *Staphylococcus. Gram-positive spheres in pairs and clusters, the cells showing variation in size and Gram positivity. Non-motile; non-sporing. Aerobic and facultatively anaerobic. Catalase positive; oxidase negative. Attack sugars by fermentation.*

6.2.2   Micrococcus (Table 6.2*b*). Hucker (1924*b*) included both staphylococci and micrococci in the genus *Micrococcus* but opinions have changed, and now the practical bacteriologist needs simple tests by which he can distinguish them. The characters that can be detected readily (Table 6.2*b*) are much less convincing than those obtained by more complex methods (base composition of DNA, chemical nature of the cell wall components, and transformations) provided by molecular biologists, biochemists, and geneticists. Micrococci themselves are so heterogeneous that we must either accept several hundred species or collect them into a few species, ignoring both the multiplicity of character permutations and the unique features, such as resistance to γ-radiation, of the few. Our predilection is to be lumpers and in Table 6.2*b* we show only three species of *Micrococcus*. The characters shown in the table are based on Shaw *et al.* (1951), supplemented by more recent descriptions by Kocur & Páčová (1970) for *M. roseus*, Kocur, Páčová & Martinec (1972) for *M. luteus*, and Kocur & Martinec (1972) for *M. varians*.

Among the micrococci pigment formation is a strong and stable character and we seldom see the pigmentless variants so common in the staphylococci. Hill (1959) and Eisenberg & Evans (1963) regard *Micrococcus roseus* as a homogeneous group, but it includes the unusual *M. agilis*, a motile coccus. Micrococci that produce pink colonies are not often isolated, and in a lifetime of bacteriology we never isolated one ourselves.

Table 6.2*b* has a footnote referring to acid production from glucose by *M. luteus*; this is needed because Kocur *et al.* (1972) proposed NCTC 2665 (Fleming's original strain of *M. lysodeikticus*) as the type of the species *Micrococcus luteus*. Many years ago we made some unpublished experiments in which we found that NCTC 2665, which did not produce acid in peptone water sugars, might do so when grown on the surface of the ammonium salt sugars (ASS) used by Smith, Gordon & Clark (1952) for the aerobic spore-formers. In our experiments about half the strains of non-saccharolytic (judged on tests in peptone water sugars) micrococci produced acid on ASS; among those consistently negative on both kinds of sugar media was ATCC 398, the strain proposed as neotype by Breed (1952) and by Evans *et al.* (1955). The significance of this taxonomic complication to the practical bacteriologist is not great, but it tends to lessen the difference between *M. luteus* and *M. varians*.

The medical bacteriologist is fortunate in that his tasks do not range into the wilderness of micrococcal speciation; the names, synonyms, and references to species with the generic name Micrococcus occupy 37 pages of *Index Bergeyana* (Buchanan, Holt & Lessel, 1966). If one has an organism that might be a micrococcus one must make sure, before discarding it, that it is not a staphylococcus. And that, fortunately, is not too difficult.

> **Minidefinition:** *Micrococcus. Gram-positive spheres in pairs, fours, and small clusters made up of cocci of uniform size. Typically non-motile and non-sporing (occasionally motile and so-called sporing forms occur). Aerobic. Catalase positive. Attack sugars oxidatively or not at all.*

6.2.3   Aerococcus (Tables 6.2a, b; 6.3a, c). A genus described and named by Williams, Hirch & Cowan (1953). The cocci, which formed the α-group of Shaw *et al.* (1951), were isolated from air samples, dust, and milking utensils, and were regarded as intermediates nearer to the streptococci than to the staphylococci. The catalase reaction is feeble and may be described in different ways by different observers; to one a result will seem to be negative, to another it will be weakly positive. Since our identification routine depends so much on the results of the catalase test, we show the characters of *Aerococcus viridans* in Table 6.2a and b among the Gram-positive, catalase-positive cocci (*Staphylococcus, Micrococcus*) and also in Table 6.3a and c with the catalase-negative streptococci. Like streptococci, the aerococci do not reduce nitrate to nitrite.

Clausen (1964) proposed to add another species, *Aerococcus catalasicus*, but as this was frankly catalase positive and reduced nitrates, we think it fits better in the genus *Micrococcus*.

> **Minidefinition:** *Aerococcus. Gram-positive spheres in pairs, fours, and small clusters. Non-motile; non-sporing. Aerobic; facultatively anaerobic. Catalase feebly positive or negative; oxidase negative. Attack sugars fermentatively without gas production.*

6.3   The streptococci

(*Streptococcus, Aerococcus, Pediococcus, and Gemella*)

Characters common to the group: Gram-positive cocci; non-motile (rare exceptions). Aerobic, facultatively anaerobic. Catalase negative; oxidase negative. Carbohydrates fermented; gas not produced. Nitrates not reduced. Indole and H_2S not produced.

With so many common characters the group is fairly homogeneous and does not include any unexpected members except the genus *Gemella*. Apart from Gemella all the other genera could be included in the genus *Streptococcus* without any violent upheaval of bacterial classification; a preliminary subdivision of the group is shown in Table 6.3a. Gemella is in a slightly different category, and the reasons for its inclusion here will be explained in Section 6.3.4.

In addition to being included in the Staphylococcus–Micrococcus group (Section 6.2.3), *Aerococcus viridans* appears here because it is an intermediate organism bridging the gap between the catalase-positive and catalase-negative Gram-positive cocci and, with characteristics of both groups, forms part of the bacterial spectrum; within that spectrum it is nearer to the streptococci than to the staphylococci.

Table 6.3a *Second-stage table for* Streptococcus, Aerococcus, Pediococcus *and* Gemella

	1	2	3	4	5	6
Motility	−	−	D	−	−	−
Catalase (in presence of boiled blood)	−	−	d	−	−	−
Haemolysis	β	α	α/β/−	α	−	(β)
Growth at 45 °C	−	D	+	−	+	−
Survives 60 °C for 30 min	−	−	+	+	−	−
Growth at pH 9.6	−	−	D	+	−	−
Growth in 40 % bile	D	D	+	+	.	−
Arabinose (acid)	−	−	D	d	+	d
Glycerol (acid)	D	−	D	+	−	.

1 **Streptococcus** (β-haemolytic subgroup) see Table 6.3b
2 **Streptococcus** (α-haemolytic subgroup) see Table 6.3b
3 **Streptococcus** (group D; enterococcus) see Table 6.3c
4 **Aerococcus** see Tables 6.2a, b; 6.3c
5 **Pediococcus** see Table 6.3c
6 **Gemella** see Tables 6.3c; 7.3

Symbols used in the table are explained in Tables 5.1 and 5.2 (facing p. 43).

6.3.1   Streptococcus (Tables 6.3a, b, c). From the 1930s to the 1960s classification of streptococci was based mainly on the groups and types determined by the polysaccharide antigens (Lancefield, 1928, 1933, 1940). Now we have swung full circle

Table 6.3b *Third-stage table for* Streptococcus *species*

	1	2	3	4	5	6	7	8	9	10	11	12	13	14
Haemolysis	β	α/β	α	β	β	β	.	(β)	α	−	α/−	α	α	α/−
Growth at 45 °C	−	−	−	−	−	−	.	−	−	+	−	d	d	−
CO_2 requirement	−	−	−	−	−	−	.	+ᵃ	−	−	−	−	−	+
Growth in 6.5 % NaCl	−	−	−	−	−	−	.	−	−	−	−	−	−	−ᵇ
Growth on 10 % bile	−	+	−	+	d	−	.	.	−	+	d	d	−	+
Growth on 40 % bile	−	+	−	−	−	−	.	−	−	d	d	d	−	d
Growth in 1/4000 tellurite	−	d	.	.	.	.	.	.	.	d	d	d	d	.
Carbohydrates; acid from:														
glycerol	−	d[O]	−	+	−	−	+	−	+	+	+	+	d	+
lactose	+	d	d	d	−	+	−	+	+	+	+	+	+	+
maltose	+	+	+	+	+	d	+	+	+	+	+	+	+	+
mannitol	−	−	−	−	−	−	+	−	−	−	−	−	−	+
raffinose	−	−	−	−	−	−	−	dᶜ	d	d	−	d	d	d
salicin	+	+	d	d	+	+	+	+		+	+	+		+
sorbitol	−	−	d	−	−	+	+	−	−	−	−	−	−	+
sucrose	+	+	+	+	+	+	+	+	+	+ᵈ	+	+ᵉ	+	+ᵉ
trehalose	+	+	+	+	−	−	+	+	d	+	+	d	d	+
VP	.	−	.	.	.	.	.	.	−	dᶠ	+	−	d	+
Aesculin hydrolysis	−	−	−	d	−	+	.	.	−	+	d	d	−	d
Litmus milk	A	AC	B	B	−	A	c/−	AB	AC	AC	NAC	AC	NAC	.
Gelatin liquefaction	−	−	−	−	−	−	.	−	−	−	−	−	−	.
Arginine hydrolysis	+	+	+	+	+	+	.	+	−	−	+	+	−	−
Hippurate hydrolysis	−	+	d	−	−	−	.	−	−	−	−	−	−	−
CAMP test	−	+	−	−	−	−	−	−	−	−	−	−	+	−
EHC (or bile) solubility	−	−	−	−	−	−	−	−	+	−	−	−	−	−
Polysaccharide antigensᵍ	A	B	C	C	C	C	E	FG1	−/O	Kʰ [Ott]	AC FG [Ott]	HK	OK M	.

1 **Streptococcus pyogenes;** *S. haemolyticus*

2 **Streptococcus agalactiae**

3 **Streptococcus dysgalactiae**

4 **Streptococcus equisimilis**

5 **Streptococcus equi**

6 **Streptococcus zooepidemicus**

7 **Group E streptococci from swine** (Deibel *et al.* 1964)

8 **Streptococcus anginosus;** 'minute haemolytic streptococci'

9 **Streptococcus pneumoniae;** *Diplococcus pneumoniae;* pneumococcus

10 **Streptococcus salivarius;** *S. hominis; S. cardioarthritidis*

11 **Streptococcus milleri;** Streptococcus MG

12 **Streptococcus sanguis;** Streptococcus s.b.e.

13 **Streptococcus mitior;** *S. viridans; S. mitis*

14 **Streptococcus mutans**

α Green zone around colonies on blood agar.

β Clear, colourless zone around colonies on blood agar.

ᵃ CO_2 needed for growth on simple media; on blood agar growth improved by 10 % CO_2.

ᵇ Positive on 4 % NaCl.

ᶜ Group G strains positive.

ᵈ Levan produced on sucrose media.

ᵉ Dextran produced on sucrose media.

ᶠ Strains that do not have group K antigen are VP positive.

ᵍ On this line capital letters in heavy type are the serological group designations; Ott = Ottens antigens, see Ottens & Winkler (1962) and Willers, Ottens & Michel (1964).

ʰ Extracts of some strains do not react in the precipitin test.

Other symbols used in the table are explained in Tables 5.1 and 5.2 (facing p. 43).

Table **6.**3*c Third-stage table for* Streptococcus (*group D and enterococci*), Aerococcus, Pediococcus *and* Gemella

	15	16	17	18	19	20	21	22	23	24
Catalase (in presence of heated blood)	+	−	−	−	−	−	−	−	−	−
Motility	−	d	−	−	−	−	−	−	−	−
Haemolysis	−/β	−/α	β	α/−	α	α	.	α	.	+ᵃ
Growth at 45 °C	+	+	d	+	+	+	+	−	+	.
Growth at 50 °C	+	+	−	.	.	.	.	.	.	.
Survives 60 °C for 30 min	+	+	+	+	−	+	.	+	−	.
Growth at pH 9.6	+	+	.	−	−	−	+	+	−	.
CO₂ requirement	−	−	.	.	.	.	.	−ᵇ	.	.
Growth in 6.5 % NaCl	+	+	+	−	−	−	+	+	.ᶜ	.
Growth on 40 % bile	+	+	+	+	+	−	.	+	.	.
Growth in 1/4000 tellurite	+	−	−	.	.	.	.	−	.	.
Citrate as C source	+	−	.	.	.	.	.	.	.	.
Carbohydrates, acid from:										
arabinose	−	+	−	d	−	−	+	d	+	w/−
glycerol	+	−	−	−	−	+	+[Ø]	+[O]	−	.
lactose	+	+	+	+	−	+	.	+	+	−
mannitol	+	+	−	d	−	+	.	d[O]	−	w/−
raffinose	−	−	−	+	−	−	.	d	+	.
salicin	+	+	d	+	+	+	.	+	+	.
sorbitol	+	−	−	−	−	+	+	d[O]	.	w/−
sucrose	d	.	−	+	+	+	.	+	+	+
trehalose	+	+	d	d	−	+	.	+	.	.
Aesculin hydrolysis	+	+	+	+	+	+	.	w/−	.	.
Litmus milk	NAC	A	AC	A	−	NAC	.	A	(A)	.
Gelatin liquefaction	d	−	.	−	−	−	.	−	.	.
Arginine hydrolysis	+	+	+	−	−	+	−	−	−	.
Hippurate hydrolysis	d	d	d	−	−	+	.	+	.	.
CAMP test	−	−	−	−	−	−ᵈ	−	.	.	.
Bile solubility	−	−	−	−	−	−	.	−	−	.
Polysaccharide antigensᵉ	**D**	**D**	**D**	**D**	**D**	−	**DQ**	−	.	.

15 Streptococcus faecalis
16 Streptococcus faecium
17 Streptococcus faecium var.
   durans; *S. durans*

18 Streptococcus bovis
19 Streptococcus equinus
20 Streptococcus uberis
21 Streptococcus avium

22 Aerococcus viridans; *Pediococcus urinae-equi*; *Gaffkya homari*
23 Pediococcus cerevisiae
24 Gemella haemolysans; *Neisseria haemolysans*

α Green zone around colonies on blood agar.
β Clear, colourless zone around colonies on blood agar.

ᵃ On rabbit blood only; negative on sheep blood.
ᵇ At 30 % may be slightly inhibitory.
ᶜ Inhibited by 8 % NaCl.

ᵈ Some strains are CAMP positive (Shuman *et al.* 1972).
ᵉ On this line capital letters in heavy type are the serological group designations.

Other symbols used in the table are explained in Tables 5.1 and 5.2 (facing p. 43).

and are almost back to the position we were in during the 1920s, when streptococci were divided into the haemolytic, by which we meant those that produced β-haemolysis in poured blood agar (Brown, 1919), the viridans (those that produced greening or α-haemolysis), and the non-haemolytic (rather foolishly labelled γ-haemolytic). For a long time we tried to correlate the serological groupings made on the basis of the Lancefield precipitin tests with arrangements based on cultural and biochemical characteristics; for example, Skadhaugh & Perch (1959) and Rifkind & Cole

(1962) found that serological group M consisted of three biotypes or groups that gave different results in biochemical tests. Allowance always had to be made for a host of exceptions, aberrant strains, and varieties. Apart from motile strains (Pownall, 1935; Langston, Gutierrez & Bouma, 1960a; Lund, 1967), other abnormalities such as catalase production (Langston *et al.* 1960b; Jones, Deibel & Niven, 1964; Whittenbury, 1964, 1965a), reduction of nitrate (Langston & Williams, 1962), and pigment production (Jones, Deibel & Niven, 1963b) can occur in group D strains; the presence of these unusual characters may, like the group D antigen itself (Medrek & Barnes, 1962), be determined by the constituents of the growth media.

New approaches to the problems of streptococcal classification have been rewarding and in the last decade better techniques in the laboratory have provided the information that in turn formed the data for new analytical methods. The result is a resurgence of the greening streptococci and the viridans group has regained the respectability it lost in the hey-day of serology. Serology still has a place in the classification of streptococci – and an even more important one in their identification – but it is no longer the final arbiter in streptococcal taxonomy; just one character to be considered with others from morphology, physiology, biochemistry and, in classification, cell wall components and genetic information.

The mass of information that has accumulated on the biochemical and serological characteristics of the various streptococci, supplemented by transformation experiments (Colman, 1968, 1969; Drucker & Melville, 1969) and cell wall composition (Colman & Williams, 1965; Gooder, 1970) have been used to develop a workable grouping of these organisms. Although Colman & Williams (1972) state that the main distinguishing characteristics of *Streptococcus mitior* are the absence of rhamnose from the cell walls and the presence of teichoic acid, it should be comforting to the diagnostician to know that in practice the identifying features remain relatively simple and within the reach of workers in any reasonably equipped laboratory. Detailed characterizations and pin-pointing (by serology and phage typing) for epidemiology remain within the province of the specialized

reference laboratory. The present position in the medical laboratory – and it could change rapidly – is that we recognize three large groups of streptococci: the first consists of the common pathogens of man and domestic animals; most, but not all, are β-haemolytic. Next we have the pneumococci and the viridans streptococci, primarily inhabitants of the respiratory tract and the oral cavity, but also associated with blood-borne infections. Finally, and these are the ones that may be split from the other streptococci, there are the enterococci, all of serological group D but with differing haemolytic propensities; generally they are more heat resistant, and also more heat tolerant, than other streptococci.

Outside the medical, dental, and veterinary fields are other streptococci, and those connected with milk and milk products are important to the cheese industry; they are not shown in our tables as they are unlikely to be isolated in laboratories where this *Manual* is used.

Exceptions to the characters shown in our tables must be expected; on suitable media dextrans may be produced by some strains of *Streptococcus bovis* (Niven, Smiley & Sherman, 1941). Some dextran-producing strains of *S. sanguis* may fail to yield group H antigen in extracts prepared from them (Porterfield, 1950); not all group H strains produce a dextran or all group K strains a levan. Group H antisera are not all alike; some are prepared against the CHALLIS strain, others against PERRYER: unfortunately these strains are serologically different so that it may be difficult to interpret results reported in the literature of group H precipitin tests. *S. sanguis* produces a dextran only in sucrose broth (Niven, Kiziuta & White, 1946); *S. salivarius* produces its levan on sucrose agar. A few strains of *S. bovis* will survive heating at 60 °C for 30 minutes. Most group D strains will grow at 45 °C but some strains of *S. faecium* var. *durans* fail to grow at this temperature.

This formidable list of exceptions makes the situation look difficult for the diagnostician, but his gloom will be lifted when he remembers that they are exceptions and that the majority of strains will behave as shown in Table 6.3b and c. Because the frequency of aberrant results in biochemical tests seems to be greatest among group D strains, the only completely reliable tests for distinguishing between *S. faecalis* and *S. faecium* are the reduction of 1% methylene blue, the reduction of 0.01% tetrazolium, and tolerance of 0.04% potassium tellurite; all these characters are positive in *S. faecalis* and negative in *S. faecium* (Barnes, 1956; Whittenbury, 1965*a*).

Some strains of *Streptococcus faecalis* are β-haemolytic and others liquefy gelatin; these abnormal forms have, at one time or another, been given varietal epithets, zymogenes and liquefaciens, but without any gain in the precision of circumscription. The durans variety of *S. faecium* is perhaps more worthy of notice, but we do not see any advantage in collecting the relatively few motile strains into a variety. The thorny subject of the varieties of *S. faecalis* and *S. faecium* was usefully reviewed by Hartman, Reinbold & Saraswat (1966).

The precipitin reactions of streptococci are not always straightforward and the difficulties that arise apply particularly to group D strains, some extracts of which will not react, unless the cells are broken up mechanically, with otherwise satisfactory antisera (Shattock, 1949; Smith & Shattock, 1962). Some strains of *Streptococcus equinus*, *S. sanguis*, and *S. salivarius* do not react with any of the grouping sera, and their identification must be made entirely on other characters.

Streptococcus pyogenes is unusual in being sensitive to bacitracin (Maxted, 1953) and disks containing the diagnostically significant amount of the antibiotic are available commercially.

Strains of *Streptococcus agalactiae* of both human and animal origin produce a substance that will lyse sheep or ox (but not human, horse, rabbit, or guinea-pig) red cells when they later come in contact with staphylococcal β-toxin (Christie, Atkins & Munch-Petersen, 1944; G. Colman, personal communication). The phenomenon, known as the CAMP reaction or test, is almost specific for group B streptococci (but see Section 4.5.5).

Streptococci may be sensitive to oxygen on first isolation and cultures of clinical material will be more successful under anaerobic conditions. Additional carbon dioxide is often advantageous for growth and some strains of pneumococci will not grow without it when first isolated (Austrian & Collins, 1966). The CO_2 dependence does not last long. *Streptococcus salivarius* will grow in media

made selective by the addition of sodium azide (0.02%) and sucrose (5%); with such media the species can be isolated from about 80% of specimens of faeces (Sherman, Niven & Smiley, 1943).

Minidefinition: *Streptococcus. Gram-positive spheres in pairs or chains. Typically non-motile (motile strains occur occasionally in one species). Non-sporing. Aerobic, facultatively anaerobic. Catalase negative; oxidase negative. Attack carbohydrates fermentatively.*

6.3.2 Aerococcus (Tables 6.2*a*, *b*; 6.3*a*, *c*). Here we deal with the strains in which the catalase reaction has been read and recorded as negative, for it is in these circumstances that aerococci must be distinguished from the streptococci, pediococci, and the gemellas. Deibel & Niven (1960) thought that aerococci resembled an organism named *Gaffkya homari* by Hitchner & Snieszko (1947) from lobsters and meat (Aaronson, 1956), and that the single species they formed should be put in the genus *Pediococcus*. *Pediococcus urinae-equi* and *Aerococcus viridans* appear to be identical (Whittenbury, 1965*b*; Sakaguchi & Mori, 1969) but there is a division of opinion on the generic allocation of the combined species. Our view (Williams *et al.* 1953), based on comparisons made of *A. viridans* and *P. cerevisiae*, that aerococci can be distinguished from pediococci seems to be shared by other workers (Günther & White, 1961; Coster & White, 1964; Whittenbury, 1965*b*; Evans & Schultes, 1969; Schultes & Evans, 1971). The resemblance between aerococci and pediococci is close and it is not surprising that the debate continues; if a change in generic allocation is needed it would seem sensible to include both aerococci and pediococci in the genus *Streptococcus*.

Minidefinition: *Aerococcus. Gram-positive spheres in pairs, fours, and small clusters. Non-motile; non-sporing. Aerobic; facultatively anaerobic. Catalase feebly positive or negative; oxidase negative. Attack sugars fermentatively without gas production. Do not produce dextran or levan on sucrose-containing media.*

6.3.3 Pediococcus (Table 6.3*a*, *c*). A genus of lactic acid producing cocci found in beer (in which they produce sarcina sickness), meat-curing brines, and fermenting vegetable juices. They are distinguished from *Leuconostoc* species by their inability to produce slimy colonies on carbohydrate-containing media or to produce CO_2 from glucose (Gibson & Abd-el-Malek, 1945). The genus is included here because some workers think that *Aerococcus viridans* should be put into the genus *Pediococcus* (Deibel & Niven, 1960; Sakaguchi & Mori, 1969), a view we do not share. Distinguishing features not shown in the tables are the microaerophilic character of *P. cerevisiae* (aerococci prefer aerobic conditions), the much greater acidity produced by pediococci in glucose broth, and the absence of tetrad formation by aerococci.

On ordinary media catalase is not produced but variable amounts appear in the presence of glucose (Felton, Evans & Niven, 1953); with a medium of low glucose content Gutekunst, Delwiche & Seeley (1957) obtained poor growth but catalase was demonstrable; in high (1%) glucose growth was better but catalase could not be demonstrated unless the pH value was first adjusted to 7.0.

Details of the characters and the different approaches to the classification of pediococci will be found in papers by Pederson (1949), Nakagawa & Kitahara (1959), Deibel & Niven (1960). Günther & White (1961), and Whittenbury (1965*b*). Whittenbury questioned the wisdom of retaining *Pediococcus* as a separate genus and favoured the inclusion of its species in the genus *Streptococcus*.

Minidefinition: *Pediococcus. Gram-positive cocci in pairs, tetrads, and short chains. Non-motile; non-sporing. Microaerophilic. Catalase negative; oxidase negative. Sugars fermented without gas production. Dextrans and levans not formed on sugar media.*

6.3.4　Gemella (Tables 6.3*a*, *c*; 7.3). Gemella is the generic name for an organism first described under the name *Neisseria hemolysans* by Thjøtta & Bøe (1938); Berger thought that it was sufficiently different from the other neisserias to be removed from that genus and he created Gemella for it (Berger, 1960*a*; 1961), describing the organism, as Thjøtta & Bøe had done, as Gram negative. In the first edition of this *Manual* we showed the charac-

ters of the species in the same table as the neisserias and did not question the Gram reaction.

On the grounds that (i) the fine structure of the cell resembled that of Gram-positive bacteria and (ii) the G+C mole per cent of the DNA was different from that of all neisserias and at the lower end of the range for streptococci (33 to 41 – Hill, 1966), Reyn (1970) thought that the genus should be placed with the Gram-positive cocci, close to the streptococci. We agree with this taxonomic reasoning and in this edition show the organism in Table 6.3*c* with some of the streptococci and with other Gram-positive cocci that, like Gemella, are fermentative, catalase negative, and do not reduce nitrates. But because it is so easily decolorized (or over-decolorized), we also show the species in Table 7.3 with *Neisseria* and *Branhamella* species, thereby hoping that the organism will not be misidentified when the decolorizing agent has been applied too zealously.

The haemolysis from which the organism derives its specific epithet occurs slowly and only on rabbit blood agar, not on media made with sheep blood. Growth is generally slow and delicate, and may be improved by serum.

Minidefinition: *Gemella. Gram-positive (but easily decolorized) spheres. Aerobic; facultatively anaerobic. Catalase negative; oxidase negative. Attack sugars by fermentation; do not produce gas.*

6.4　The anaerobic cocci
(*Peptococcus, Peptostreptococcus*)
Characters common to members of the group: Gram-positive cocci. Microaerophilic or strictly anaerobic. Catalase negative (rare exceptions).

6.4.1　Peptococcus and **Peptostreptococcus** are genera of anaerobic cocci that do not need fermentable carbohydrate. Like *Veillonella*, their Gram-negative counterpart, their pathogenicity is doubtful. They have been isolated from clinical material (when looked for) and they seem to be part of the normal flora of man and animals, especially of the colon and vagina and, in herbivorous animals, of the rumen. Identification presents serious practical problems to the clinical bacteriologist

Table 6.4 *Second-stage table for* Peptococcus, Peptostreptococcus *and* Leuconostoc

	1	2	3
Carbohydrates, acid from:			
glucose	+	+	+
lactose	−	+	+
maltose	−	+	d
sucrose	−	−	+
Gas production	+	+	+
Gelatin liquefaction	−/w	−/w	−

1 **Peptococcus** spp. (7 spp. in ALM)
2 **Peptostreptococcus** spp. (5 in ALM); *P. putridus*; *Streptococcus putridus*
3 **Leuconostoc** spp.

Symbols used in the table are explained in Tables 5.1 and 5.2 (facing p. 43).

unless he happens also to be a biochemist with the knowledge and equipment for analysing metabolic products, which play a disproportionate part in the characterization of the non-sporing anaerobes.

The non-sporing anaerobes have provided a free-for-all for the splitters and the most trivial character difference seems to justify the creation of a new species. We show in Table 6.4 some easily discernible characters of Peptococcus species (the *Anaerobe Laboratory Manual* (ALM, 1972) lists seven species) and Peptostreptococcus (ALM lists five species). ALM does not name *Peptostreptococcus putridus* (*Streptococcus putridus*) among its five species, but it is believed to be the commonest potential pathogen of the group (Thomas & Hare, 1954). Those who wish to attempt to identify these anaerobes should consult reference works such as ALM (1972) or Willis (1964).

> **Minidefinitions:** *Peptococcus. Gram-positive spheres, often in clusters. Strict anaerobes. Feeble fermentative power.*
>
> *Peptostreptococcus. Gram-positive spheres in chains. Strict anaerobes. Fermentative attack on sugars and gas may be produced.*

6.4.2 **Leuconostoc** species are heterofermentative and, when tested under suitable conditions of medium, pH value, temperature of incubation, and a heavy inoculum, will produce CO_2 from glucose (Gibson & Abd-el-Malek, 1945). Garvie's review (1960) of the dairy organisms of the genus will be useful for those who wish to subdivide the group into species. Whittenbury (1966) thought that the division into species on the basis of the fermentation of pentoses and sucrose, and dextran formation from sucrose was not satisfactory but he could not find a workable alternative. The most useful characteristics seemed to be the ability to form detectable amounts of H_2O_2 from glucose, dextran production from sucrose, the production of catalase and pseudocatalase, and the ability to grow at various temperatures.

> **Minidefinition:** *Leuconostoc. Gram-positive cocci in pairs or short chains. Microaerophilic. Attack sugars fermentatively and may form dextran from sucrose.*

6.5 **The diphtheroids**
(Corynebacterium, Listeria and Kurthia)
Characters common to members of the group: **Gram-positive rods, not spore-forming. Aerobic, facultatively anaerobic. Catalase positive; oxidase negative.**

There is a similarity in morphology between members of the group; all members might be labelled 'diphtheroid' in a medical laboratory or 'coryneform' in one with a greater regard for scientific accuracy. Most of the bacteria in the group grow better on media enriched by serum or blood, but none requires X or V factor(s). '*Haemophilus*' *vaginalis* will be found in Table 6.5b among the diphtheroids, and some notes on the species are given in Section 6.5.1 on *Corynebacterium*. Jayne-Williams & Skerman (1966) report *C. bovis* to be oxidase positive.

6.5.1 **Corynebacterium** (Table 6.5a, b) is a genus in which are included animal pathogens and commensals, plant pathogens, and soil bacteria. The cell wall composition and antigens of the plant pathogenic corynebacteria are unlike those of the animal strains (Cummins, 1962). Conn (1947) and others (e.g. Clark, 1952) have protested against the inclusion of motile or branched Gram-positive rods in the genus; in the non-medical fields the confusion was so great that Conn & Dimmick (1947) stated that Krassilnikov's *Mycobacterium* was the same as Jensen's *Corynebacterium*. For a review of the coryneform bacteria in fields other than medicine see Jensen (1952) and Keddie, Leask & Grainger

(1966). Abd-el-Malek & Gibson (1952) describe the corynebacteria of milk and with them include the genus *Microbacterium*, a group of thermophilic organisms (Doetsch & Pelczar, 1948). We limit our consideration to the human and other animal strains, pathogenic and saprophytic, and will not deal with the more widely distributed coryneform bacteria (Harrington, 1966; Lazar, 1968; Davis & Newton, 1969).

In Table 6.5*b* we show the characters of *Corynebacterium vaginale* (Zinnemann & Turner, 1963) but these represent only some of the strains that have been labelled 'Haemophilus' vaginalis, which is a heterogeneous group (Vickerstaff & Cole, 1969). According to Redmond & Kotcher (1963) at least two organisms masquerade under the name *Haemophilus vaginalis*; one is Gram negative and needs X and V factors and can correctly be described as haemophilic – it is probably one of the recognized species of *Haemophilus*. The other consists of bacteria that need neither of these factors, that have cell walls of the Gram positive type, and on inspissated serum have cells that are not only Gram positive but also show metachromatic granules (Zinnemann & Turner, 1963). Some strains need CO_2 and grow best under microaerophilic conditions (10 % oxygen) + 10 % CO_2.

In the medical field there are bacteria in the genus *Corynebacterium* that should be excluded. One such is *C. acnes* which produces propionic acid from the breakdown of carbohydrates and is now classified in the genus *Propionibacterium* (Douglas & Gunter, 1946). We deal with it in Section 6.7.

The corynebacteria, and particularly *Corynebacterium diphtheriae*, are rewarding to the microscopist; older bacteriologists recall that when diphtheria was a common disease a smear of the growth on a Loeffler slope from a throat swab was sufficiently characteristic for the experienced worker to report not only that *C. diphtheriae* was present, but also identify the variety of the species. Each worker had his preferred staining method (we used a polychrome methylene blue that took six months to ripen) and soon developed considerable skill in recognizing the different varieties (then called types) described by Anderson, Happold, McLeod & Thomson (1931) and Anderson, Cooper, Happold & McLeod (1933). Typically, the gravis variety produces the club-shaped and dumb-bell forms, and while metachromatic granules are few there are always areas in each cell stained in different shades of blue. One gravis serotype (Robinson & Peeney, 1936) may be difficult to identify microscopically because it does not produce clubs. The mitis types are the easiest of all to recognize for they show the typical textbook picture of *Corynebacterium diphtheriae*: pleomorphic rods with numerous metachromatic granules, the contiguous cells arranged in Vs and Ws, thus resembling cuneiform characters. The inappropriately named intermediate variety (from the clinical severity of the disease in Leeds in the early 1930s, not from the bacteriological characteristics of the organisms) is least like the textbook description; it consists of short rods which stain with alternating bands of light and dark blue; metachromatic granules are not seen in this variety and their absence makes it resemble a 'barred diphtheroid'; the true nature of the organism is indicated by the variation in the size of the cells and in their cuneiform arrangement. Of the diphtheroids found in the human throat, *C. xerosis* may mimic the gravis type of diphtheria bacillus but in a single culture it will be more uniform in shape and, like other diphtheroids, tend to form compact bundles, the palisade arrangement. Of the animal pathogens, *C. murium* and *C. ovis* are, in morphology, very similar to the mitis variety of *C. diphtheriae*.

The characteristic colony forms of the *Corynebacterium diphtheriae* varieties are best seen on

Table 6.5*a Second-stage table for* Corynebacterium, Listeria *and* Kurthia

	1	2	3
Motility	−	+	+
Catalase	D	+	+
Carbohydrate attack	F/−	F	−
VP	−	+	−
H_2S	−	−	d

1 Corynebacterium
2 Listeria; *Listerella*
3 Kurthia

Symbols used in the table are explained in Tables 5.1 and 5.2 (facing p. 43).

58

Table 6.5b *Third-stage table for* Corynebacterium, Listeria *and* Kurthia

	1	2	3	4	5	6	7	8	9	10	11	12	13	14	15
Motility	+	−	−	−	−	−	−	−	−	−	−	−	+	+	+
Catalase	+	+	+	+	+	+	+	+	+	+	−	−	+	+	+
Metachromatic granules	−	D	−	±ᵃ	+	+	+	.	−	d	d	d	−	−	−
Haemolysis	−	D	+	−	−	d	d	−	−	+	+	+	+	−	−
Growth improved by blood/serum	−	+	+	+	+	+	+	+	+	+	+	−ᵇ	+	.	+
Carbohydrate breakdown [F/O/−]	−	F	F	F	F	F	F	?ᶜ	−	F	F	F	F	F	F
Carbohydrates, acid from:															
glucose	−	+	+	+	+	+	+	−ᶜ	−	+	+	+	+	+	+
lactose	−	−	−	−	−	d	d	−	−	+	+	−	(d)	+	+
maltose	−	+	+	+	+	d	+	−ᶜ	−	+	+	+	+	+	+
mannitol	−	−	−	−	−	−	.	−	−	−	−	−	−	+	+
salicin	−	−	−	−	−	−	−	−	−	−	−	+	+	+	+
starch	−	D	+	−	+	d	+	−	−	d	+	+	(d)	+	+
sucrose	−	−	−	+	+	−	d	−	−	+	d	d	(d)	−	−
trehalose	−	−	+	−	+	−	−	−	−	−	−	−	+	+	+
xylose	−	−	−	−	.	.	−	.	−	+	d	−	−	−	−
VP	−	−	−	−	−	−	−	−ᶜ	−	−	−	−	+	+	+
Aesculin hydrolysis	.	.	.	.	.	.	.	.	−	.	.	.	+	+	+
Nitrate reduced	−	+	−	+	+	+	d	−ᶜ	+	−	−	−	−	−	−
Gelatin liquefaction	D	−	+	−	−	−	d	−	−	+	+	−	−	−	−
Urease	d	−	+	−	d	+	+	−ᶜ	+	−	−	−	−	.	.
Arginine hydrolysis	−	−	−	−	−	+	+	−	−	.	−	−	−	.	.

1 **Kurthia** spp.
2 **Corynebacterium diphtheriae**
3 **Corynebacterium ulcerans**
4 **Corynebacterium xerosis**
5 **Corynebacterium murium;**
 C. pseudotuberculosis-murium;
 C. kutscheri
6 **Corynebacterium renale**

7 **Corynebacterium ovis; C.**
 pseudotuberculosis-ovis; Preisz-
 Nocard bacillus
8 **Corynebacterium bovis**
9 **Corynebacterium hofmannii;**
 C. pseudodiphtheriticum (and
 variant spellings of both specific
 epithets)

10 **Corynebacterium haemolyticum**
11 **Corynebacterium pyogenes**
12 **Corynebacterium vaginale;**
 Haemophilus vaginalis
13 **Listeria monocytogenes;**
 Listerella monocytogenes
14 **Listeria grayi**
15 **Listeria murrayi**

ᵃ ± indicates few granules.
ᵇ Needs blood but not X/V factors (Dunkelberg & McVeigh, 1969).

ᶜ Positive when Tween 80 added to medium (see p. 60).

D Different results in the varieties (gravis, mitis, and intermediate) of *C. diphtheriae.*

Other symbols used in the table are explained in Tables 5.1 and 5.2 (facing p. 43).

McLeod's chocolate tellurite agar (described in Anderson *et al.* 1931); most gravis strains produce the 'daisy head' colony (but one serotype – not found in England – has a different colony form); mitis has a smooth-surfaced colony, black in the centre but surrounded by a clear grey zone; intermedius produces the smallest colony, grey in colour, with a smooth glistening surface.

Cummins & Harris (1956) showed that the cell wall composition of *Corynebacterium pyogenes* differed from that of other corynebacteria and was very like that of streptococci; moreover, Barksdale *et al.* (1957) reported that extracts of S forms of the species reacted with several group G streptococcus antisera, and showed that *C. pyogenes* could give rise to mutants indistinguishable from *C. haemolyticum* (Maclean, Liebow & Rosenberg, 1946). The picture is complicated by the fact that some streptococci (especially group H strains) in artificial culture tend to elongate and produce bacillary forms so that in a stained smear they have the appearance of a chain of short rods. Two

biochemical reactions of *C. pyogenes* (catalase negative and failure to reduce nitrates) are unusual in
corynebacteria but are characteristic of streptococci.
As with streptococci, occasional strains of *C.
pyogenes* are catalase positive; the catalase activity
is inhibited by azide and is, therefore, a true catalase
(Cummins, 1971).

Corynebacterium ulcerans (Gilbert & Stewart,
1926–7) is a starch-fermenting corynebacterium
that in some respects resembles *C. diphtheriae* var.
gravis. It can, however, be distinguished by gelatin
liquefaction, urease production, and its inability
to reduce nitrates (Cook & Jebb, 1952; Henriksen
& Grelland, 1952).

Corynebacterium equi produces a pink pigment;
it is misplaced in this genus and is probably a
member of the '*Mycobacterium*' *rhodochrous* group,
described with the nocardias in Section 6.10.1.

Corynebacteria may not grow well enough in
peptone water sugars to show their fermentative
capabilities. Calf serum (Cobb, 1963, 1966), Tween
80, and aeration (Jayne-Williams & Skerman, 1966)
improve growth of *C. bovis* so that acid may be produced from carbohydrates and the VP becomes
positive. The basal medium for carbohydrate tests
may be more critical for corynebacteria than for some
other organisms; Lovell (1946) found that in peptone water sugars, glucose was the only sugar to be
attacked regularly by *C. renale*.

Apart from the plant and soil corynebacteria
(some of which are motile), members of the genus
show great variety both within the genus and
within the species. In medical laboratories it is not
now sufficient to isolate and identify a diphtheria
bacillus on cultural and morphological characters
alone; it is essential to determine the virulence of
the isolate. The test in the guinea-pig (see Okell &
Parish, 1926) is still the most reliable test for
virulence but toxigenicity can be shown without
loss of accuracy by a modification of the Elek plate
(see, for example, Jameson, 1965).

Minidefinition: *Corynebacterium. Gram-
positive rods which, under most conditions
of growth do not branch. Typically non-
motile; non-sporing; not acid fast. Aerobic
and facultatively anaerobic. Usually catalase
positive; oxidase negative. Attack sugars
fermentatively or do not attack them.*

6.5.2 Listeria (Tables 6.5*a, b*; 6.6*a, b*). Described
by Murray, Webb & Swann (1926) as *Bacterium
monocytogenes*, the generic name later became
Listerella but as this name had been used for genera
in botany and zoology the bacterial genus was
renamed once again and became *Listeria*. The Lister
element of the name is derived from the name of
Lord Lister the surgeon, not from the name of the
South African bacteriologist, Sir Spencer Lister.
The name Listerella used by zoologists and
botanists honours Lord Lister's father and younger
brother (Gibbons, 1972).

The organism was first isolated from laboratory
animals at Cambridge but since the genus became
better known it has been isolated from a variety of
animals including man, and its distribution seems
to be world-wide. Characteristic of the genus is
survival and growth at 5 °C, a temperature at
which many other organisms will die; advantage
of this unusual quality is taken in the isolation of
the organism; if its presence is suspected, the specimen is kept in a refrigerator and cultures made from
it at intervals. Another characteristic of the genus
is that strains produce acetylmethylcarbinol. The
disease listeriosis and its bacteriology has become
much better known since Seeliger produced his
monograph in 1961.

Within the last few years two new species of
Listeria have been proposed; although the distinguishing features seem to us to be trivial we show the
characteristics of the three species in Table 6.5*b*.

Minidefinition: *Listeria. Gram-positive rods;
motile; non-sporing; not acid fast. Aerobic
and facultatively anaerobic. Catalase positive; oxidase negative. Attack sugars by
fermentation.*

6.5.3 Kurthia (Table 6.5*a, b*) is not usually
regarded as a pathogen, but Elston (1961) isolated
three strains from clinical material and this
suggested a possible pathogenic role. We record
it so that it may be identified, should it be isolated
by users of this *Manual*.

Proteolytic activity (inspissated serum and
gelatin are liquefied) and a weak urease activity
distinguish *Kurthia bessonii* (positive in these
characters) from *K. zopfii* (negative).

Minidefinition: *Kurthia. Gram-positive pleomorphic rods. Motile. Not spore-forming; not acid fast. Aerobic. Catalase positive; oxidase negative. Acid not produced from the breakdown of carbohydrates.*

6.6 Coryneform-actinomycete intermediates

(*Lactobacillus, Listeria, Erysipelothrix, Arachnia, Actinomyces*)

Characters common to the group: **Gram-positive rods; non-sporing. Not acid fast. Fermentative.**

The members of this large group have relatively few common characters but most of the taxa are microaerophilic. The group is divisible into two subgroups: (i) the lactic acid producing bacilli, and (ii) the branching rods (actinomycetes); between these two subgroups there are organisms with intermediate characters. *Lactobacillus* can be split into three subgenera (*Thermobacterium, Streptobacterium*, and *Betabacterium*) and these are shown in columns 3 to 5 in Table 6.6*a*; two of the subgenera are homofermentative (sugars are fermented mostly to lactic acid) and the third, *Betabacterium*, is heterofermentative (sugars fermented partly to lactic acid and partly to volatile acids including CO_2). Species characteristics of the lactic acid bacilli will be found in Table 6.6*b*.

Though normally regarded as catalase negative some strains of lactobacilli (also some leuconostocs and pediococci) have been reported as being able to produce catalase in media containing only low concentrations of glucose. These catalases are insensitive to sodium azide (Johnston & Delwiche, 1962) and are 'pseudocatalases' which do not appear when the organisms are grown on media containing 1 % glucose (Whittenbury, 1964).

The genus *Erysipelothrix* has some resemblance to *Lactobacillus*, and as it has often been compared with *Listeria*, and indeed combined with it, these organisms are shown in adjacent columns in Table 6.6*a, b. Erysipelothrix rhusiopathiae* is also shown in Table 6.7, which includes the medically significant propionibacteria.

Some species are shown in more than one of these tables, and some also in Table 6.7; this arrangement has the advantage that by it we can introduce additional characters and make direct comparisons between a greater number of similar or possibly similar organisms.

We should perhaps remind readers that our minidefinitions of genera, especially of these genera that are seldom seen in medical laboratories, are drawn up only with the medically interesting species in mind, and our definitions do not necessarily apply to all species of the genus.

6.6.1 Lactobacillus (Table 6.6*a, b*). Of Orla-Jensen's (1919) three subgenera of *Lactobacillus*, one (*Betabacterium*) is heterofermentative and, under suitable conditions, will produce gas from glucose (Gibson & Abd-el-Malek, 1945). This gas production is not likely to be confused with gas production by clostridia and their non-sporing variants, which is vigorous and occurs in a variety of media when cultures are incubated anaerobically. Heterofermentative lactobacilli (and *L. leichmannii*) produce ammonia from arginine when grown in a tomato juice basal medium containing glucose, yeast extract, and Tween 80 (Briggs, 1953*a, b*). Man, Rogosa & Sharpe (1960) recommended a special medium (Section A2.6.7) for testing the sugar reactions of lactobacilli, and Whittenbury (1963) showed that a soft agar medium was advantageous.

The characters of lactobacilli likely to be found in a medical laboratory are shown in Table 6.6*b* but we do not show the division of *Lactobacillus casei* and *L. plantarum* into varieties. Quite specialized methods are used in the thorough and detailed characterization of lactobacilli, and as these are outside the scope of this *Manual* we refer readers for information to papers by G. H. G. Davis (1955, 1960), Sharpe (1955), Rogosa & Sharpe (1959, 1960), J. G. Davis (1960), Rogosa, Franklin & Perry (1961) and Sharpe, Fryer & Smith (1966). It seems clear that there are many and varied views on the classification of the lactobacilli, and that these views change rapidly and repeatedly.

Döderlein's bacillus is not a bacteriological entity; most lactobacilli from the human vagina seem to be *Lactobacillus acidophilus* (Rogosa & Sharpe, 1960). The acidophilic bacteria isolated from carious teeth by McIntosh, James & Lazarus-Barlow (1922) were not adequately described and are not shown in Table 6.6*b*.

Motile lactobacilli have been found (Harrison &

Hanson, 1950; Gemmell & Hodgkiss, 1964), as have sporing forms (and a new subgenus described for them), but the taxonomic significance of these observations is obscure.

> **Minidefinition:** *Lactobacillus. Gram-positive rods, typically non-motile and not producing spores. Not acid fast. Aerobic and facultatively anaerobic. Catalase negative. Grow best at about pH 6. Attack sugars fermentatively.*

Table 6.6a *Second-stage table for* Lactobacillus, Listeria, Erysipelothrix, Arachnia *and* Actinomyces odontolyticus

	1	2	3	4	5	6	7	8
Motility	+	−	−	−	−	−	−	−
Growth at 5 °C	+	−	−	−	−	−	−	−
Growth at 15 °C	+	+	−	+	D	.	.	.
Gas from glucose	−	−	−	−	+	−	−	+
Carbohydrates, acid from:								
arabinose	−	+	−	d	D	w	−	−
maltose	+	−	+	+	+	+	−	+
melezitose	+	−	−	+	−	−	−	−
salicin	+	−	+	+	−	−	−	−
VP	+	−	−	−	−	−	−	.
Nitrates reduced	−	−	−	−	−	+	+	+

1 **Listeria** spp.
2 **Erysipelothrix** sp.
3 **Lactobacillus** subgenus *Thermobacterium*
4 **Lactobacillus** subgenus *Streptobacterium*
5 **Lactobacillus** subgenus *Betabacterium*
6 **Arachnia propionica**
7 **Actinomyces odontolyticus**
8 **Clostridium welchii** (asporogenous variants)

Symbols used in the table are explained in Tables 5.1 and 5.2 (facing p. 43).

6.6.2   Listeria (Tables 6.5*a*, *b*; 6.6*a*, *b*) was at one time considered to be closely related to Erysipelothrix and both were put in the same genus (*Erysipelothrix*) in the earlier editions of *Topley & Wilson's Principles of Bacteriology and Immunity*. Barber (1939) always maintained the separation of the two genera, and in this she has been supported by the numerical taxonomic work of Davis & Newton (1969), Davis, Formin, Wilson & Newton (1969), and of Stuart & Pease (1972). The last pair of authors thought that *Listeria* most closely

resembled the enterococci, and *Erysipelothrix* the other streptococci.

The minidefinition for *Listeria* is repeated here; for the derivation of the name Listeria see the paragraph in Section 6.5.2.

> **Minidefinition:** *Listeria. Gram-positive rods; motile; non-sporing; not acid fast. Aerobic and facultatively anaerobic. Catalase positive; oxidase negative. Attack sugars by fermentation.*

6.6.3   Erysipelothrix (Tables 6.6*a*, *b*; 6.7). Although veterinarians seem to agree that one species causes swine erysipelas, erysipeloid, and mouse septicaemia, that species has at one time or another been placed in eleven different genera and given fourteen different specific epithets (Shuman & Wellmann, 1966). The nomenclatural problem was resolved when Opinion 32 (1970) was issued declaring *Erysipelothrix rhusiopathiae* to be a conserved name, that is, the officially approved name for future use.

The organisms grow well in the presence of crude bile salts (0.1–0.2%) which seem to act as a serum substitute; purified bile salts are inactive but the serum need can be satisfied by oleic acid (Hutner, 1942) or by Tween 80 (Ando, Moriya & Kuwahara, 1959). White & Shuman (1961) showed that the fermentation patterns of erysipelothrix strains varied with the medium and the indicator, but most strains had a consistent pattern under the same growth conditions; they recommended a basal medium containing peptone, meat extract, and 10% horse serum.

Erysipelothrix strains have several characters in common with both listerias and streptococci. From a numerical analysis Stuart & Pease (1972) suggest that streptococci may be the connecting link, Listeria resembling the faecal streptococci and Erysipelothrix being more like the non-faecal streptococci.

> **Minidefinition:** *Erysipelothrix. Gram-positive rods; not branching. Non-motile; non-sporing. Catalase negative. Not acid fast. Attack sugars by fermentation.*

6.6.4   Arachnia (Tables 6.6*a*, *b*; 6.7) is an actinomycete capable of growing in air (especially

Table 6.6*b Third-stage table for* Lactobacillus, Listeria, Erysipelothrix, Arachnia *and* Actinomyces odontolyticus

	1	2	3	4	5	6	7	8	9	10	11	12	13
Growth at 15 °C	−	−	−	−	+	+	+	d	−	+	+	.	.
Growth at 45 °C	+	+	+	+	d	−	−	−	+	+	−	.	.
Gas from glucose	−	.	−	−	−	−	+	+	+	−	−	−	−
Carbohydrates, acid from:													
arabinose	−	−	−	−	−	d	+	+	d	−	+	w	−
galactose	+	d	−	+	+	+	(w)	+	+	−	+	d	−
lactose	+	−	d	+	d	+	d	d	+	(d)	+	+	+
maltose	+	+	+	+	+	+	+	+	+	+	−	+	−
mannitol	−	−	−	+	+	+	d	−	−	−	−	w	d
melezitose	−	−	−	−	+	+	−	−	−	+	−	−	−
melibiose	d	−	−	+	−	+	+	+	+	d	+	w	.
raffinose	d	−	−	+	−	+	d	+	+	−	−	+	−
salicin	+	+	+	d	+	+	−	d	−	+	−	−	−
sorbitol	−	−	−	+	+	+	−	−	−	−	−	−	.
trehalose	+	+	+	+	+	+	−	+	−	+	−	+	−
Aesculin hydrolysis	+	+	+	d	+	+	d	+	−	+	−	−	.
Nitrate reduction	−	−	−	−	−	−	−	−	−	−	−	+	+
Arginine hydrolysis	−	+	d	−	−	−	+	+	+	−	+	.	.

1 **Lactobacillus acidophilus**
2 **Lactobacillus jensenii**
3 **Lactobacillus leichmannii**
4 **Lactobacillus salivarius**
5 **Lactobacillus casei**

6 **Lactobacillus plantarum**
7 **Lactobacillus brevis**
8 **Lactobacillus cellobiosus**
9 **Lactobacillus fermenti**
10 **Listeria monocytogenes;**
   Listerella monocytogenes

11 **Erysipelothrix rhusiopathiae;**
   E. insidiosa
12 **Arachnia propionica;**
   Actinomyces propionicus
13 **Actinomyces odontolyticus**

Symbols used in the table are explained in Tables 5.1 and 5.2 (facing p. 43).

in an air $+ CO_2$ mixture) and, being catalase negative, will in our first-stage table (6.1) be included in the same major group as *Lactobacillus* and *Erysipelothrix*, and hence in Table 6.6*a* and *b*.

Morphologically *Arachnia* resembles the actinomycetes, physiologically the propionibacteria; hence its characters will also be found in Table 6.7 and additional information in Section 6.7.2.

> **Minidefinition:** *Arachnia. Non-motile, Gram-positive branched rods; short or filamentous. Aerobic; facultatively anaerobic. Catalase negative. Attack sugars fermentatively, with propionic and acetic acids as the main end products.*

6.7   The actinomycetes

(*Actinomyces, Propionibacterium, Arachnia, Rothia* and *Bifidobacterium*)

Characters common to members of the group: Gram-positive rods with branching, even if only rudimentary. Non-motile; not acid fast. Aerial mycelium not produced. Attack sugars fermentatively.

Many of the organisms of this group – which can loosely be called the actinomycetes – appreciate an increase in CO_2 concentration, and with it some species will grow in air. The cultural characters of the organisms do not appear to be very stable, and this probably reflects differences in media rather than in biochemical techniques. When media and methods are better standardized it should be possible to draw up more reliable specifications for the different species; until that time comes all we can do is to sift the evidence (much of it conflicting) and hope that we draw the right conclusions, but it is rather like trying to pick a winner with a pin.

Characters of members of the group are shown in Table 6.7 but we warn against relying too much on individual characters; identification in this group, more than in most, should be based on a summation of characters.

6.7.1   Propionibacterium (Table 6.7). A genus of bacteria that produce propionic acid as one of the end products of metabolism, and of only limited interest to those working in a clinical laboratory. The anaerobic acne bacillus was obviously ill placed in *Corynebacterium*; from the finding that it produced propionic and acetic acids Douglas & Gunter (1946) recognized that it was one of the propionic acid bacteria better known in industrial microbiology, and they proposed its translation to *Propionibacterium* as *P. acnes*. Although this was supported by Moore & Cato (1963) there developed a curious debate about whether *C. acnes* represented all the anaerobic diphtheroids (Zierdt, Webster & Rude, 1968; Moore, Holdeman & Cummins, 1968; Zierdt, 1970).

The characterization of the species *C. acnes* has been conflicting and confusing; Puhvel (1968) summarized the findings of seven groups of authors, gave his own results and came to the conclusion that, although some characters showed strain variation, the species seemed to be fairly homogeneous. Zierdt *et al.* (1968) noticed that in about 10% of strains four biochemical characters (indole, nitrate reduction, gelatin, and the clotting of milk) were negative when first isolated but on further sub-culture strains might acquire these characters. Brzin (1964) found an inverse correlation between indole production and maltose fermentation and thought that the species *Corynebacterium acnes* could be divided into two biotypes, the indologenic and the saccharolytic; his conclusions were confirmed by Voss (1970) who added a partial correlation with sensitivity to a bacteriophage. A comparison of the characters of Voss's group II organism with those of *Propionibacterium granulosum* in the *Anaerobe Laboratory Manual* (1972) suggests to us that these are the same organism. If we are correct – and our opinion seems to be supported by the DNA homology work of Johnson & Cummins (1972) – it is merely a matter of opinion whether the organism should be labelled *P. acnes* group II or *P. granulosum*; in this case we prefer the species to the group.

Minidefinition: *Propionibacterium. Unbranching (anaerobic) or club-shaped and branching (aerobic) Gram-positive rods. Non-motile; non-sporing. Anaerobic and facultatively aerobic. Catalase positive.*

Attack sugars fermentatively and produce propionic acid as a breakdown product.

6.7.2   Arachnia (Tables 6.6*a, b*; 6.7), a genus of actinomycete that produces propionic acid from the fermentative breakdown of glucose and has diaminopimelic acid as one of the constituents of its cell wall (Johnson & Cummins, 1972). These characters, which distinguish it from species of *Actinomyces*, are unlikely to be looked for or detected in a medical bacteriological laboratory, and we do not know of any way of identifying this organism without enlisting the help of a biochemist; this is unfortunate as the species has been isolated from clinically typical actinomycosis (Gerencser & Slack, 1967). For full details of the single species see Pine & Georg (1969) and for characters that help to distinguish it from *Actinomyces* species see Buchanan & Pine (1962) and Table 6.7.

Minidefinition: *Arachnia. Non-motile, Gram-positive branched rods or filaments. Aerobic and facultatively anaerobic. Catalase negative. Attack sugars fermentatively, with propionic and acetic acids as the main end products.*

6.7.3   Actinomyces (Table 6.7) species are microaerophilic rather than anaerobic, and after a few subcultures many strains will grow aerobically; growth is often improved by carbon dioxide. Classically, *Actinomyces bovis* is isolated from lumpy jaw in cattle, *A. israelii* from actinomycotic infections in man, *A. naeslundii* from tonsils and the mouth of man, *A. odontolyticus* from carious teeth, and *A. viscosus* (the 'hamster organism') from the teeth of hamsters; in fact, the organisms are widely distributed and may be isolated from both healthy and diseased tissues and from secretions. Apart from producing a dark red colony (Batty, 1958), *A. odontolyticus* is very similar to *A. bovis* and its acceptance as a distinct species may not be justified (Melville, 1965).

Problems of the pathogenicity of the actinomycetes arise continually but inoculation of laboratory animals does not help. The more pigmented the growth, the less likely is the strain to be pathogenic. On pigments, Conn & Conn (1941) warned that although production may be constant, the colours –

Table 6.7 *Second-stage table for* Propionibacterium, Arachnia, Actinomyces, Rothia, Bifidobacterium, Erysipelothrix

	1	2	3	4	5	6	7	8	9	10	11	12
Growth in air	−	−	+	−[a]	−[a]	+	−[a]	d[a]	−	+	−	+
Growth anaerobically	+	+	+	+	+	+	+	+	+	−	+	+
Catalase	+	+	−	−	−	−	+	−	−	+	−	−
CO$_2$ required	−	−	−	−	−	−	+	−	−	−	−	.
CO$_2$ improves growth	.	.	+	+	+	+	+	+	−	−	−	.
Carbohydrates, acid from:												
glycerol	+	+	−	−	−	d	d	−	d	w	.	−
lactose	−	−	+	+	+	+	+	+	+	−	+	+
maltose	d	+	+	+	+	+	+	−	+	+	.	−
mannitol	d	−	w	+	−	−	−	d	+	−	D	−
raffinose	−	d	+	+	−	+	+	−	+	−	+	−
salicin	−	−	−	+	−	+	+	−	+	−	D	−
sorbitol	d	−	−	−	−	−	−	.	.	−	D	−
sucrose	d	d	+	+	+	+	+	+	+	+	+	−
trehalose	+	w	+	+	−	+	d	−	+	+	D	−
xylose	−	−	−	+	d	−	w	−	+	−	D	+
VP	−	−	−	−	−	−	−	−	−	+	.	−
Aesculin hydrolysis	.	.	.	.	.	+	+	.	.	+	.	−
Starch hydrolysis	−	−	−	w/−	+	−	+	−	+	−	.	.
Nitrates reduced	d	d	+	d	−	+	+	+	−	+	−	−
Indole	+	−	−[b]	−[b]	−[b]	−[b]	−	−	d	−	.	−
Gelatin liquefaction	+	d	−	−	−	−	−	−	.	(+)	.	−

1 **Propionibacterium acnes;** *Corynebacterium acnes;* Voss' *C. acnes* group I; *C. parvum* (Cummins & Johnson, 1974)
2 **Propionibacterium granulosum;** Voss' *C. acnes* group II
3 **Arachnia propionica;** *Actinomyces propionicus*

4 **Actinomyces israelii**
5 **Actinomyces bovis**
6 **Actinomyces naeslundii**
7 **Actinomyces viscosus;** *Odontomyces viscosus;* the 'hamster organism'
8 **Actinomyces odontolyticus**

9 **Actinomyces eriksonii**
10 **Rothia dentocariosa;** *Nocardia dentocariosa*
11 **Bifidobacterium spp.;** *Lactobacillus bifidus*
12 **Erysipelothrix rhusiopathiae;** *E. insidiosa*

[a] Positive in air+CO$_2$.   [b] Contrary reports by different (but reliable) authors.

Symbols used in the table are explained in Tables 5.1 and 5.2 (facing p. 43).

influenced by the pH value of the medium – vary and are most intense in the alkaline range. Information on the characteristics of actinomycetes is unsatisfactory; it comes from a few groups of workers and it seems that their methods differ. Attempts are being made to standardize methods (Slack, 1968).

> **Minidefinition:** *Actinomyces. Non-motile Gram-positive rods which may show true branching. Non-sporing; not acid fast. Microaerophilic and anaerobic. Catalase negative (one exception). Attack sugars fermentatively.*

6.7.4   Rothia (Table 6.7). This group of aerobic, catalase-forming, Gram-positive rods was at one time part of the genus *Nocardia*. It differs from that genus in several ways (the organisms ferment carbohydrates, and never produce a mycelium or conidia) and a new genus was created for it by Georg & Brown (1967). The rods show branching filaments but as the culture ages fragmentation occurs and after a few days the culture seems to consist of masses of coccoid forms.

Rothias have been isolated from carious dentine. They grow under microaerophilic conditions, but feebly or not at all, under strict anaerobic conditions. There is one species, *Rothia dentocariosa*.

> **Minidefinition:** *Rothia. Non-motile, filamentous Gram-positive rods; pleomorphic but do not form a mycelium or produce*

aerial hyphae. Aerobic and microaerophilic. Catalase positive. Attack sugars by fermentation. Reduce nitrite to ammonia.

6.7.5   Bifidobacterium (Table 6.7) species are characterized by their crudely branching forms, often Y-shaped. *Bifidobacterium bifidum (Lactobacillus bifidus)* is probably the best known and, because of its limited ability to attack sugars, is the easiest to identify (Scardovi *et al.* 1971).

Bifidobacteria are found in the faeces of infants and adults, in the human vagina, and in the faeces (or rumen contents) of animals and birds (Reuter, 1971; Scardovi *et al.* 1971). A wide range of sugars is attacked and, based on the differences in fermentation reactions, sixteen species have been named; we do not attempt to show species characteristics in Table 6.7.

> **Minidefinition:** *Bifidobacterium. Gram-positive rods with a tendency to form rudimentary branches. Non-sporing and not acid fast. Anaerobic. Catalase negative. Sugars attacked fermentatively.*

6.8   The anaerobic bacilli
(*Clostridium, Eubacterium*)
***Characters common to members of the group:* Gram-positive rods; not acid fast. Anaerobic; do not grow under aerobic conditions.**

The degree of anaerobiosis required by members of the group varies from the strict (*Eubacterium* spp., *Clostridium tetani, C. chauvoei*) through the less exacting species (*C. welchii*) to the aerotolerant (*C. histolyticum*). The techniques used to deal with anaerobes have become more specialized and some workers who deal with them in large numbers do not now consider that reliance should be placed on anaerobic jars (McIntosh & Fildes or Brewer's, or the newer forms using a cold catalyst). The *Anaerobe Laboratory Manual* (ALM, 1972), which describes methods used in the Virginia Polytechnic Institute that are based on those of R. E. Hungate, should be consulted by those who intend to set up a special anaerobe laboratory, but general bacteriological laboratories can do a great deal of good work with simpler techniques and anaerobic jars (Willis, 1964). To those who think that flushed cabinets are necessary, a design from the National Institute for Medical Research at Mill Hill may appeal (Leach, Bullen & Grant, 1971).

The anaerobes, both sporing and non-sporing, are the splitter's paradise. We are not of their company for in our view the only justification for excessive splitting (or speciation) is epidemiological, and anaerobes are not causes of what are usually regarded as infectious or epidemic diseases. Epidemics of food-poisoning are commonly due to certain toxin types of *Clostridium welchii* (*C. perfringens*) and rarely to *C. botulinum*; epizootics due to clostridial infections cause considerable losses in flocks and herds; in both man and animals anaerobes are responsible for clinical enteritis in individuals. The identification of specific toxin types is possible but is work for a reference laboratory. Food-poisoning strains of *Clostridium welchii* are often known as 'heat-resistant *C. welchii*', in contrast to the more usual strains of the species, which have a lower resistance to heating (boiling) than most clostridia. Paradoxically, although cultures of the heat-resistant strains resist boiling for at least an hour, it is very difficult to find stainable spores in smears from the cultures.

A point in favour of putting the two anaerobic genera together is to have their characters recorded in the same table, for on paper it might seem that non-sporing variants of clostridia could be mistaken for eubacteria. In practice this is an unlikely event; the swarming of the motile clostridia, which seldom produce discrete colonies, is so characteristic that even a novice would see that it is different from the growth of eubacteria, though that same novice might not detect the fine and almost invisible growth of *Clostridium tetani*. The clostridium isolated most frequently (*C. welchii*) grows so vigorously that it could hardly be confused with the less robust eubacteria.

We think we should repeat the advice given by Reddish & Rettger (1924) in connexion with the identification of clostridia, which is also applicable to eubacteria. They stressed that undue emphasis should not be put on the results of fermentation tests, for the results may be inconstant. They thought that the shape and position of spores could be characteristic but motility was not of much help in identifying anaerobes. We hope that

Table 6.8 *Second-stage table for* Clostridium

	1	2	3	4	5	6	7	8	9	10
Motility	−	+	+	+	+	+	+	−	+	+
Spore	UX	UX	TX	VX	VX	VX	VX	TX	TX	VX
Microaerophilic	−	−	+	+	−	−	−	−	−	−
Haemolysis	+	−	−	+	+	+	+	−	−	+
Growth at 37 °C	+	+	+	+	+	+	+	+	+	+
Carbohydrates, acid from:										
glucose	+	+	+	+	+	+	+	+	+	+
lactose	+	+	+	+	+	+	+	−	+	+
salicin	−	+	+	+	+	+	−	+	+	−
sucrose	+	+	+	+	+	−	+	+	−	−
Milk	AGC	AGC	AC	AC	A(C)	A(C)	AGC	E	−	GC
Nitrates reduced	+	+	+	−	+	+	+	−	−	+
Indole	−	−	−	−	−	−	−	−	−	d
Gelatin	+	−	−	−	−	+	+	−	+	+
Meat (digestion)	−	−	−	−	−	−	−	−	−	−
Urease	−	−	−	.	.	−	.	.	.	−
H₂S	+	−	−	−	−	+	+	.	+	+
Egg-yolk (pearly layer)	−	−	−	−	−	−	−	−	−	d
LV (lecithinase)	+	−	−	−	−	−	−	−	−	d

	11	12	13	14	15	16	17	18	19	20	21	22
Motility	+	+	+	+	+	+	+	+	−	−	−	−
Spore	UX	UX	VX	UVX	UVX	TY	TY	VX	TY	−	−	−
Microaerophilic	−	−	−	−	−	−	−	+	−			
Haemolysis	+	+	−	+	+	d	+	+	−	−	−	−
Growth at 37 °C	+	+	+	+	+	+	+	+	−	+	+	+
Carbohydrates, acid from:												
glucose	+	+	+	+	+	+	−	−	−	+	+	−
lactose	−	−	−	−	−	−	−	−	−	−	+	−
salicin	−	−	−	+	−	−	−	−	−	−	+	−
sucrose	−	−	−	−	−	−	−	−	−	−	+	−
Milk	A	M	M	CM	CM	−	E	M	−	−	A	−
Nitrates reduced	−	−	+[a]	+[a]	+[a]	+[a]	+[a]	−	−	−	−	+
Indole	−	−	−	+	+	+	+	−	−	−	−	
Gelatin	−	+	+	+	+	−	(w)	+	−	−	−	
Meat (digestion)	−	+	+	+	+	−	−	+	−	−	−	
Urease	−	d	−	−	+	−	d	+	.	.	.	
H₂S	+	+	+	+	+	+	−	+	w	.	.	.
Egg-yolk (pearly layer)	+	+	+	−	−	−	−	−	−	−	−	−
LV (lecithinase)	+	+	+	+	+	−	−	−	−	−	−	−

1 **Clostridium welchii;** *C.*
  perfringens; *Welchia perfringens*
2 **Clostridium butyricum**
3 **Clostridium tertium**
4 **Clostridium carnis**
5 **Clostridium fallax**
6 **Clostridium septicum**
7 **Clostridium chauvoei;** *C. feseri*
8 **Clostridium innocuum**

9 **Clostridium difficile**
10 **Clostridium oedematiens;** *C. novyi*
11 **Clostridium botulinum** types
  C, D, E (non-proteolytic)
12 **Clostridium botulinum** types A, B, F
13 **Clostridium sporogenes**
14 **Clostridium bifermentans**
15 **Clostridium sordellii;** *C.*
  bifermentans

16 **Clostridium tetanomorphum**
17 **Clostridium tetani;** *Plectridium*
  tetani
18 **Clostridium histolyticum**
19 **Clostridium putrefaciens**
20 **Eubacterium limosum**
21 **Eubacterium aerofaciens**
22 **Eubacterium lentum**

[a] May be reduced beyond nitrite.

Symbols used in the table are explained in Tables 5.1 and 5.2 (facing p. 43).

users of our *Manual* will bear this advice in mind when they compare the results of their own tests with the characters recorded in our table(s), for the characterizations in them are often based on our judgement of conflicting data, and we cannot claim infallibility.

6.8.1   Clostridium (Table 6.8). In choosing species for inclusion in Table 6.8 we took into account the likelihood of isolating them; some (e.g. *Clostridium hastiforme*) have seldom, if ever, been isolated since their original description and naming; these we regard as a burden on the literature and we do not propose to add to it by including the species here. We are reminded of the adage 'do not describe a new disease on one case' which in the field of anaerobic bacteriology is reflected in Willis' (1964) aphorism 'At all costs the publication of single isolations must be avoided', a sentiment with which we heartily concur. *Clostridium difficile* and *C. innocuum* are species that are not well known but were isolated and studied intensively by Smith & King (1962*a, b*) and we think are now well enough characterized to justify inclusion. King *et al.* (1963) isolated *Clostridium tertium* from the blood of two patients, an event sufficient to justify a place in a table such as ours. *Clostridium putre-faciens* is a neglected anaerobe (Ross, 1965) that seems to be responsible for the souring of brine-cured hams, and has also been isolated from animal sources. We hesitated about putting *Clostridium fallax* in Table 6.8. Willis (1964), to whom we refer readers for information on the pathogenic anaerobes, says that spores are rarely produced, and this statement is amply confirmed by others. The original workers (Weinberg & Séguin, 1915) who characterized the species (and named it *Bacillus fallax* at a time when all rod-shaped bacteria, whether sporing or not, were labelled Bacillus) reported that it did not produce spores in media with or without glucose, and that old cultures did not resist boiling for a minute. It seems possible that *Bacillus fallax* Weinberg & Séguin was a non-spore-forming anaerobe and should not be in the genus *Clostridium*; our inclusion of the species in that genus is made with considerable reserve.

In compiling Table 6.8 we consulted papers and

books by various authors (see Table 6.11) but, as in the first edition of this *Manual*, relied most on the results obtained by Miss H. E. Ross during her work in the National Collection of Type Cultures and elsewhere. We follow Brooks & Epps (1959) in keeping separate *Clostridium bifermentans* from *C. sordellii*; in showing reduction of nitrates our results appear to contrast with those of Brooks & Epps and others who did not test the medium for residual nitrate and thus wrongly assumed that nitrate had not been reduced. Unlike Moussa (1959) we do not combine *Clostridium chauvoei* (*C. feseri*) with *C. septicum*. The only significant difference between *C. botulinum* and *C. sporogenes* is toxin production and this is not shown in our table. The similarity between *C. sporogenes* and proteolytic *C. botulinum* types extends to genetic relationships (Lee & Riemann, 1970).

It is well known that *Clostridium welchii* does not spore readily, either in culture or in the animal body; indeed, Willis (1964) goes so far as to say that the absence of spores is one of the characteristic features of the species; as a consequence, he recommends omission, for primary isolation, of the heating technique (see below) which is likely to kill any *C. welchii* present. Because the species does not produce spores readily detectable in culture and does not need strict anaerobic conditions for growth, we have included it also in Table 6.6*a*, which characterizes other Gram-positive bacteria whose growth is favoured by anaerobic conditions.

Many species of clostridia can be subdivided into varieties (or even species, as *C. welchii* var. *agni* or *C. agni*) or toxin types (Sterne & Warrack, 1964) by the different toxins produced. However, few bacteriologists have available the specific antitoxins or the experience to carry out the tests, and we have not thought it necessary or advisable to draw up third-stage tables to show these toxin types. Those interested in the finer subdivisions we refer to papers by Brooks, Sterne & Warrack (1957) for *C. welchii*, and Oakley, Warrack & Clarke (1947) and Oakley & Warrack (1959) for *C. oedematiens*. The anaerobes of wound infections are dealt with extensively by Willis (1964, 1969).

The isolation of clostridia is not unusually difficult but their purification is one of the best tests of a bacteriologist's patience and skill, and may take several weeks or even months. Isolation techniques usually involve putting a liberal inoculum into freshly boiled (and cooled) cooked meat medium; always do this in duplicate, the first tube should be seeded with some unheated specimen, the second with a part of the specimen that has been heated at 80 °C for 10 minutes to destroy vegetative organisms. After incubation of the cooked meat cultures for 24–48 hours, subculture to other media (e.g. blood agar plates) and, if *Clostridium tetani* is suspected, adopt Fildes' tip and inoculate the condensation water of a long thin slope. Keep the tube upright and after incubation for 6–18 h subculture from the thin, perhaps drying, top edge of the slope. *C. tetani* swarms more rapidly than other bacteria and the advancing edge of the very fine growth may be seen with a hand lens; from it, *C. tetani* can often be isolated in pure culture. Another useful technique (from the Fildes era) for the isolation, identification, and purification of toxigenic clostridia is to inoculate a part of the specimen into guinea-pigs, some protected with antisera, others unprotected. Cultures of the heart blood and the surface of the liver of those that die may yield a pathogen, and surprisingly often in pure culture. The protective action of monospecific antitoxins enables an infecting organism (but not atoxic secondary invaders) to be identified. More than one anaerobe may be present in a wound and will add to the difficulties of identification. The isolation in pure culture and the identification of a clostridium is one of the most satisfying achievements of a bacteriologist.

Some comment on the tests used for the characters shown in Table 6.8 is needed. The motility of anaerobes is not easy to detect and cannot be done by the usual hanging-drop technique; only a positive result has any significance. The capillary tube method is the most satisfactory and, since there is evidence of negative aerotaxis, the examination should be made away from the air/liquid meniscus. Anaerobes from a solid medium (though flagellated) suspended in water, buffer, or broth are non-motile (Stanbridge & Preston, 1969). The shape and surface of the spore may be bizarre (Hodgkiss & Ordal, 1966); the spore position in the cell calls for a subjective judgement and it may well be making too fine a distinction to describe one spore as

subterminal and another as central. In our earlier tables (Cowan & Steel, 1961) we avoided this issue by indicating only those species that produced terminal spores, and assumed that all others produced central or subterminal spores. A few clostridia are microaerophilic, but even these species grow better under anaerobic conditions.

> **Minidefinition:** *Clostridium. Rods, Gram-positive in young cultures; typically motile (non-motile forms occur). Not acid fast. Produce spores that are usually heat resistant. Anaerobic; some species facultatively microaerophilic. Catalase negative. Some species attack sugars fermentatively, others not at all.*

6.8.2   Eubacterium (Table 6.8). These non-sporing anaerobic rods are probably quite unimportant in clinical bacteriology; they seem to be part of the normal intestinal flora and have not been incriminated as pathogens. ALM (1972) characterizes eighteen species but if weak reactions are ignored (as we think they should be, particularly with anaerobes) only two or three patterns show sufficient differences to justify consideration as species; we remind our readers of the advice given by Reddish & Rettger (see p. 66). We have been liberal and in Table 6.8 show characters of three eubacteria; these seem to be enough to indicate the range of the reactions obtained and are sufficient to distinguish them from the non-sporing variants of clostridia.

> **Minidefinition:** *Eubacterium. Gram-positive rods; do not branch. Non-sporing; not acid fast. Anaerobic. Split sugars fermentatively or not at all.*

6.9   The aerobic spore-formers
(Bacillus)
Characters common to members of the group: Gram-positive rods. Not acid fast. Grow under aerobic conditions. Produce heat-resistant spores.

Members of the Bacillus group have the unique character among the aerobic Gram-positive rods of producing endospores. But it is not a homogeneous group, especially in those characters by which we make our first-stage (primary) subdivision (Table 6.1); the variable characters include (i) the Gram reaction, (ii) motility, (iii) ability to grow under anaerobic conditions, (iv) the oxidase reaction, and (v) the method by which carbohydrates are broken down. Of these, the variable Gram reaction is the most disturbing to the neatness of our identification scheme, for this is based on the division of bacteria into the Gram positives and the Gram negatives. Both Dr T. Gibson and Dr Ruth Gordon insist that the Gram reaction of *Bacillus* species may be 'positive, indefinite or negative' and Dr Gordon tells us that of 163 strains of her group II bacilli, 46% were Gram variable after 6 hours of incubation, and 20% were Gram negative. Commenting on a draft of Table 6.9 she says that our footnote J is 'not [good] enough' and she wants 'to root out the fallacy that all strains of *Bacillus* spp. are Gram positive'. We justify our more rigid but less scientific treatment of *Bacillus* as a genus of Gram-positive bacilli on the grounds that the interest of medical bacteriologists is centred on group I, primarily on *Bacillus anthracis* and how to distinguish it from the other species that are less important in the medical field. The identification of *B. anthracis* is a matter of some urgency; it does not matter if the identification of other species takes weeks or even months. Perhaps once again we should remind readers and users of this *Manual* that out minidefinitions apply to species likely to be identified in a medical laboratory, and are not necessarily applicable to all the species of a genus.

In spite of the different reactions to our primary criteria by Bacillus species or strains, the variables themselves are not satisfactory for making further subdivisions. Those who have tried to subdivide *Bacillus* have used many distinguishing characters, but the results do not seem to have been very successful or useful. Ford (1916) listed nine groups (mostly named after the best-known species) among the non-pathogenic aerobic spore-formers, and Buchanan (1918) recognized three subgenera, *Eu-Bacillus* [sic], motile by peritrichous flagella; *Bacteridium*, non-motile; and *Astasia*, motile rods, spores oval with longitudinal stripes. Another approach divides the group into the psychrophilic, mesophilic, and thermophilic subgroups, but the dividing lines are far from clear, most workers

disregard them, and spore-formers with different temperature requirements are retained in *Bacillus*.

Other methods have been applied to the characterization of *Bacillus* species; Knight & Proom (1950) and Proom & Knight (1955) used nutritional requirements, and Jayne-Williams & Cheeseman (1960) applied chromatographic techniques to the thermophils, but no one has yet produced a tidy subdivision to rival the arrangement of Smith, Gordon and Clark (1946, 1952) and brought up to date by Gordon, Haynes & Pang (1973).

6.9.1   Bacillus (Table 6.9). We have included most of the species recognized by Smith, Gordon & Clark (1952) but have excluded *Bacillus pasteurii*, an organism that does not grow on ordinary media and which is therefore not likely to be isolated in a medical laboratory. The characters chosen are those which most readily distinguish the different species; they are based on our standard tests carried out at a slightly lower temperature (28–30 °C). When determining the maximum temperature for growth (not shown in Table 6.9) tests should be carried out in water baths in incubators at appropriate temperatures (N. R. Smith, 1947). *Bacillus stearothermophilus* cultures will not grow at 28 °C and should be incubated at 45–60 °C. Except for *Bacillus coagulans*, which prefers organic nitrogen, the sugar tests should be made in a medium with an ammonium salt as nitrogen source (Section A2.6.5).

Smith *et al.* (1952) regarded *Bacillus anthracis* as a pathogenic variety of *Bacillus cereus*, and *Bacillus mycoides* as another variety of *Bacillus cereus*. If they had followed the principles and precepts of the Bacteriological Code *Bacillus anthracis* would have been the species and *B. cereus* the variety as the epithet anthracis antedated the epithet cereus, but they gave sensible and adequate reasons for regarding *Bacillus cereus* as the parent form, and for disregarding the less scientific requirements of the Bacteriological Code. As bacteriologists working primarily with pathogens we do not follow the logical course taken by Smith and his colleagues, but like Leise, Carter, Friedlander & Freed (1959) and Burdon & Wende (1960), we retain *Bacillus anthracis* as a separate species. Among the features of *Bacillus anthracis* used by Leise *et al.* to distinguish it from *B. cereus*

Table 6.9 *Second-stage table for* Bacillus

	1	2	3	4	5	6	7	8	9	10	11	12	13	14	15	16	17	18	19
Gram reaction	+	+	+	+	+	+	+	+	+	J	J	J	J	J	J	J	J	J	J
Motility[a]	−	+	+	+	+	+	+	+	+	+	+	+	+	+	+	+	+	+	+
Morphological group (see text)	1	1	1	1	1	1	1	1/2	2/3	2	2	2	2	2	2	2	2	2	3
Spore shape	X	X	X	X	X	X	X	X	XY	X	X	X	X	X	X	X	X	X	Y
Spore position	U	U	U	U	U	U	U	UVT	T	UVT	UVT	UVT	U	T	UVT	T	T	T	T
Swelling of bacillary body	−	−	−	−	−	−	−	d	+	+	+	+	+	+	+	w	+	+	+
Growth at 45 °C	−	d	d	+	d	+	+	+	+	d	d	d	d	d	−	+	+	+	d
Growth at 65 °C	−	−	−	−	−	−	−	d[b]	−	−	−	−	−	−	−	+	w	+	−
Growth at pH 5.7	+	+	−	+	+	+	+	−	−	d	d	.	+	+	.	.	.	−	d
Growth in 7 % NaCl	+	d	+	+	+	+	+	−	+	−	−	d	−	−	−	−[c]	.[d]	−[c]	d[e]
Utilization of citrate	d	+	−	+	+	+	+	d	−	−	d	−	−	−	−	.	.	−	d
Anaerobic growth in glucose broth	+	+	−	+	−	−	−	+	+	+	−	d	+	+	+	−	−	+	−
Carbohydrates, acid from:																			
glucose	+	+	w	+[f]	+	+	+	+	+	+	d	+	+	+[f]	+[f]	+	+	+	−
arabinose	−	−	d	+	d	+	+	d	−	−	−	+	−	+	+	d	−	−	−
mannitol	−	−	+	+	d	+	+	d	−	−	d	+	+	+	+	d	+	−	−
xylose	−	−	d	+	d	+	+	d	−	−	−	+	−	+	+	d	+	−	−
VP test	+	+	−	+	−	+	+	d	−	+	−	−	+	−	+	−	−	−	−
Starch hydrolysis	+	+	+	+	+	−	+	+	+	+	−	+	−	+	+	−	−	+	−
Nitrate reduction	+	+	d	+	d	−	+[g]	d	d	−	d	d	+	+	+	+[h]	−	d	−
Indole	−	−	−	−	−	−	−	−	+	−	−	d	−	−	−	−	−	−	−
Gelatin hydrolysis	+	+	+	+	+	+	+	−	+	+	+	+	+	+	+	d	−	d	+
Casein hydrolysis	+	+	+	+	+	+	+	d	d	+	+	d	+	−	+	−	−	d	d
Urease	−	d	−	d	d	−	d	−	−	−	−	−	−	−	.	.	.	.	d
LV	+	+	−	−	−	+	−	−	−	−	−	−	+	−	−	.	.	d	.
Lysozyme sensitivity	r	r	s	d	s	d	d	s	s	r	d	d	r	s	d	.	.	s	d

1 Bacillus anthracis	**8 Bacillus coagulans**	**15 Bacillus polymyxa**
2 Bacillus cereus; *B. anthracoides*	**9 Bacillus pantothenticus**	**16 Bacillus sp. Wolf & Barker group I**
3 Bacillus firmus	**10 Bacillus alvei**	**17 Bacillus sp. Wolf & Barker group II**
4 Bacillus licheniformis	**11 Bacillus brevis**	**18 Bacillus stearothermophilus;** Wolf & Barker group III
5 Bacillus megaterium	**12 Bacillus circulans**	**19 Bacillus sphaericus**
6 Bacillus pumilus	**13 Bacillus laterosporus**	
7 Bacillus subtilis	**14 Bacillus macerans**	

[a] All species may produce non-motile variants.
[b] Some strains grow at 65 °C at pH 6.2 (Wolf & Barker).
[c] Negative in 3 % NaCl.
[d] Positive in 3 %; unknown 7 %.
[e] Positive in 5 %; unknown 7 %.
[f] Gas may be produced on suitable medium.
[g] Often negative in strains that have survived severe heating.
[h] Under anaerobic conditions reduced to nitrogen gas.
J positive in young cultures; inconstant in older cultures.

r resistant.
s sensitive.
T terminal spore.
U central spore.
V subterminal spore.
X spore oval.
Y spore round.

Other symbols used in the table are explained in Tables 5.1 and 5.2 (facing p. 43).

were (i) lysis by specific (gamma) bacteriophage, (ii) its failure to produce haemolysis on blood plates (*B. cereus* is haemolytic), and (iii) the production of mucoid colonies by virulent strains growing on bicarbonate agar in an atmosphere of CO_2 (avirulent strains and strains of *B. cereus* did not do so).

We do not show *Bacillus mycoides* in Table 6.9; in the characters listed it does not differ from *B. cereus* but examination of a colony on a plate would show clearly the main difference between them – the rhizoid nature of the *B. mycoides* colony. Dr Gordon tells us that *B. cereus* var. *mycoides* strains and their non-rhizoid variants are usually non-motile, and thus differ from *B. anthracis* only in pathogenicity.

We do not include in our table the insect pathogen *Bacillus thuringiensis* but we show *B. stearothermophilus*, a useful organism for checking the efficiency of hospital sterilizers. Wolf & Barker (1968) recognize three varieties (or possible species) of this thermophilic organism (or group of organisms), and recommend 55 °C as a suitable temperature for the biochemical tests; a water bath is preferable to an air incubator. We have not included the psychrophilic species (Larkin & Stokes, 1967) which, theoretically at least, might be met in sterility tests on stored blood.

The differences between *Bacillus subtilis* and *Bacillus licheniformis* do not appear great in Table 6.9, and in the first edition of their monograph Smith *et al.* (1946) did not recognize *B. licheniformis*. Gibson (1944) has pointed out that *B. licheniformis* colonies adhere to the medium and are difficult to pick off, and in our limited experience of this genus we have found that *B. licheniformis* spores are more heat resistant than those of *B. subtilis*. *B. licheniformis* is a facultative anaerobe and, in fact, was first described as an anaerobic species and named *Clostridium licheniforme*. Detectable gas may be produced by *Bacillus licheniformis*, *B. macerans*, and by *B. polymyxa* when grown under an oil seal in a glucose medium containing peptone and meat (or yeast) extract. Neotype strains of many *Bacillus* species were proposed by Smith *et al.* (1964), who hoped that this step would avoid the confusion that surrounded the correct identity of *Bacillus subtilis* for so many years (see,

for example, Conn, 1930; Soule, 1932) and had to be ended by the issue of Opinion A (1958).

The morphological groups in Table 6.9 are those of Smith *et al.* (1952), and are as follows:

Group 1   Spores oval or cylindrical; central, subterminal or terminal. Bacillary body only slightly swollen or not at all.

Group 2   Spores oval, rarely cylindrical; central, subterminal or terminal. Bacillary body definitely swollen.

Group 3   Spores spherical; terminal or subterminal. Bacillary body swollen.

Some atypical characters may be found; for example, three strains of *Bacillus stearothermophilus* we examined were catalase negative at the temperature (60 °C) at which we grew the cultures.

Minidefinition: *Bacillus. Rods typically Gram-positive in young cultures; motile (non-motile forms occur); not acid fast. Produce spores that are usually heat resistant. Aerobic; some species facultatively anaerobic. Catalase positive; oxidase variable. Species differ in the manner in which they attack sugars; some do not attack them.*

6.10   The acid-fast rods

(*Mycobacterium*, *Nocardia*, the rhodochrous group)

Characters common to members of the group: Gram-positive rods; non-motile. Acid fast. Aerobic. Attack sugars oxidatively.

The characteristic acid fastness of members of the group varies from the slight to the strong, from *Nocardia* to *Mycobacterium* with the rhodochrous group ('*Mycobacterium*' *rhodochrous*) between the two extremes. Like most intermediates, the rhodochrous group is more like one pole (in this case *Nocardia*) than the other. Nocardias are distinguished from streptomycetes by the *meso*-diaminopimelic acid contained in the cell walls and in cell extracts (Becker *et al.* 1964).

6.10.1   Nocardia (Table 6.10*a*). Although mainly soil organisms, nocardias are isolated occasionally in medical laboratories and are sometimes incrimi-

nated (with doubtful justification) as infecting agents. As a consequence we give them more than a passing mention but we give our attention only to those species that are regarded as potential pathogens. There will be a taxonomic revision of the group within the next decade and we do not intend to anticipate it. We have not worked with this group ourselves and we have obtained most of our facts from one reliable source, Dr Ruth E. Gordon; we have supplemented this from publications of other workers who have examined large numbers of strains and analysed their results by numerical methods (Tsukamura, 1969; Goodfellow, 1971). But wherever the facts came from, the opinions expressed are our own and we hope that they will not embarrass the original sources.

In general the nocardias are rather slow-growing organisms and accurate identifications may take months rather than days, but as the infections with which they may be associated are chronic, this delay will not be of much consequence.

A new genus, *Actinomadura*, has been proposed on chemotaxonomic grounds for the species *Nocardia madurae*; for all practical purposes the organism remains a nocardia and we show it as such in Table 6.10*a*; the characters in the table are from Gordon (1966*a*, *b*) and Goodfellow (1971). Another new genus, carved out of Nocardia on the basis of chemistry and motility, is *Oerskovia*, but its interest is more taxonomic than of concern to the diagnostician.

Gordon & Mihm (1957) and Gordon (1966*a*) provisionally designated the rhodochrous organism as a mycobacterium, but the mycobacteriologists do not seem eager to accept it (Kubica *et al.* 1972). Tsukamura (1971) created a new genus, *Gordona*, as an intermediate between *Nocardia* and *Mycobacterium* and included the rhodochrous group in it; Goodfellow, Fleming & Sackin (1972) were unable to accept *Gordona* as a new home for the problem species (in search of a genus) '*M.*' *rhodochrous*. Kanetsuna & Bartoli (1972) and Mordarska, Mordarski & Goodfellow (1972), using chemical methods for analysis of lipids, thought that the rhodochrous organisms should be classified as nocardias. Goodfellow (1971) had earlier divided the members of the rhodochrous group into eight subgroups and had speculated on the probability

Table 6.10*a Second-stage table for* Nocardia *and* 'Mycobacterium' rhodochrous

	1	2	3	4	5
Acid fast	d	d	d	–	d
Aerial hyphae	+	+	+	+	–
Carbohydrates, acid from:					
glucose	+	+	+	+	+
adonitol	–	–	–	+	.
arabinose	–	–	–	+	–
inositol	–	+	+	d	d
maltose	–	d	–	d	d
mannitol	–	+	+	+	d
rhamnose	d	–	–	+	–
sorbitol	–	–	–	–	d
xylose	–	–	–	+	d
ONPG[a]	+	+	+	d	–
Nitrate reduced	+	+	+	+	d
Decomposition of:					
casein	–	–	+	+	–
tyrosine	–	–	+	+	d
xanthine	–	+	–	–	–
urea	+	+	+	–	d

1 **Nocardia asteroides**
2 **Nocardia caviae**
3 **Nocardia brasiliensis**; *N. mexicana*; *N. pretoriana*
4 **Nocardia madurae**; *Actinomadura madurae*
5 **'Mycobacterium' rhodochrous**

[a] Tsukamura (1974).

Symbols used in the table are explained in Tables 5.1 and 5.2 (facing p. 43).

that the group will become a new genus. Our guess, inspired by experience that the creation of a new genus is the easy way out of this kind of difficulty, is that Goodfellow's forecast will prove correct. In this book for medical bacteriologists we confess that we do not regard this organism as important or its classification as a vital issue. On the other hand, we should be honest and admit that we like these taxonomic enigmata for they bear out our contention that bacteria cannot be arranged in neat genera, as if they were in pigeon-holes, but blend into each other and are akin to the bands of a spectrum.

Minidefinition: *Nocardia. Gram-positive rods and filaments which sometimes show branching. May be weakly acid fast. Non-motile (rare exceptions). Produce aerial hyphae. Aerobic. Catalase positive. Attack sugars by oxidation.*

6.10.2 Mycobacterium (Table 6.10*b*). The genus has been and continues to be the subject of intense studies by workers in various countries who have formed themselves into the International Working Group on Mycobacterial Taxonomy (IWGMT); members examine the same cultures by methods used in their different laboratories and eventually the group hopes to be able to advise on the most suitable tests and the best methods to use. Two reports have been published and others are awaited; this means that our table and characterizations should be regarded as provisional and likely to be changed when further reports of the co-operative studies are available. The two IWGMT reports (Wayne *et al.* 1971; Kubica *et al.* 1972) and Kubica's paper (1973) have been used freely in revising our diagnostic table for mycobacteria, but compression has been necessary; many of the characters used differ from those of the corresponding table of the first edition of this *Manual*, and for the methods the monograph by Kubica & Dye (1967) should be consulted. Kubica (1973) strongly recommends that in making an identification all the characters used in his diagnostic table should be determined by the approved methods. We have not given details of these methods in our Appendix C because we accept Kubica's contention that his methods should be followed in detail. An exception is made of the catalase test on which we rely so much in this *Manual* to make the primary sorting before going on to the second-stage tables; as carried out by our methods 1 and 2 the results are qualitative, but mycobacteriologists use (or prefer) a semiquantitative method that is pitched at a level that takes notice only of greater catalase activity. For example, our method 1 will show catalase activity by strains of *Mycobacterium tuberculosis*, but by the mycobacteriologist's rating this is too feeble to count and their diagnostic tables record the character as negative. To avoid confusion, we show the character as negative in Table 6.10*b*, but we have to specify method 3 and give details of that method in Section C3.9. The catalase of *M. tuberculosis* and *M. bovis* is heat labile, whereas that of other mycobacteria is stable at 68 °C for 20 minutes (Kubica & Pool, 1960).

During treatment and especially when it becomes isoniazid resistant, the infecting strain may become catalase negative by our method 1; Kubica & Silcox (1973) do not think that this causes difficulty or confuses the taxonomist. We follow our usual practice and do not record resistance to isoniazid or other drugs.

In the animal tissues mycobacteria at first occur alone, but later secondary infection with organisms of lower pathogenicity is liable to occur. The isolation of slowly growing mycobacteria from sputum and other material containing bacteria capable of rapid growth requires measures to kill, or at least inhibit multiplication of the quickly growing organisms. We make use of the greater resistance to chemical agents possessed by the mycobacteria and treat the material either with acid or alkali for 10 to 30 minutes, after which we adjust the reaction and inoculate the neutralized material on media suitable for the growth of mycobacteria. These media contain bacteriostatic dyes such as malachite green, or antibiotic(s) to inhibit growth of surviving non-mycobacterial organisms. Incubation will be prolonged (from 1 to 8 weeks) and the medium must not be allowed to dry.

We should warn the unwary that the identification of mycobacteria is specialist's work, but we can comfort him with the information that mycobacterial reference laboratories exist in many countries, and these are staffed by people willing and able to help.

Although mainly concerned with tubercle bacilli (*M. tuberculosis*, *M. bovis*, and *M. avium*), medical and veterinary bacteriologists also take an intelligent interest in other species that have been seen in or isolated from clinical material. *M. leprae* and *M. lepraemurium* will not grow on 'lifeless' media but may multiply after inoculation into the footpads of mice (Pattyn, 1965). The vole bacillus (*M. murium, M. microti*) does not appear in Table 6.10*b* as too little is known of its characters. Johne's bacillus (*M. johnei, M. enteritidis, M. paratuberculosis*) is also excluded; its isolation and propagation need special media containing killed acidfast bacilli or extracts from them (Taylor, 1950; Smith, 1953). Many of the slowly growing species are regarded as causal agents of some chronic infections, but fast-growing mycobacteria, for which 'too many species have been suggested' (Goodfellow *et al.* 1972), are regarded as non-pathogenic.

Table **6.10***b Second-stage table for* Mycobacterium

	1	2	3	4	5	6	7	8	9	10	11	12	13
Catalase (method 3: > 45 mm)	−	−	−	+	+	+	+	−	+	+	+	+	+
Pigment in light	−	−	−	+	−	−	−	+	−	−	−	−	−
Pigment in dark	−	−	−	−	+	−	−	−	−	+	−	+	−
Growth < 3 days	−	−	−	−	−	+	−	−	+	+	+	−	+
Growth at 25 °C	−	−	d	+	+	+	d	+	+	+	+	+	+
33 °C	+	.	+	+	+	+	+	+	+	+	+	+	+
37 °C	+	+	+	+	+^{a}	+	−	d	+	+	+	+^{b}	+
45 °C	−	−^{c}	d^d	−	−	−^{a}	−	−	−^{c}	+	+	−	d
52 °C	−	−	−	−	−	−	−	−	−	+	−	−	−
Growth on MacConkey	−	−	−	−	−	+	−	−	+	−	−	−	−
Growth on 5 % NaCl	−	−	−	−	−	+	.	−	D^e	+	+	−	−
Nitrate reduced	+	−	−	+	−	+	−	−	−	+	+	−	d
Urease	+	+	−	+	+	+	.	+	+	+	+	d	d
Tween hydrolysed	d	−	−	+	−	d	−	+	−	+	+	d	.
Niacin produced	+	−	−	−	−	−	+	−	−	−	−	−	−

1 **Mycobacterium tuberculosis;** human type of tubercle bacillus
2 **Mycobacterium bovis;** bovine type of tubercle bacillus
3 **Mycobacterium avium;** *M. intracellulare*; avian type of tubercle bacillus
4 **Mycobacterium kansasii**

5 **Mycobacterium scrofulaceum;** *M. marianum*
6 **Mycobacterium fortuitum;** *M. minettii*; *M. peregrinum*
7 **Mycobacterium ulcerans**
8 **Mycobacterium marinum;** *M. balnei*
9 **Mycobacterium chelonei;** *M. borstelensis*

10 **Mycobacterium phlei**
11 **Mycobacterium smegmatis**
12 **Mycobacterium gordonae;** *M. aquae*; tap-water scotochromogen
13 '**Mycobacterium**' **rhodochrous;** *Jensenia canicruria*; *Corynebacterium equi.*

^{a} Positive at 39 °C.
^{b} Negative at 39 °C.

^{c} Negative at 42 °C.
^{d} Positive at 42–43 °C.

^{e} *M. chelonei* divided into two varieties; one NaCl +, the other NaCl −.

Symbols used in the table are explained in Tables 5.1 and 5.2 (facing p. 43).

In the identification of mycobacteria we depend to a large extent on the acid fastness of the organisms; in tissues they stain well, but it has long been known that false positives may occur in stained smears and sections, and that the error can be introduced by acid-fast organisms in the staining reagents (see, for example, Keilty, 1917; Wilson, 1933; Carson, Kingsley, Haberman & Race, 1964). Some older textbooks gave the impression that a useful distinction could be made between bacilli that were acid fast and those that were acid and alcohol fast. This distinction cannot be substantiated in practice and many workers in the field use, as a decolorizing agent, a mixture of acid and alcohol as this gives the most reliable and consistent results. We use and recommend such a mixture, and consequently in Table 6.10*b* do not have a line for alcohol fastness.

In identifying the mycobacteria we make use of the temperatures at which the different species will grow. The tests involve the use of several water baths which may impose a strain on the resources of a routine laboratory that does not do much mycobacterial identification. We show the results to indicate how helpful these tests can be when the facilities are available. *Mycobacterium phlei* is unusual in being able to grow at 52 °C; *M. marinum* (*M. balnei*) in having a narrow temperature range for growth when first isolated, after it has been in subculture for some time it may be able to grow at 37 °C.

There are two geographical variants of *Mycobacterium chelonei* which show differences in ability to grow in 5 % NaCl and in utilizing citrate as C source (Stanford, Pattyn, Portaels & Gunthorpe, 1972).

We do not stress pigment formation which, in mycobacteria, may show great variability (Gordon

& Rynearson, 1963; Hauduroy, Hovanessian & Roussianos, 1965). Other characters, not shown in our table, may be important; these include colonial consistency, emulsifiability and texture; bacillary length, 'cord' formation (tendency to parallel alignment) and other manifestations of virulence (Middlebrook, Dubos & Pierce, 1947), and, of course, virulence for laboratory animals (especially rabbits) and birds.

> **Minidefinition:** *Mycobacterium. Non-motile Gram-positive rods that do not branch. Typically acid fast. Non-sporing, and do not produce aerial hyphae. Aerobic. Catalase positive* (method 1) *or variable* (method 3). *Attack sugars by oxidation.*

6.11 Source material for the tables

For the compilation of the tables many sources were consulted; all started with the corresponding table in the first edition of this *Manual* for those tables were based on results obtained in the National Collection of Type Cultures between 1947 and 1963. For the present edition additional information was obtained from correspondents who wrote about particular points in the earlier tables, from colleagues who let us use their (sometimes unpublished) results, and from published papers and monographs. These papers are referred to in the text of this chapter; sources not referred to in the text are given in Table 6.11. We were also helped and encouraged by many personal communications on the organisms dealt with in this chapter, and we are especially grateful to A. C. Baird-Parker, G. Colman, R. H. Deibel, the late T. Gibson, R. E. Gordon, G. Kubica, and R. E. O. Williams.

The reports of international working groups have been particularly useful for in many instances the groups have dealt with conflicting results obtained by different techniques. Where such groups have

Table 6.11 *Additional sources consulted for Tables* 6.1 *to* 6.10

Author(s)	Table
Bojalil *et al.* (1962)	6.10
Colman (1968)	6.3
Colman & Williams (1967)	6.3
Deibel *et al.* (1963, 1964)	6.3
Dunkelberg & McVeigh (1969)	6.5
Engbaek *et al.* (1971)	6.10
Gasser (1970)	6.6
Gasser *et al.* (1970)	6.6
Georg *et al.* (1965)	6.7
Gordon *et al.* (1973)	6.9
Gordon & Mihm (1959, 1961, 1962)	6.10
Gordon & Smith (1953, 1955)	6.10
Hansen (1968)	6.6
Holmberg & Hallander (1973)	6.7
Howell & Jordan (1963)	6.7
Howell *et al.* (1959)	6.7
Julianelle (1941)	6.5
Karlson & Lessel (1970)	6.10
Mirick *et al.* (1944)	6.3
Moore *et al.* (1966)	6.8
Nowlan & Deibel (1967)	6.3
Pine (1970)	6.7
Pine *et al.* (1960)	6.7
Reed & Orr (1941)	6.8
Roberts (1968)	6.5
Rogosa (1970)	6.6
Rogosa & Hansen (1971)	6.6
Slack *et al.* (1969)	6.7
Stanford & Beck (1969)	6.10
Street & Goldner (1973)	6.3
Stuart (1970)	6.5
Topley & Wilson's Principles of Bacteriology and Immunity	6.5
Walker & Wolf (1971)	6.9
Wayne *et al.* (1971)	6.10
Welshimer & Meredith (1971)	6.5
Wetzler *et al.* (1968)	6.5
Williams, R. A. D. & Bowden (1968)	6.3
Williams, R. E. O. (1956)	6.3
Wolf & Chowdhury (1971)	6.9

reported, their conclusions have been followed in principle; where such guidance was not available we have exercised our own judgement in assessing the relative merits of conflicting results and views.

7
Characters of Gram-negative bacteria

The Gram reaction is not ideal for making a major subdivision of bacteria but it is convenient because everyone uses Gram's method of staining (in one of its many modifications) when characterizing a bacterium. There is an unfortunate tendency to omit this step, especially when dealing with cultures isolated on selective media, for an old wives' tale has it that the staining reactions are upset by the selective or inhibitory substances included in the medium; the assumption is that colonies on selective media have the appropriate (or expected) tinctorial and shapely qualities. We must all have seen or read papers by water bacteriologists in which are described the characters of so many thousand strains of Gram-negative bacilli, and we know from observing them at work that water bacteriologists seldom use a microscope. Their work is accepted and acceptable because it is primarily concerned with pollution and the potability of water supplies, and statements about the characters of organisms are, in the words of W. S. Gilbert, 'merely corroborative detail, intended to give artistic verisimilitude to an otherwise bald and unconvincing narrative'. As diagnosticians, our objectives are not artistic and we want to know what our organisms are; we need accurate characterizations and we cannot afford to omit making smears and staining them by Gram's method, even if we do not pursue our microscopy any further.

7.1   Division into major groups
Our first steps into the world of the Gram-negative bacteria must take notice of those organisms that seem to be on the borderline between the Gram positives and the Gram negatives. We shall meet *Gemella*, a genus which until recently was thought to be made up of Gram-negative cocci; we shall find other bacteria that show an unusual phenomenon in that they develop some Gram positivity as cultures age, in contrast to the Gram-positive bacteria, which become Gram negative as the cells age and degenerate.

7.2   The Gram-negative anaerobes
(*Bacteroides*, *Veillonella*)
Characters common to members of the group: **Gram-negative bacteria; do not form spores. Strictly anaerobic.**

In this *Manual* all Gram-negative, non-spore-forming, anaerobic rods are collected into one genus, *Bacteroides* and all the Gram-negative anaerobic cocci into *Veillonella*. The label Bacteroides means different things to different men, and Holdeman & Moore (1972) warn that the genus *Bacteroides* of Beerens & Tahon-Castel (1965) is not the genus *Bacteroides* recognized in the VPI Anaerobe Laboratory. And this is not the end of the differences, which extend to approaches to classification and details of characterization of the organisms. The classification of these anaerobic rods has been made on two (not exclusive) criteria: (i) morphological, paying particular attention to the ends of the rods (pointed ends = Fusiformis, Fusobacterium; rounded ends = Bacteroides), or (ii) fermentation products (butyric acid = Fusobacterium; do not produce butyric acid = Bacteroides). From this it follows that different names do not necessarily indicate different organisms, or the same name refer to the same organism.

As with all anaerobes, the techniques used in different laboratories are likely to produce different descriptions (see *Veillonella*, Section 7.2.2). If we compare the tables of diagnostic characters given in the *Anaerobe Laboratory Manual* (ALM, 1972) and by Willis (1964), and bear in mind that

Table 7.1 *First-stage table for Gram-negative bacteria*

	1	2	3	4	5	6	7	8	9	10	11	12	13	14	15	16	17	18
Shape	R	S	S	S	S/R	R	R	R	R	R	R	R	R	R	R	R	R	R
Motility	−	−	−	−	−	−	+	+	−	+	−	−	+	D	−	−	+	−
Growth in air	−	−	+	+	+	+	+	+	+	+	+	+	+	+	+	−*	−†	+
Growth anaerobically	+	+	−	−	−	−	−	−	−	+	+	+	+	+	+	+	−	+
Catalase	d	D	+	+	+	+	+	+	+	+	+	−	+	+	D	−	D	−
Oxidase	−	×	+	+	−	+	+	+	+	+	+	+	+	−	−	+	+	−
Glucose (acid)	D	−	+	−	+	−	+	−	+	+	+	+	+	+	D	−	−	+
Carbohydrates [F/O/−]	F/−	−	O	−	O	−	O	−	O	O	F	F	F	F	NT	−	−	F

Bacteroides   7.2

Veillonella

Neisseria

Branhamella   7.3

Acinetobacter

Moraxella

Brucella   7.4

Bordetella

Chromobacterium lividum   7.5

Alcaligenes

Flavobacterium   7.6

Pseudomonas

Actinobacillus

Pasteurella   7.7

Necromonas

Cardiobacterium

Chromobacterium violaceum

Beneckea

Vibrio   7.8

Plesiomonas

Aeromonas

Enterobacteria   7.9

Haemophilus

Eikenella

Campylobacter

Streptobacillus‡   7.10

Mycoplasms

*   No growth in air; growth in air+CO_2.

†   No growth in air or anaerobically; growth in 5–6% O_2.

‡   Also *Shigella dysenteriae* 1 (Shiga's bacillus).

▓   Typical form

×   Not known.

⌐ ¬ Cultural characters of these organisms can be found in tables with the number indicated.

NT Not testable by usual methods. Fermentative (Sneath & Johnson, 1973).

Symbols used in the table are explained in Tables 5.1 and 5.2 (facing p. 43).

Bacteroides in ALM generally equals Fusiformis in Willis, the only descriptions that agree reasonably well are those for *Bacteroides melaninogenicus* and *Fusiformis melaninogenicus*, organisms easily recognized by the black pigment produced. On the other hand, *Fusobacterium necrophorum* in ALM is an asaccharolytic organism, variable in gelatin liquefaction; in Willis the organism with a similar name, *Fusiformis necrophorus*, is saccharolytic but non-liquefying. It seems to us that it is necessary to accept *in toto* the descriptions and classification of a particular school and to work in splendid isolation from the rest of the anaerobic world. We do not have much regard for any of the classifications of the Gram-negative anaerobes we have seen, but we prefer the simple approach in which all the rods are placed in one genus and the cocci in another. The conflicting characterizations given by different authors make the construction of a useful diagnostic table well-nigh impossible, and since we do not think that much progress has been made in the last ten years in the descriptions of these anaerobes, we repeat with only slight modifications the diagnostic table of *Bacteroides* from our first edition, based as it was on the works of Prévot (1961), Willis (1964), and our colleague, Miss H. E. Ross. The organism named *Bacteroides corrodens* by Eiken (1958) will be found in Section 7.10.2 under the name *Eikenella corrodens*.

Readers are referred to the *Anaerobe Laboratory Manual* (1972) for details of techniques developed at the Virginia Polytechnic Institute, where workers have made a determined effort to overcome the manipulative problems associated with the growth and subculture of strict anaerobes, and with the tests needed for their characterization. New characterizations based on the results of applying these methods will be found in ALM.

Collee & Watt (1972) are encouraging: they note that Bacteroides–Fusiformis organisms will tolerate transient manipulation under the relatively aerobic conditions of working at the bench; that CO_2 has such a marked effect on their growth that it should be included as part of the standard procedure for isolating and maintaining the non-sporing anaerobes. On a more pessimistic note they conclude that on first isolation members of this group can only be reported as GNABs (Gram-

negative anaerobic bacteria) because identification – if possible at all – will take a long time.

7.2.1   Bacteroides (Table 7.2). We show the characters of four anaerobic species in our table and also show a species that was thought to be an anaerobe (Eiken, 1958) and indeed may be on first isolation, but it will grow in air supplemented with CO_2; this organism has been moved to a new genus *Eikenella* (Jackson & Goodman, 1972).

Table 7.2 *Second-stage table for* Bacteroides *and* Veillonella

	1	2	3	4	5	6
Shape	R	R	R	R	R	S
Motility	−	−	−	+	−	−
Growth in air + CO_2	−	−	−	−	+	−
Catalase	d	d	−	−	−	D
Oxidase	−	−	−	−	+	.
Black pigment	−	−	+	−	−	−
Haemolysis	+	−	+	−	−	−
Carbohydrates, acid from:						
glucose	+	+	+[a]	+	−	−[b]
lactose	d	−	+	+	−	−
maltose	+	−	+	+	−	−
mannitol	d	−	+	−	−	−
sucrose	+	+	+	−	−	−
Indole	+	−	+	−	−	−
Gelatin liquefaction	−	−	d	(+)	−	−
H_2S	d	−	+	−	−	−

1 **Bacteroides necrophorus**
2 **Bacteroides fragilis**
3 **Bacteroides melaninogenicus**
4 **Bacteroides serpens**
5 **Eikenella corrodens**; *Bacteroides corrodens*
6 **Veillonella** spp.

[a] Acid may be produced from the basal medium (Willis, 1964).
[b] May be positive in some media.

Symbols used in the table are explained in Tables 5.1 and 5.2 (facing p. 43).

The production of catalase, on which our scheme of identification depends so much, is usually given as negative for these anaerobic bacteria, and such a character would fit our scheme very well. Unfortunately, bacteroides are no more accommodating than P. R. Edwards' traditional salmonellas and, like them, have not read their literature. Beveridge (1934) found that *Bacteroides necrophorus* was catalase positive, and Miss Ross found *B. fragilis* also positive; we record the catalase reactions of these species as 'd' to indicate that some strains may vary in their ability to produce the enzyme. Once again we draw attention to the differences in characterization shown in our table and in those of ALM; we do not attempt to point out any synonymy.

Minidefinition: *Bacteroides. Gram-negative rods; non-sporing. Usually non-motile. Anaerobic. Attack sugars fermentatively.*

7.2.2   Veillonella (Table 7.2) is a group of Gram-negative anaerobic cocci; for a general discussion on anaerobic cocci the reader is referred to Hare *et al.* (1952) and Thomas & Hare (1954). In spite of a good deal of work by Prévot the systematics of these bacteria have not been worked out satisfactorily. Two technical difficulties seem to stultify progress; the first concerns the purity of cultures; either these organisms mutate with great rapidity or, more likely, they exist mostly as mixed cultures, perhaps growing synergistically. The second difficulty in working with these organisms is that they tend to die out quickly in artificial culture; possibly they are intolerant of air for they do not seem to survive being left on the bench for more than a few minutes. It is for organisms such as these that the VPI Anaerobe Laboratory has worked out elaborate techniques to maintain the reduced state of media by flushing tubes and areas with oxygen-free gases.

As with *Bacteroides*, the characters ascribed to *Veillonella* species by different authors are conflicting (cf. the descriptions of *Veillonella parvula* in *Bergey's Manual* (1957) with that in the VPI *Anaerobe Laboratory Manual* (1972)); the contrasting characters may be due to different media or anaerobic methods, but it hardly seems possible that the authors in the two manuals are describing the same species. Pelczar in *Bergey's Manual* describes six species, the ALM – whose editors are not noted for a lumping policy – describe only two species, and these differ only in their ability to produce catalase (*V. parvula* is negative and *V. alcalescens* is positive). Conflicts such as these make life difficult for the identifier and for the compiler of diagnostic tables. Characteristics that

are agreed are few and are given in the minidefinition below.

Minidefinition: *Veillonella. Gram-negative cocci; non-motile. Anaerobic.*

7.3   The Gram-negative cocci
(*Neisseria, Branhamella, Veillonella*)
Characters common to members of the group: Gram-negative cocci or coccobacilli. Non-motile.

Although one species of *Neisseria* elongates under the influence of penicillin, other members of the genus and those of *Branhamella* (which might be described as ex-*Neisseria*), and *Veillonella* (a genus of anaerobes) are all Gram-negative cocci and share that morphological characteristic with the coccal forms of *Acinetobacter*. To American bacteriologists acinetobacters started life as mimeas, a group of ill-described Gram-negative cocci that could be confused with gonococci. The morphological resemblance is a real one, especially in direct smears from clinical specimens, but in culture the acinetobacters soon become slightly elongated and coccobacillary; finally, they assume a true rod-like form. Clinical bacteriologists meet and see the coccal form of acinetobacters and we think it will be helpful to have the characters included in a table of the neisserias and branhamellas; systematically their proper place is undoubtedly with the Gram-negative rods and we shall show them again in Table 7.4*a*.

At the generic level veillonellas are not an identification problem; by their strictly anaerobic habit they are readily distinguished from neisserias, branhamellas, and acinetobacters, all of which are fairly exacting aerobes. Although not really a member of the group, *Gemella haemolysans* was first described as a neisseria and as it usually appears to be Gram negative, it is shown in Table 7.3 for comparison with *Neisseria* species. It is an organism with a poor-quality Gram-positive coat, and its rightful place is in Chapter 6 (see Section 6.3.4).

7.3.1   Neisseria (Table 7.3). In this genus there has been a proliferation of species and, when the unsatisfactory responses to biochemical tests are taken into account, this seems to be unwarranted. In the opposite direction molecular biological and

Table 7.3 *Second-stage table for* Neisseria, Branhamella, Veillonella, Gemella *and* Acinetobacter anitratus

	1	2	3	4	5	6	7	8	9	10	11	12	13
Gram reaction	−	−	−	−	−	−	−	−	−	−	±^a	−	−
Growth under anaerobic conditions	−	−	−	−	−	−	−	−	−	−	w	+	−
Catalase	+	+	+	+	+	+	w	+	+	+	−	D	+
Oxidase	+	+	+	+	+	+	+	+	+	+	−	.	−
Carbohydrate breakdown [F/O/−]	O	O	?	O	O	.	−	−	−	−	F	−	O
Pigment	−	−	+	+	−	−	−	−	+	−	−	−	−
Haemolysis	−	−	−	−	−	−	−	−	α	β	β	−	−/β
Growth at 22 °C	−	−	+	+	+	(+)	+	w	w	w	+	w	+
Growth on nutrient agar	−	−	+	+	+	+	+	+	+	+	w	+	+
Requirement for blood or serum	+	+	−	−	−	−	−	−	−	−	−	−	−
Carbohydrates, acid from:													
glucose	+	+	−^b	+	+	d	−	−	−	−	+	−^c	+
lactose	−	−	−	−	(+)	−	−	−	−	−	−	.	+
maltose	−	+	−^b	+	−	−	−	−	−	−	+	.	d
sucrose	−	−	−^b	d	−	(+)	−	−	−	−	+	.	−
Nitrates reduced	−	−	−	−	+	+	−	d	+	+	−	+	−

1 **Neisseria gonorrhoeae**; gonococcus
2 **Neisseria meningitidis**;
 N. intracellularis; meningococcus
3 **Neisseria flavescens**
4 **Neisseria pharyngis**; *N. flava*;
 N. perflava; *N. subflava*; *N. sicca*

5 **Neisseria mucosa**; *Diplococcus mucosus*
6 **Neisseria animalis**
7 **Neisseria elongata**
8 **Branhamella catarrhalis**;
 Neisseria catarrhalis

9 **Branhamella caviae**; *Neisseria caviae*
10 **Branhamella ovis**; *Neisseria ovis*
11 **Gemella haemolysans**; *Neisseria haemolysans*
12 **Veillonella** spp.
13 **Acinetobacter anitratus**

^a Gram positive but easily decolorized.

^b Negative on isolation; after some time in artificial cultivation may be positive.

^c May be positive in some media.

Symbols used in the table are explained in Tables 5.1 and 5.2 (facing p. 43).

genetical techniques show the heterogeneous nature of the constituent species of *Neisseria*, and indicate that the genus as circumscribed in the late 1960s needs revision (Kingsbury, 1967; Henriksen & Bøvre, 1968b; Baumann, Doudoroff & Stanier, 1968a; Kingsbury, Fanning, Johnson & Brenner, 1969; Bøvre, Fiandt & Szybalski, 1969). There has been a sloughing of species. Catlin (1970) proposed that *Neisseria catarrhalis* should form the type of a new genus, *Branhamella*, and she thought that other species might follow; we agree, and show in the new genus two other species, *N. caviae* and *N. ovis* which, by gas–liquid chromatography, form a homogeneous group with *Branhamella catarrhalis* (Lambert, Hollis, Moss, Weaver & Thomas, 1971).

Neisseria flavescens, a species that caused a limited epidemic of meningitis in Chicago (Bran-

ham, 1930), has not with certainty been isolated since (personal communication from the late Dr Sara Branham), though Prentice (1957) thought that the organism he isolated from a patient with meningitis might be *N. flavescens*. At first none of the strains isolated in Chicago attacked any sugars but after many years in artificial culture our strains (originally received from Dr Branham) and those kept by Dr Branham herself, developed the ability to produce acid from glucose, maltose, and sucrose. We include *N. flavescens* in Table 7.3 and show its original characters in the hope that someone will isolate it again and recognize it. The exclusion of *N. catarrhalis*, *N. caviae*, and *N. ovis* from *Neisseria* leaves us with a genus (excluding *N. elongata* which is based on one strain) made up of bacteria that attack carbohydrate by oxidation; as usually described *N. flavescens* is said not to attack carbohydrates but, in view of the experience of Dr Branham and ourselves, the truth of this statement seems doubtful, though the ability may be masked on first isolation. In the minidefinition below we shall deliberately omit mention of species that do not attack any sugars.

Several different organisms have been described under the name of *Neisseria mucosa* but none fits exactly the earlier description of *Diplococcus mucosus* by von Lingelsheim (1906, 1908). The characters shown in Table 7.3 are mainly from Cowan (1938a) and are based on strains isolated post-operatively from the cerebro-spinal fluids of two patients with cerebral tumours; we repeat the characterization with some hesitation as the original strains were lost and similar organisms do not seem to have been isolated again.

Neisserias grow better on the surface of a solid medium than in an equivalent liquid medium; most strains grow better in an atmosphere with increased CO_2; it is doubtful if any will grow under strictly anaerobic conditions. They are not organisms easy to characterize for freshly isolated strains grow feebly in artificial culture. Some species are described as Gram variable or are said to resist decolorization; this may seem to be a difference due to technical variation in different laboratories, but it is reported so frequently that notice should be taken of it. Henriksen & Bøvre (1968b) describe the tendency to resist decolorization as a characteristic of the family Neisseriaceae which, in their view at that time, comprised the genera *Neisseria* and *Moraxella*. Bacillary forms may occur in *N. elongata* (Bøvre & Holten, 1970) and, judged by the G+C content of DNA and the results of transformation experiments, the generic allocation seems to be correct. The neisserian pathogens grow feebly or not at all in media prepared for the usual biochemical characterizing tests, and they seem to be worthy candidates for the rapid single-substrate tests in which multiplication of the organism is not essential, the reaction being between preformed enzymes and the substrate without interference from metabolic by-products. But, to our knowledge, no one has applied these methods to the characterization of gonococci and meningococci.

It is often impossible to decide, on purely laboratory information, whether the organism isolated is a gonococcus or a meningococcus; the sugar reactions of these organisms are quite unreliable and, although most meningococci will produce acid from both glucose and maltose, some undoubted meningococci may attack glucose only and, occasionally, neither sugar (Arkwright, 1909). Neisserias normally do not produce acid from lactose, but Mitchell, Rhoden & King (1965) reported that they had collected thirty-five lactose-positive strains of meningococcus-like bacteria over a period of fifteen years. Hollis, Wiggins & Weaver (1969) named these organisms *Neisseria lactamicus*, but as they showed fermentation in oxidation-fermentation media they must be excluded from *Neisseria* as defined in this *Manual*, namely, as an oxidative bacterium.

Bøvre & Holten (1970) argue that the definition of the genus *Neisseria* should be amended to allow the inclusion of rod-shaped organisms. We resist this suggestion because we regard neisserias as basically coccal organisms; at the same time we admit the ability of all cocci to elongate under adverse conditions. It should be noted that spheres and short rods are the normal forms of *N. elongata*, and that long filaments appear only under the influence of penicillin.

The species *Neisseria animalis* (Berger, 1960b), *N. caviae* (Pelczar, 1953) – as *Branhamella caviae*, and *N. ovis* (Lindqvist, 1960) – as *Branhamella ovis*, are shown in Table 7.3; the characters recorded are mostly from the papers of the original authors. In Table 7.3 we also show the classical nasopharyngeal commensals, *N. flava*, *N. perflava*, *N. subflava*, and *N. sicca*, collected in the umbrella species *Neisseria pharyngis* (Wilson & Smith, 1928; Warner, Faber & Pelczar, 1952) as there seems little to be gained from maintaining their independent status.

Minidefinition: *Neisseria. Gram-negative spheres. Aerobic; carboxyphilic. Catalase positive; oxidase positive. Attack sugars by oxidation.*

7.3.2 Branhamella (Table 7.3) is a genus that was created on the basis of one set of characters but, because these were of the research laboratory kind, it is recognized in day-to-day work on the basis of different characters. The genus was split from

Neisseria by removing species that were distinguished from neisseria (*sensu stricto*) by differences in the base composition of the DNA; in *Branhamella* the G + C mole per cent varies between 40 and 44, and in *Neisseria* this is about 50; the two genera also differ in the fatty acid composition of the bacterial cells (Catlin, 1970). Unfortunately these characteristics are not among those on which differentiations are made in clinical laboratories, but as will be seen from Table 7.3, the distinction between the genera can be made on tests that are part of the normal routine.

Catlin transferred one species, *Neisseria catarrhalis*, to the new genus, but indicated that she thought others should also be moved to it. Several workers showed that *N. caviae* and *N. ovis*, like *N. catarrhalis*, were out-of-place in the genus *Neisseria* (for references see Section 7.3.1); as they have physiological characters in common and show mutual transformations with *B. catarrhalis* (Bøvre et al. 1969) we show these two species in Table 7.3 as *Branhamella caviae* and *B. ovis*.

Like neisserias, but possibly to a greater degree, the bacterial cells of the branhamellas tend to resist decolorization when Gram's method of staining is applied to them. *Gemella*, a Gram-positive coccus that shows the opposite characteristic (a Gram-positive organism that is easily overdecolorized), is shown in Table 7.3 so that its characters can be compared with those of *Branhamella* and *Neisseria* species.

Of the usual characterizing tests we recommend particularly tests for the reduction of nitrate, and the production of acid from carbohydrates. In the species so far translated to *Branhamella*, the first of these tests is positive and the second negative; among the species left in *Neisseria* (excluding *N. elongata*, which has yet to justify its place there), most fail to reduce nitrate and all attack carbohydrate(s) (but see Arkwright, 1909, and Section 7.3.1).

Minidefinition: *Branhamella. Spheres; Gram-negative but may resist decolorization. Aerobic. Catalase positive; oxidase positive. Do not produce acid from carbohydrates. Reduce nitrate to nitrite.*

7.3.3 **Acinetobacter** is a genus in which we now recognize two species, in contrast to the seventeen listed by Prévot (1961). These two species have a coccal or coccobacillary morphology, and in smears may show a superficial resemblance to the gonococcus or meningococcus. In a series of papers De Bord (1939, 1942, 1943, 1948) emphasized this morphological similarity but confused the picture by giving brief (and inadequate) descriptions of several different organisms, including two new species of *Neisseria*, and he placed all except his two new neisserias into a new tribe which he named Mimeae. The species that most mimicked the gonococcus is now known as *Acinetobacter anitratus* or *A. calcoaceticus*, and this species is show in Table 7.3 for comparison with *Neisseria gonorrhoeae* and *N. meningitidis*.

The acinetobacters have much in common with the moraxellas and there have been suggestions that the two genera should be united; both genera will be described in greater detail in Table 7.4.

Minidefinition: *Acinetobacter. Non-motile, Gram-negative rods. Aerobic. Catalase positive; oxidase negative. Attack sugars by oxidation or not at all. Do not produce pigment. Arginine test negative.*

7.3.4 **Gemella**, an organism that is easily decolorized and usually appears to be Gram negative (as it was first described). In cell structure and mode of division it resembles the Gram-positive bacteria (Reyn, 1970) and in its cultural characters it seems to be close to the streptococci. We describe this organism in Table 6.3*a*, *c* and Section 6.3.4 with the Gram-positive cocci, but because of the ease with which it is decolorized, we also show it with the Gram-negative cocci in Table 7.3.

Minidefinition: *Gemella. Gram-positive cocci (but easily decolorized). Aerobic; facultatively anaerobic. Catalase negative; oxidase negative. Attack sugars by fermentation; do not produce gas.*

7.3.5 **Veillonella** is shown in Table 7.3 for comparison with *Neisseria* and *Branhamella*, and by including it there we show some characters of all the Gram-negative cocci in one table. Veillonellas are organisms of uncertain characterization (see Section

7.2.2) but are easily distinguished from the neisserias and branhamellas by their strictly anaerobic requirements.

> **Minidefinition:** *Veillonella. Gram-negative cocci; non-motile. Anaerobic.*

7.4   The Moraxella–Acinetobacter group
(*Moraxella, Acinetobacter, Achromobacter, Brucella, Bordetella*)
Characters common to members of the group: **Gram-negative coccobacilli or short rods. Strictly aerobic. Catalase positive. Do not ferment carbohydrates.**

There have been suggestions that the genera *Moraxella* and *Acinetobacter* should be combined, and it is true that they have much in common. Indeed, species have been translated from one genus to the other (e.g. *Moraxella lwoffii →Acinetobacter lwoffii*) and confusion has arisen because a species and its 'variety' were equated with species in different genera (*Mima polymorpha = Acinetobacter lwoffii* and *Mima polymorpha* var. *oxydans = Moraxella nonliquefaciens*). Both *Moraxella* and *Acinetobacter* were created for species thrown out of other genera but like unwanted children placed in better surroundings, both have flourished and proved themselves to be good and useful taxa. *Moraxella* took care of organisms that had been wrongly placed (because they were not haemophilic) in the genus *Haemophilus*; the genus *Acinetobacter* was made for non-motile members of *Achromobacter*, itself an unsatisfactory collection of non-pigmented Gram-negative rods. A note on Achromobacter appears in Section 7.4.3.

7.4.1   Moraxella (Table 7.4) was created by Lwoff (1939) for non-haemophilic bacteria that had previously been placed in *Haemophilus*; these bacteria did not need X and/or V factor(s), and did not attack carbohydrates. Most of the organisms placed by Lwoff in the genus had been isolated from the conjunctiva, but other workers added strains from other sources (*M. lwoffii* from soil) and also strains that attacked carbohydrates (*M. lwoffii* var. *glucidolytica*); the last organism was later shown to be *Bacterium anitratum* (Brisou & Morichau-Beauchant, 1952). Brisou (1953), Floch (1953) and others excluded *M. lwoffii* and the sugar-attacking

species from *Moraxella*; Henriksen (1960) also excluded *M. lwoffii* and restricted the genus to oxidase-positive organisms. The debate about what should be included and what excluded from the genus was prolonged (it may not have ended) and complicated, but most workers (see Baumann *et al.* 1968a; Henriksen & Bøvre, 1968b; Samuels *et al.* 1972; Lautrop in *Bergey's Manual*, 1974) agree that only oxidase-positive, non-saccharolytic organisms should go into *Moraxella*.

An organism resembling *Moraxella lacunata* may be isolated from the conjunctiva of guinea-pigs (Ryan, 1964), and *Moraxella bovis* causes pink eye in cattle. Scandinavian workers report that *Moraxella bovis* is unable to reduce nitrates and that the catalase test is positive; in the USA, Pugh, Hughes & McDonald (1966) found that all their strains reduced nitrates but were catalase negative; because of these discrepancies (and the possibility that we are dealing with an example of 'geographical races') these characters are shown as 'd' in Table 7.4a.

Moraxella osloensis (Bøvre & Henriksen, 1967a) might be difficult to distinguish from *Moraxella nonliquefaciens*; a relative insensitivity to penicillin (Baumann *et al.* 1968a) was thought to help but Gilardi (1972a) found that his strains were sensitive. *Moraxella phenylpyruvica* (Bøvre & Henriksen, 1967b) is distinguished by its unique deamination of phenylalanine and tryptophan when suitable methods are used; the Clarke & Shaw test (Section C3.41) is insufficiently sensitive and Snell & Davey (1971) recommend the Goldin & Glenn method (1962).

Of two organisms provisionally placed in the genus and labelled 'Moraxella', one, '*M.*' *urethralis* (Lautrop, Bøvre & Frederiksen, 1970), is said to resemble *M. osloensis*; the other, '*M.*' *kingii* (Henriksen & Bøvre, 1968a), is saccharolytic on media enriched with ascitic fluid, and probably should be excluded.

The proposal by Henriksen & Bøvre (1968b) to include the so-called 'false neisserias' (*Neisseria catarrhalis, N. ovis,* and *N. caviae*) in the genus *Moraxella* has not been followed in this *Manual*; *N. catarrhalis* will be found in *Branhamella* (Section 7.3.2).

Cultures of *Moraxella* species are sensitive to

drying and some strains will not grow at 37 °C unless they are in a moist atmosphere; they grow best when plates are put in a closed jar (Henriksen, 1952).

Minidefinition: *Moraxella. Gram-negative rods; non-motile. Aerobic. Catalase positive; oxidase positive. Sugars not attacked. Growth improved by the addition of blood or serum but specific growth factors are not known.*

7.4.2   Acinetobacter (Tables 7.3, 7.4*a*). A genus proposed by Brisou & Prévot (1954) for non-motile species that, apart from their lack of motility, would have fitted into *Achromobacter* as that genus was defined at that time; they included in it, as *Acinetobacter anitratum* (sic), two species, *Bacterium anitratum* (Schaub & Hauber, 1948) and *Moraxella lwoffii* var. *glucidolytica*, which had previously been shown to be identical (Brisou & Morichau-Beauchant, 1952). In 1961 Prévot listed seventeen species in the genus, but as a taxonomic entity *Acinetobacter* had a chequered career, with much debate about the species to be included, and whether it should be a separate genus or included in *Moraxella*. The first good descriptions of organisms in the taxon were published by Schaub & Hauber (1948) for *Bacterium anitratum* and by Stuart, Formal & McGann (1949) for the B5W group. Ewing (1949*a*) recognized that these organisms bore some resemblance to a poorly described tribe Mimeae with genera *Mima*, *Herellea*, and *Colloides* (De Bord, 1939, 1942, 1943, 1948), some strains of which simulated gonococci. Henriksen (1963) and Pickett & Manclark (1965) showed that these names were being misapplied and that because the original descriptions had been vague and ambiguous, bacteriologists and their literature were becoming confused.

We (Steel & Cowan, 1964) put a finger in this stew-pot and stirred it by modifying the definition of the genus to allow inclusion of bacteria that did not produce acid from carbohydrates; this was an improvement and allowed the inclusion of *Moraxella lwoffii*, an organism that was misplaced in *Moraxella*. But we were imprudent, and in our paper suggested the translation to *Acinetobacter* of the glanders bacillus, which has since found a better resting place in another genus (*Pseudomonas*).

After considerable bibliographical research, which must have taken almost as long as their bench work, Baumann, Doudoroff & Stanier (1968*b*) unearthed an organism labelled *Micrococcus calcoaceticus* which had the characteristics of *Acinetobacter anitratus*, and thus inflicted yet another name on long-suffering bacteriologists. Because it is the oldest, *calcoaceticus* becomes the nomenclaturally correct specific epithet and produces a combination that is a labial exercise, *Acinetobacter calcoaceticus*. However, we continue to think and write about the species under its better known name, *Acinetobacter anitratus*, and shall resist this example of logomachy.

Thornley (1967) added to the genus strains (isolated from poultry carcases) that grew at 0 °C but not at 37 °C, and as many of them were oxidase positive she amended the definition of the genus. But Samuels and her colleagues (1972), working in a medically oriented laboratory where cultures are presumably not incubated as a routine at 0 °C, found the 'inclusion of oxidase-positive organisms in the genus *Acinetobacter* … unacceptable' and with this statement we agree, even though our reasons for doing so may not be as (taxonomically) pure.

One of the characteristics of *Acinetobacter anitratus* is its ability to attack monosaccharides but not higher saccharides in peptone water sugars. When the sugar concentration is raised to 5 or 10 % the organism can attack lactose. The oxidative production of acid from several carbohydrates in complex media is the work of a non-specific aldose dehydrogenase (Baumann *et al.* 1968*b*); from this it follows that in this genus it is a waste of time and material to put up conventional tests for acid production from more than one sugar, and the one we normally test is glucose.

Biotypes of *Acinetobacter anitratus* occur and these may vary in soap tolerance (Billing, 1955), gelatin liquefaction, and ability to grow at 44 °C (Ashley & Kwantes, 1961). In the characterization of the species there is general agreement on the main points but some disagreement on detail; urease, for example, has been reported as negative, variable, and positive for the two species we recognize here. The differences may be explained by Henderson's (1967*a*) finding that urease production by members of the genus is suppressed by ammonia from peptone and other nitrogenous constituents of the media. Reports on acid production from carbohydrates vary, and again the anomalies may be due to peptone breakdown (Henderson, 1967b).

> **Minidefinition:** *Acinetobacter. Non-motile, Gram-negative coccobacilli or short rods. Strictly aerobic. Catalase positive; oxidase negative. Attack sugars by oxidation or not at all. Do not produce pigment. Arginine test negative.*

7.4.3 Achromobacter. This was an ill-defined genus of motile Gram-negative rods whose main distinguishing feature was the negative one of not producing pigmented colonies. The genus was never adequately defined and Achromobacter became the name of the dump-heap left unnamed by the rejection of the generic name *Bacterium* by the Judicial Commission (Opinion 4 (revised), 1954).

The similarity between bacteria placed in *Achromobacter* and those in *Alcaligenes* was noticed by Conn, Wolfe & Ford (1940), and species that at one time or another were included in *Achromobacter* are now placed in more closely defined genera such as *Acinetobacter, Alcaligenes,* and *Pseudomonas*.

7.4.4 Brucella (Tables 7.4a, b) is a group of bacteria whose cultural and serological characters blend into each other so that some workers regard the whole as one species, while others see them as three not-too-well-defined species; others will accept the three species without question and are willing to consider other candidates for inclusion in the genus. In 1963 the international Brucella Subcommittee (Stableforth & Jones) decided in favour of three species, each divided into biotypes, and then accepted a new species, *Brucella neotomae*, only seven strains of which had then been isolated. Other species have been proposed and *B. ovis* and *B. canis* provisionally accepted by the Subcommittee (Jones & Wundt, 1971).

Some distinguishing features of the classical species (*Brucella melitensis, B. abortus,* and *B. suis*) are shown in Table 7.4b; details of the various biotypes are given in the 1971 report of the Subcommittee, and the technical methods will be found in Morgan & Gower (1966). The tests used to separate the biotypes require investigation of the oxidative metabolism (Meyer & Cameron, 1961a, b), testing for sensitivity to Tbilisi bacteriophage (which is not specific for any species – Parnas, 1961), and serological tests using monospecific sera (which are not available commercially and are quite troublesome to prepare).

Differentiation kits and fluorescent antibody available commercially are not adequate for distinguishing between the various biotypes, and their use does not improve on the results of tests given in Table 7.4b. The performance of the tests must be well controlled at all stages and, since their interpretation is subjective they can only be relied upon when carried out in a laboratory doing large numbers of tests; in other words, the breakdown to biotypes is work for reference laboratories.

In Table 7.4b we show H_2S production by *Brucella suis* as 'D', indicating differences between the main biotypes; American strains produce H_2S and Danish strains do not; these may be more examples of geographical races of species.

Brucella neotomae differs from classical brucellas in that acid production from various sugars can easily be shown in peptone-containing media. We are not impressed with the minor antigenic overlapping that occurs with classical strains, and from our examination of a few strains we did not (and still do not) accept the species as a brucella; it is oxidase negative and oxidizes carbohydrates, and if we showed it in our tables (which we do not) it would be included with the acinetobacters. *Brucella ovis* also is oxidase negative; it needs CO_2 for isolation, does not produce H_2S; it does not reduce nitrates. We do not show this species in any of our tables.

Except for *Brucella neotomae*, brucellas do not produce acid from carbohydrate in peptone-containing media, but by using methods that avoid the peptone, acid production from carbohydrate can be shown by the classical *Brucella* species (Pickett & Nelson, 1955).

> **Minidefinition:** *Brucella. Short, Gram-negative rods; non-motile. Aerobic or carboxyphilic. Catalase positive; oxidase positive (doubtful species are oxidase negative). Do not show acid production from sugars in peptone-containing media. Urease positive.*

Table 7.4a *Second-stage table for* Acinetobacter, Moraxella, Brucella *and* Bordetella

	1	2	3	4	5	6	7	8	9	10	11	12	13	14
Catalase	+	+	+	+	+	d	+	+	−	+	+	+	+	+
Oxidase	−	−	+	+	+	+	+	+	+	+	+	+	.	−
Carbohydrate breakdown [F/O/−]	O	−	−	−	−	−	−	−	O	−^{a}	−^{a}	−^{a}		−
PHB accumulation	.	.	−	−	+	−	.	+	.	.	.	.	.	.
Haemolysis	−/β	−/β	−	−	−	β	−	−	−/β	−	−	−	.	.
Growth at 42 °C	+	+	−	d	+	−	d	−	−	−	−	−	.	−
Growth on nutrient broth/ agar	+	+	−	d	+	+	+	+	+	+	+	+	−	+
Serum requirement	−	−	+	d	−	−	−	−	−	−	−	−	.	−
Growth on MacConkey	+	+	−	d	d	−	+	.	−	−	−	−	−	+
Citrate as C source	+	d	−	d	w	−	−	d	−	−	−	−	−	(d)
Carbohydrates, acid from:														
glucose	+	−	−	−	−	−	−	−	−^{b}	−^{a}	−^{a}	−^{a}	.	−
lactose	+	−	−	−	−	−	−	−	−	−	−	−	.	−
maltose	d	−	−	−	−	−	−	−	(+)	−	−	−	.	−
xylose	+	−	.	−^{c}	−^{c}	−	−	−	−	−^{a}	−^{a}		.	−
Nitrate reduced	−	−	+	d	d	d	+	−	d	+	+	+	.	−
Gelatin liquefaction	d	−	+	−	−	+	−	−	d	−	−	−	.	−
Urease	d	−	−	−	d^d	−	+	−	−	+	+	+	.	+
Phenylalanine	−	−	−	−	−	−	+	−	+	.	.	.	.	.

1 **Actinobacter anitratus**; *A. calcoaceticus*; B5W; *Moraxella lwoffii* var. *glucidolytica*; *M. glucidolytica*; *Herellea vaginicola*
2 **Acinetobacter lwoffii**; *Moraxella lwoffii*; *Mima polymorpha*
3 **Moraxella lacunata**; *M. duplex*; *M. liquefaciens*
4 **Moraxella nonliquefaciens**; *Mima polymorpha* var. *oxidans*
5 **Moraxella osloensis**
6 **Moraxella bovis**
7 **Moraxella phenylpyruvica**
8 **'Moraxella' urethralis**
9 **'Moraxella' kingii**
10 **Brucella melitensis**; *Alcaligenes melitensis*; *Brucella brucei*
11 **Brucella abortus**; Bang's bacillus
12 **Brucella suis**
13 **Bordetella pertussis**; *Haemophilus pertussis*
14 **Bordetella parapertussis**; *Haemophilus parapertussis*; *Alcaligenes parapertussis*

^{a} Positive in the open tube of Hugh & Leifson's medium = oxidative.
^{b} Positive on ascitic agar + glucose.
^{c} May be positive when carried out as a buffered single substrate test.
^{d} Some strains positive on first isolation; the property is soon lost.
^{β} clear zone of haemolysis around colonies.

Other symbols used in the table are explained in Tables 5.1 and 5.2 (facing p. 43).

7.4.5 **Bordetella** (Table 7.4a). The two species of this genus have little in common except a clinical association, which is a poor criterion for inclusion in the same genus. They are included here because they (i.e. both species) have little in common with any other genus or group of bacteria. Our suggestion (Steel & Cowan, 1964) that the parapertussis organism should be placed in *Alcaligenes* was received with horror by at least one expert and was also described by another as a 'monstre taxonomique' (Piechaud & Szturm-Rubinsten, 1965). We regret this, for we still do not think that the parapertussis organism should be in the same genus as the whooping cough bacillus; moreover, we never cease to preach that the similarity of clinical manifestations is of no taxonomic significance. We must admit that during our experience of clinical bacteriology we never isolated the organism, or if we did, we labelled it *Alcaligenes faecalis*.

The whooping cough bacillus does not grow on ordinary media until it has been in artificial culture for some time, and a medium rich in blood has usually been considered essential for its isolation. Bordet-Gengou (Section A2.4.3) is the medium

Table 7.4*b* *Third-stage table to distinguish the classical species of* Brucella

	1	2	3
CO₂ requirement	−	+	−
H₂S produced	−	+ (early)	D*a*
Growth in:			
thionin*b* 1/25 000	−	−	+
1/50 000	+	−	+
basic fuchsin 1/50 000	+	+	−
safranin O 1/5000	+	d	−

1 Brucella melitensis
2 Brucella abortus
3 Brucella suis

a American strains positive; produce H₂S over several days. Danish strains do not produce H₂S. See note in text on geographical races.
b Dyes should be obtained from the National Aniline Division, Allied Chemical and Dye Company, New York.

Symbols used in the table are explained in Tables 5.1 and 5.2 (facing p. 43).

most often chosen, and many attempts have been made to improve its selectivity (see, for example, Lacey, 1951).

The characteristic nutritional requirements seem to justify a special genus for the whooping cough bacillus, but this argument does not extend to the parapertussis organism, which is much less exacting. Turner (1961) has shown that the whooping cough organism is not an organism that demands a rich medium but it is nutritionally exacting; peptones contain substances that are inhibitory to *Bordetella pertussis*, but a meat extract agar without peptone is suitable for isolation of the organism. The nutritional requirements and the metabolism of the species were reviewed by Rowatt (1957), its isolation and identification by Lautrop (1960).

> **Minidefinition:** *Bordetella. Gram-negative rods; non-motile. Aerobic. Catalase positive; oxidase positive. Do not grow in simple media containing peptone. Do not attack sugars in peptone-containing media.*

7.5   The apparently asaccharolytic group
(*Alcaligenes, Flavobacterium, Chromobacterium lividum*)
Characters common to members of the

group: Gram-negative rods. Strict aerobes. Catalase positive; oxidase positive. Do not ferment sugars.

Bacteria that produce pigmented colonies are easy to recognize but some produce non-pigmented variants, and these can be useful for biochemical tests that involve a colour reaction. Media have been devised to encourage pigment production and one that is especially useful for *Chromobacterium* species is mannitol yeast-extract agar (Section A2.5.2). The temperature of incubation is at least as important as the medium and stronger pigments are usually produced at the lower end of the growth range; 20–25 °C is a good range for pigment production by most mesophilic organisms.

The group is heterogeneous but all species come within the descriptive term non-fermentative; they do not usually show acid production from glucose in peptone-containing media. Many of the species oxidize carbohydrates and this is best seen in basal media with a low peptone content or better, in BSS (buffered single substrate – Pickett & Pedersen, 1970*b*) tests.

In our survey of the literature for the tables of this chapter (and particularly for Table 7.5) we have been surprised at the frequency of failure to check the nitrate medium for residual nitrate after negative nitrite tests (see Section 4.5.30); the test for nitrite can be negative when nitrate has been reduced, and the test for residual nitrate is an essential part of the nitrate reduction test (see Table 4.1).

A characteristic of the group is its lack of positive characters, or even information about many reactions; in the absence of information, shown by dots (stops, periods) in our tables, one assumes that the results of the test(s) to determine the character are negative, but it is equally possible that the appropriate tests have not been made. The absence is understandable for organisms such as *Bordetella pertussis* which are unable to grow in/on the media used for so many tests, but Johnson & Sneath (1973) have recently added to the characterization of these bacteria.

7.5.1   Chromobacterium (Tables 7.5; 7.8*a*, *b*) is characterized by the production of violet pigments which make determination of the oxidase reaction difficult by those methods that depend on the production of a purple colour in the test. Snell (1973) was able to find non-pigmented variants which he used for the oxidase test; in their absence, very young cultures are less pigmented and should be used. To encourage pigment production use mannitol yeast-extract agar and incubate the cultures at 20–25 °C (20 °C is optimal for *Chromobacterium lividum* and 25 °C for *C. violaceum*). *Chromobacterium violaceum* will be dealt with in Section 7.8.6.

Chromobacterium is a genus created around a colour and seems to be as unsuccessful as other genera confined to a particular colour, such as *Albococcus* and *Aurococcus* (Winslow & Rogers, 1906). Both species of *Chromobacterium* are made up of Gram-negative rods but there are several important differences between them: *C. lividum* grows between 4 and 30 °C, *C. violaceum* between 10 and 37 °C. *C. lividum* oxidizes carbohydrates and its characters are shown in Table 7.5; *C. violaceum* ferments sugars and is shown in Table 7.8a, b with the fermenting Gram-negative rods. The characters of the two species are shown alongside each other in Table 7.8b. At one time or another both species have been labelled *Chromobacterium violaceum*, and in consulting the older literature (before 1958) the names should be received with caution.

Chromobacteriosis is a rare disease of man and is caused by the mesophilic species (Sneath, 1960); the psychrophil is unlikely to be isolated from clinical material but may arise as an infrequent contaminant.

Minidefinition: *Chromobacterium lividum. Gram-negative rods; motile. Produce a violet pigment. Aerobic; psychrophilic. Catalase positive; oxidase positive. Sugars may be oxidized.*

7.5.2 Alcaligenes (Table 7.5).

Nyberg (1934–5) divided the Gram-negative rods that did not produce acid from carbohydrates into two subgroups: (i) *B. faecalis alcaligenes* was a short thick rod, non-motile or feebly motile by peritrichate flagella, and (ii) *Vibrio alcaligenes*, a long thin rod, actively motile by a polar flagellum: the second

group would probably now be classified as a pseudomonad, *Pseudomonas alcaligenes* (Ikari & Hugh, 1963) or *Comamonas percolans* (Davis & Park, 1962).

Conn (1942) reviewed the changes that had occurred in our ideas on the genus and pointed out that the non-fermenting bacteria may be of two kinds (Conn used the term fermenting to mean acid producing from carbohydrate media): (i) those unable to use carbohydrate, and (ii) those that break it up so completely that the end-products do not give an acid reaction in ordinary media, CO_2 being so feeble an acid that it cannot be detected in media of even a low buffer content. Moore & Pickett (1960) pointed out that strains that fail to show acid production in conventional sugar media may do so in tests designed to show oxidation of the sugar, or in rapid tests in which alkali production is kept to a minimum (see also Section 4.5.6).

We include in *Alcaligenes* motile strains of Gram-negative rods that fail to produce acid in conventional media, and as we do not take notice of the type of flagellation, we do not distinguish between Nyberg's subgroups. We return *Alcaligenes bronchisepticus* to what we think is its rightful place in the genus; it is distinguished from *A. faecalis* by its ability to break down urea (Ulrich & Needham, 1953); judged by analysis of the DNA-base composition, De Ley (1968) thinks that the relationship is remote.

The autotrophic species, *Alcaligenes eutrophus* and *A. paradoxus*, although facultatively heterotrophic (Davis *et al.* 1969) are unlikely to be isolated in medical laboratories and are not shown in Table 7.5.

Alcaligenes odorans (Málek, Radochová & Lysenko, 1963) was first isolated from stools and urine and named *Pseudomonas odorans*; descriptions of the odour have been typically subjective – from valerian to jasmine – and from strawberry in young cultures to ammoniacal in old ones. The species reduces nitrate and then reduces the nitrite quickly so that it gives a negative nitrite test. A variant of the species, *Alcaligenes odorans* var. *viridans*, has a fruity smell and produces a bright green zone around colonies on blood agar (Mitchell & Clarke, 1965; Gilardi & Hirschl, 1969); we do not think that the differences warrant the status of

Table 7.5 *Second-stage table for* Chromobacterium lividum, Alcaligenes *and* Flavobacterium

	1	2	3	4	5	6	7
Motility	+	+	+	+	−	−	−
Pigmentation	+[a]	−	−	−	+[b]	+[b]	+[b]
Growth at 42 °C	−	+	+	+	−	−	+
Growth on SS agar	.	+	+	+	−	−	−
Growth on MacConkey agar	d	+	+	+	+	+	−
KCN (growth on)	−	+	+	−	−	.	.
Citrate as C source	+	+	+	+	−	−	−
Carbohydrates [in peptone media], acid from:							
glucose	−[c]	−	−	−	(+)	−[c]	−
lactose	−	−	−	−	−[d]	−	−
sucrose	−[c]	−	−	−	−	−	−
xylose	−[c]	−	−	−	−	−	−
Aesculin hydrolysis	+	−	−	−	+	+	.
Nitrate reduced	+[e]	d	+	+[e]	−	−	.
Indole	−	−	−	−	+	+	+
Gelatin liquefaction	(+)	−	−	−	+	+	+
Urease	−	−	+	−	−	−	.

1 **Chromobacterium lividum**
2 **Alcaligenes faecalis**
3 **Alcaligenes bronchisepticus**; *Bordetella bronchiseptica*;
  Haemophilus bronchisepticus
4 **Alcaligenes odorans**; *A. odorans* var. *viridans*
5 **Flavobacterium meningosepticum**; Pickett's group I
6 **Flavobacterium**, Pickett's group II
7 **Flavobacterium**, Pickett's group III

[a] Violet pigment.
[b] Yellow pigment.
[c] Positive in open tube of OF medium (Section A 2.6.1)
  = oxidative.
[d] Positive in ONPG test (Lapage *et al.* 1973).
[e] Gas detected, indicating further breakdown of nitrite.

Symbols used in the table are explained in Tables 5.1 and 5.2 (facing p. 43).

variety and in Table 7.5 we show only the characteristics of the species.

> **Minidefinition:** *Alcaligenes. Gram-negative rods; motile. Aerobic. Catalase positive; oxidase positive. Do not produce acid from sugars in peptone-containing media.*

7.5.3   Flavobacterium (Table 7.5). Pessimists tolerate *Flavobacterium* as a genus for Gram-negative, rod-shaped bacteria that produce yellow colonies but fail to qualify for other, better defined genera (Hendrie, Mitchell & Shewan, 1968); it is made up of a heterogeneous collection (*Index Bergeyana* lists 129 species) and the type species is no longer regarded as a flavobacterium!

We often find that colonies of *Enterobacter cloacae* have a yellow pigment, and *Erwinia herbicola* (known in medical laboratories as *Bacterium typhiflavum*) characteristically produces yellow colonies. In other fields some species of *Pseudomonas*, *Vibrio*, *Aeromonas*, and *Xanthomonas* produce yellow pigments, and those who neglect to determine the Gram reaction of their isolates may have some difficulty with a few Gram-positive species.

The definition of Pickett & Pedersen (1970*b*) covers all the flavobacteria shown in Table 7.5; their group I corresponds reasonably well with King's (1959) *Flavobacterium meningosepticum*, a homogeneous species divisible into several serotypes. We have not attempted to fit all the species listed by Buchanan *et al.* (1966), Hatt & Zvirbulis (1967), and Zvirbulis & Hatt (1969) into the other two groups of Pickett & Pedersen.

Indole, reported negative by Cabrera & Davis (1961) and weakly positive by Gilardi (1972*a*), is produced slowly and King (1964) advised extraction with xylol before adding the test reagents. Pickett & Pedersen (1970*a*) regard indole production as definitive of the genus.

> **Minidefinition:** *Flavobacterium. Gram-negative rods; usually non-motile. Aerobic. Catalase positive; oxidase positive. Colonies have a yellow colour. Sugars attacked slowly by oxidation or not at all.*

7.6   The pseudomonads of medical importance
(*Pseudomonas*)

7.6.1   Pseudomonas (Table 7.6*a*) is a genus that includes pathogens for both animals and plants, but because specimens from animal and plant tissues are studied in different laboratories they are submitted to different tests and techniques; this results in a separation into animal and plant species which is quite unjustified, for it is possible that strains pathogenic for plants might also be pathogenic for animals. Species studied by both groups of workers are *Pseudomonas aeruginosa*

Table 7.6a *Second-stage table for* Pseudomonas

	1	2	3	4	5	6	7	8	9	10
Motility	+	+	+	+	+	+	+	+	−	+
Oxidase	+	+	+	+	+	d	+	+	d	+
PHB accumulation in cells	−	−	−	+	+	−	−	+	+	+
Pigment	+^{a}	+^{b}	.	+^{c}	d^d	+^{c}	.	+^{c}	−	−
Fluorescence in u.v. light	+	+	+	−	−	−	−	−	−	.
Growth at 5 °C	−	+	d	−	−	−	d	−	−	.
Growth at 42 °C	+	−	−	−	d	−	d	+	−	.
Growth on MacConkey	+	+	+	+	+	+	+	+	−	.
Growth in KCN	+	d	−	.	−	+	−	+	d	.
Utilization of citrate as C source	+	+	+	−	+	−^{e}	+	+	−	+
Carbohydrates,^{f} acid from:										
glucose	+	+	+	−	+	(w)^g	+	+	+	+
lactose	−	−	−	−	+	−	−	+	−	−
maltose	−	−	d	−	+	+	d	+	d	−
mannitol	+	+	d	−	+	−	d	+	+	−
salicin	−	−	.	.	+	−	−	−	−	−
sucrose	−	d	−	−	+	−	−	+	d	−
xylose	+	+	+	−	+	−	+	+	−	+
Starch hydrolysis	−	−	−	−	−	−	+	d	−	−
Nitrate reduced to nitrite	+	d	d	−	d	+^{h}	+	+	+	+
Nitrite reduced to N gas	d	−	−	−	−	−	+	d	−	+
Gelatin hydrolysis	+	+	−	+	+	+	−	+	d	.
Casein hydrolysis	+	+	−	+	+	+	−	+	.	.
Urease	+	d	d	−	+	−	(d)	d	d	.
Arginine dihydrolase	+	+	+	−	−	−	d	+	+	−
Lysine decarboxylase	−	−	−	−	+^{j}	+	−	−	−	.
Ornithine decarboxylase	−	−	−	−	d	−	−	−	−	.
Egg-yolk reaction	−	d	−	−	+	−	+	+	d	−
Tween 80 hydrolysis	+	d	−	−	+	−	+	+	d	+

1 **Pseudomonas aeruginosa**; *P. pyocyanea*
2 **Pseudomonas fluorescens**
3 **Pseudomonas putida**
4 **Pseudomonas diminuta**
5 **Pseudomonas cepacia**; *P. multivorans*; *P. kingii*
6 **Pseudomonas maltophilia**
7 **Pseudomonas stutzeri**
8 **Pseudomonas pseudomallei**; *Loefflerella pseudomallei*; *L. whitmor(e)i*; *Pfeifferella whitmori*; *Malleomyces pseudomallei*
9 **Pseudomonas mallei**; *Loefflerella mallei*; *Pfeifferella mallei*; *Malleomyces mallei*
10 **Pseudomonas pickettii**

PHB Poly-β-hydroxybutyrate.
^{a} Pyocyanin.
^{b} Fluorescin.
^{c} Yellow.
^{d} Positive on Kligler's iron agar and TSI.
^{e} Positive on Christensen's citrate medium and in BSS tests.
^{f} Hugh & Leifson base (A 2.6.1)+ 1 % sugar; ASS sugars (Section A 2.6.5).
^{g} Weak on H & L medium; negative on ASS.
^{h} Cannot use nitrate as N source.
^{j} Positive by Richard's method; d by Møller's method.

Symbols used in the table are explained in Tables 5.1 and 5.2 (facing p. 43).

(often named *Pseudomonas pyocyanea* in medical laboratories) and *P. fluorescens*, and until recently, that was the extent of the common ground.

Pseudomonas aeruginosa produces two water-soluble pigments: pyocyanin which gives the green–blue appearance to the area surrounding the colony or confluent growth, and fluorescin, yellow in colour but, as its name implies, its main characteristic is fluorescence in u.v. light. While pyocyanin is formed only by *P. aeruginosa*, another green pigment, chlororaphin, is produced by a plant pseudomonad; this pigment is not water soluble

Table 7.6b *Buffered single substrate (BSS) tests* (Pickett & Pedersen, 1970*b*, *c*)

	1	2	3	4	5	6	7	8
Acid from:								
glucose	+	+	+	−	+	+	+	+
fructose	+	+	+	−	+	+	+	+
lactose	−	d	−	−	+	+	−	+
maltose	−	+	−	−	+	+	+	+
mannitol	+	d	−	−	+	−	d	+
salicin	−	−	−	.	+	d	−	+
sucrose	−	d	−	.	d	+	−	−
xylose	+	+	+	−	+	d	+	+

1 **Pseudomonas aeruginosa**
2 **Pseudomonas fluorescens**
3 **Pseudomonas putida**
4 **Pseudomonas diminuta**
5 **Pseudomonas cepacia**
6 **Pseudomonas maltophilia**
7 **Pseudomonas stutzeri**
8 **Pseudomonas pseudomallei**

and is seen as crystals in the agar medium. Other pseudomonads may produce the fluorescent pigment.

An organism that has much in common with the fluorescent pseudomonads is Whitmore's bacillus. Wetmore & Gochenour (1956) found that this organism was inhibited on media such as SS agar, deoxycholate agar, and cetrimide (CTAB) agar, on which the fluorescent species would grow. The flagella of Whitmore's bacillus were first described as peritrichate by Legroux & Genevray (1933), but later as polar by Brindle & Cowan (1951) and by Wetmore & Gochenour (1956); all these workers showed that the organism had much in common with the pseudomonads but none suggested translating it to that genus. It was included in *Pseudomonas* by Haynes in *Bergey's Manual* (1957) as *Pseudomonas pseudomallei*. Redfearn, Palleroni & Stanier (1966) included the glanders bacillus in their survey of *Pseudomonas* species, and regarded it as a typical but permanently non-motile member of that genus.

Fortunately, glanders is almost a disease of the past and few of us have the opportunity (or the risks) of working with recently isolated cultures. Meliodosis is a disease of tropical countries but occasionally occurs in temperate climates in

people who were probably infected abroad. *Pseudomonas pseudomallei* may be confused with other pseudomonads and although its wrinkled colony form may be characteristic, it is not diagnostic and its appearance can be simulated by *P. aeruginosa*. Zierdt & Marsh (1971), who have recent experience of isolating the organism, say that after three or four days colonies of *P. pseudomallei* have an aromatic odour that is distinctive (but until one has experienced it we do not think that this subjective characteristic can be of much help in making the identification). Other diagnostic features are the development of bright red colonies on MacConkey agar (and on the basal medium without lactose) and an ability to grow on deoxycholate agar. Zierdt & Marsh recommend that in laboratories in which the isolation of *Pseudomonas pseudomallei* is a rare event (and that means most laboratories), confirmation should be sought in serology, using a specific antiserum that has been well tested against *Pseudomonas aeruginosa* and other pseudomonads. The difficulty, of course, is to find such an antiserum, and the use of fluorescent-antibody methods should be considered. While *P. mallei* may be regarded as the most dangerous organism to work with in a laboratory, *P. pseudomallei*, though probably less dangerous, should be treated with the same respect.

Many other pseudomonads have been isolated from clinical material and the hospital environment (see, for example, Gilardi, 1970, 1971*a*, *b*, 1972*b*; Lapage, Hill & Reeve, 1968; Pickett & Pedersen, 1970*a*, *b*, *c*) and there has been intense activity to find distinguishing features and to assess the potential pathogenicity of the different species. Undoubtedly some strains are 'opportunistic pathogens' and as many of them are resistant to antiseptic solutions they may cause low-grade infections from contaminated catheters, wash-out fluids, and drip lines. Media for the selective isolation of pseudomonads have been reviewed by Park & Billing (1965). Thom, Stephens, Gillespie & Alder (1971) found that the addition of nitrofurantoin to King's B medium was easier to prepare than cetrimide media and was equally good for the selective isolation of *Pseudomonas aeruginosa*. On this medium most strains of *Proteus* spp., *Escherichia coli*, *Streptococcus faecalis*, and staphylococci were either inhibited completely or grew only feebly after overnight incubation at 37 °C.

Tests to identify the many species are becoming more complex; for example, one of the distinguishing characters is to show by phase-contrast microscopy the presence or absence of poly-β-hydroxybutyrate (PHB) in the cells of a culture grown preferably in a medium with DL-β-hydroxybutyrate as carbon source, and to confirm by staining with Sudan Black B. Apart from the accumulation of PHB in the bacterial cells, the characters shown in Table 7.6a are ones that are examined in most laboratories and do not call for exceptional knowledge or skill in biochemistry. The growth of *P. aeruginosa* is often accompanied by iridescence; the mechanism of this phenomenon is still unknown, but it occurs independently of phage sensitivity (Zierdt, 1971). Strains of *P. aeruginosa* are usually lysogenic but phage typing schemes – and there are many of them – have not become popular. For epidemiological work the species can be 'fingerprinted' by determining the production of and sensitivity to bacteriocins and phages (Farmer & Herman, 1969) but these are methods for the reference laboratory and are not described here.

The acid production from carbohydrates shown in Table 7.6a is that observed when organisms are grown in media containing small amounts of peptone (e.g. Hugh & Leifson base, Section A2.6.1) or none at all (ASS, Section A2.6.5). Acid may be produced from more carbohydrates in the BSS (buffered single substrate) tests of Pickett & Pedersen (1970b, c) in which a heavy suspension of the test organism is added to the carbohydrate + buffer + indicator + bacteriostat. The difference between the results of the two kinds of test can be seen by comparing Table 7.6a and b.

Pseudomonas aeruginosa produces alkali on Christensen's urea medium and, rather more slowly, on the base without urea; in Stuart, van Stratum & Rustigian's (1945) urea medium, alkali is not produced. Many pseudomonads break down arginine but Møller's method is not satisfactory with these organisms; Sherris *et al.* (1959) and Thornley (1960) have described suitable methods. For detecting lysine and ornithine decarboxylases of pseudomonads, Richard's (1968) methods are more sensitive than those of Møller (Snell *et al.* 1972).

Nutritional requirements can provide diagnostic characters for some pseudomonads: *Pseudomonas maltophilia* requires methionine, and *P. diminuta* needs cystine.

Pseudomonas maltophilia, described by Hugh & Ryschenkow (1961) as an Alcaligenes-like species, is unusual in producing acid from maltose in H and L sugars before acid is seen in glucose, and glucose remains negative in ASS media. Park (1967) found that even when acid was not produced the glucose was attacked. *P. maltophilia* is unusual for a pseudomonad in being variable in the oxidase test. Hugh & Ryschenkow found 10 of 26 strains positive but Pickett & Pedersen (1970b) had only 3 positives among their 27 strains; the variability may be due to differences in sensitivity of the reagents used for the test (Snell, 1973).

A new species (*Pseudomonas pickettii*) made up of strains from clinical material and hospital equipment has been described by Ralston *et al.* (1973) and its characters are shown in Table 7.6a. What is now needed is a description suitable for use in a clinical laboratory.

> **Minidefinition:** *Pseudomonas. Gram-negative rods; motile. Aerobic. Catalase positive; oxidase positive. Attack sugars by oxidation. Fluorescent, diffusible yellow pigment may be produced.*

7.7 Pasteurellas and the pasteurella-like group
(*Pasteurella, Actinobacillus, Cardiobacterium, Necromonas*)
Characters common to members of the group: Gram-negative rods; non-motile at 37 °C. Aerobic and facultatively anaerobic. Oxidase positive. Attack sugars fermentatively.

Actinobacillus and *Pasteurella* (*sensu stricto*) have so much in common that their fusion has been suggested, and it is convenient to show their characters in the same table so that the comparison can be made easily. Three species formerly placed in *Pasteurella* have several important differences from the pasteurellas (*sensu stricto*) and resemble more closely the enterobacteria; we describe them as *Yersinia* species in Section 7.9.16 and in Table 7.9a, b; we also show them in Table 7.7a, b so that readers may judge for themselves the wisdom of the translation to *Yersinia*.

Table 7.7a *Second-stage table for* Pasteurella, Actinobacillus, Cardiobacterium *and* Yersinia

	1	2	3	4	5	6	7	8	9	10	11	12	13	14	15	16	17
Motility at 22 °C	–	–	–	–	–	–	–	–	–	–	–	–	–	–	+	+	–
Catalase	+	+	+	+	–	+	w	+	+	+	+	–	–	+	+	+	+
Oxidase	d	+	+	+	+	+	+	+	+	.	–	–	+	–	–	–	+
Growth on MacConkey agar	–	–	–	+	+	–	+	+	+	+	–	–	–	+	+	+	.
Growth improved by CO₂	.	.	.	.	.	.	–	–	–	+	+	+	+	.	.	.	.
Growth on KCN	+	–	–	d	–	–	.	.	.	.	.	.	.	–	–	–	–
Carbohydrates, acid from:																	
arabinose	d	d	–	d	–	–	d	–	+	+	–	.	–	+	+	+	+
lactose	d	(d)	–	d	–	d	(+)	+	+	–	–	+	–	–	–	(d)	–
maltose	d	+	+	+	+	+	+	+	+	–	+	+	+	+	+	+	+
mannitol	+	–	+	+	+	–	+	+	–	+	d	–	d	+	+	+	+
raffinose	–	+	–	+	+	.	–	+	+	–	–	+	.	–	–	–	.
salicin	–	–	–	–	+	–	–	–	+	–	–	–	–	+	+	–	+
sorbitol	d	–	d	+	+	–	d	–	–	.	–	–	+	–	–	+	–
sucrose	+	+	+	+	+	+	+	+	+	–	+	+	+	–	–	+	–
trehalose	d	+	–	–	+	+	–	+	+	–	–	+	–	+	+	+	d
xylose	d	d	–	+	–	d	+	+	+	+	d	–	–	+	+	(+)	–
ONPG	d	+	–	d	–	d	+	+	+	.	–	.	–	+	+	+	.
Aesculin hydrolysis	–	–	–	d	+	–	–	–	+	.	–	–	–	+	+	–	+
Nitrate reduced	+	+	+	+	+	+	+	+	+	+	+	+	–	+	+	+	+
Nitrite reduced	d	–	+	+	+	–	.	.	.	.	.	.	.	.	.	.	–
Indole	+	+	–	–	–	–	–	–	–	–	.	–	–	+	–	d	–
Gelatin hydrolysis	–	–	–	–	(+)	–	–	(+)	–	–	–	–	–	–	–	–	+
Urease	d	+	+	–	–	–	+	+	+	+	–	–	–	–	+	+	–
H₂S	–	–	–	–	(+)	–	+	+	+	+	+	+	+	–	–	–	–
Ornithine decarboxylase	+	d	–	–	–	d	–	–	–	.	.	.	–	–	–	+	–

1 **Pasteurella multocida**; *P. septica*
2 **Pasteurella pneumotropica**
3 **Pasteurella ureae**; *P. haemolytica* var. *ureae*
4 **Pasteurella haemolytica** type A
5 **Pasteurella haemolytica** type T
6 **Pasteurella gallinarum**
7 **Actinobacillus lignieresii**
8 **Actinobacillus equuli**; *Shigella equuli*; *S. equirulis*; *Bacterium viscosum-equi*; *B. nephritidis-equi*
9 **Actinobacillus suis**
10 Actinobacillus from sow's vagina (Ross *et al.* 1972)
11 **'Actinobacillus' actinomycetemcomitans**
12 **Haemophilus aphrophilus**
13 **Cardiobacterium hominis**
14 **Yersinia pestis**; *Pasteurella pestis*; plague bacillus
15 **Yersinia pseudotuberculosis**; *Pasteurella pseudotuberculosis*
16 **Yersinia enterocolitica**; Pasteurella X
17 **Necromonas salmonicida**; *Aeromonas salmonicida*

Symbols used in the table are explained in Tables 5.1 and 5.2 (facing p. 43).

Also shown in Table 7.7a are two organisms that are difficult to allocate to genera; these are *Actinobacillus actinomycetemcomitans* and *Haemophilus aphrophilus* which are more like each other than like the genera whose names they bear (King & Tatum, 1962). In morphology both organisms are small Gram-negative coccobacilli; in broth they grow as granules adherent to the side of the tubes. On plates, the actinobacillus colonies are the smaller and stick to the medium. Growth of both organisms is improved by CO₂; neither needs X nor V factors, except perhaps, on first isolation, when *Haemophilus aphrophilus* seems to be X

dependent. King & Tatum found that most strains produced a small amount of gas when tested by the unusual technique of Hormaeche & Munilla (1957) of plunging a red-hot wire into the medium. In the OF test, sugars are fermented. King & Tatum did not make any recommendation about the taxonomic position of this pair and, as far as we know, none has been made from any other quarter. *Haemophilus aphrophilus* is also shown in Table 7.10b for comparison with the X- and V-requiring bacilli.

Cardiobacterium is a new genus that has some resemblance to the pasteurellas; it was first described as a pasteurella-like organism by Tucker *et al.* (1962). Table 7.7a seems to be the best place for the genus in this *Manual*.

Necromonas is an organism from fish and has not been described as pasteurella-like but its characters make it fit quite well into Table 7.7a, where we show it. It is doubtful if it has any medical importance but it seems to have figured in medical journals and it certainly appears in medical laboratories for identification. It has been placed in *Aeromonas* but was never at home there; it may not like its present company any better but here its presence does not upset the definitions.

7.7.1 Pasteurella (Table 7.7a, b). The name is used here in its strict sense, and the genus described does not include those organisms, formerly in *Pasteurella*, that have been removed and made into another genus, *Yersinia*. *Pasteurella multocida* is an umbrella species and includes strains that were originally named after animals from which they had been isolated. In this genus there has been a sensible disregard for rules of priority in the name(s) used for the commonest species, and a single epithet is used for strains that produce haemorrhagic septicaemia in animals of all kinds. Once a unified species had been accepted a start was made to break it up into various subdivisions; *Pasteurella haemolytica* (Newsom & Cross, 1932) and *P. pneumotropica* (Jawetz, 1950; Henriksen, 1962) were two early ones, and *P. haemolytica* var. *ureae* (Henriksen & Jyssum, 1960) was elevated to specific rank (Jones, 1962; J. E. Smith & Thal, 1965). The biochemical characters of these species are shown in Table 7.7a. The principles of the CAMP test have been used by Bouley (1965) for making a quick distinction between *P. multocida* (negative) and *P. haemolytica* (positive). It is also possible to divide pasteurellas into species by sensitivity to dyes (Table 7.7b) and the method clearly distinguishes between *Pasteurella* and *Yersinia* (Midgley, 1966).

Pasteurella haemolytica was divided into serotypes by Biberstein, Gills & Knight (1960) and into biotypes A (arabinose fermenters) and T (trehalose fermenters) by G. R. Smith (1961). Biberstein & Gills (1962), who correlated the two typing systems, found that not all strains of *P. haemolytica* were catalase positive, but catalase-negative strains seemed to be confined to type T.

J. E. Smith & Thal (1965) thought that the differences between the A and T types, though mainly in fermentation reactions, might justify the recognition of two separate species.

Several serological schemes for the subdivision of *Pasteurella multocida* have been proposed and these were reviewed by Steel (1963). Frederiksen (1971), mainly on biochemical characters, subdivided *Pasteurella multocida* into six biotypes, and *P. pneumotropica* into three. There is a close resemblance between *P. multocida* and *P. pneumotropica* (Smith & Thal, 1965; Midgley, 1966) and it seems likely that *P. pneumotropica* is the product of over-enthusiasm for the creation of new taxa.

Midgley found that among her subgroup *a* only the human strains of *Pasteurella multocida* fermented lactose and produced β-galactosidase (ONPG positive); human strains of subgroup *c* were unusual in fermenting maltose, and in this respect resembled *P. pneumotropica*. Midgley (1966) thought that *P. ureae* could be a human pathogen; it was the only pasteurella in her collection that needed an enriched medium for growth.

> **Minidefinition:** *Pasteurella. Gram-negative rods; non-motile. Aerobic and facultatively anaerobic. Catalase positive (a few exceptions); oxidase positive (a few exceptions). Attack sugars by fermentation but do not produce gas.*

7.7.2 Actinobacillus (Table 7.7a) is made up of species for which no obvious home can be found and at least two kinds of organism seem to be represented; the actinobacilli proper (based on the type *Actinobacillus lignieresii*) and another organism usually, but not always, associated with *Actinomyces israelii* in material from patients with actinomycosis, which was put in the genus by Topley and Wilson in the first edition of their book as *Actinobacillus actinomycetemcomitans*. Our impression, which may be wrong, is that neither Topley nor Wilson could think where to put it but, having put it in Actinobacillus, it has stuck. We agree with King & Tatum (1962) that it more closely resembles *Haemophilus aphrophilus* than *Actinobacillus lignieresii*, but as its only growth requirement is CO_2 it would be illogical to place it in *Haemophilus* as we define that genus. To indicate our uncertainty and our dissatisfaction with the disposal of the organism we shall adopt the convention established for 'Mycobacterium' rhodochrous of putting the generic name within quotation marks (quotes) as 'Actinobacillus' actinomycetemcomitans.

Actinobacillus lignieresii is found in cattle and sheep, in lesions and in rumen contents; it is said to cause infections occasionally in man. In comparisons made by Phillips (1960, 1961) the rumen strains were more frequently positive in the catalase, VP, and urease tests, but Phillips did not suggest that the species should be divided into biotypes; it can be divided into serotypes. Colonies of A. lignieresii are sticky and difficult to remove from an agar surface; this stickiness is relative and is much less than in A. equuli.

Actinobacillus equuli is the name now given to the organism that causes joint-ill and nephritis in foals; in bacteriological systematics it has migrated from Bacillus (in the old sense of a rod-shaped organism), through Bacterium, Eberthella, and Shigella. It is an organism that produces a copious slimy covering, but this is not capsular material (as in pneumococci or klebsiellas); the mucoid material of which it is composed makes broth cultures viscid and colonies sticky and very difficult to remove from an agar surface.

Other organisms have been placed in Actinobacillus and, like Achromobacter, it has been a dump-heap for Gram-negative rods that were difficult to place in a genus. Temporary residents have included the glanders bacillus, now so rare that few bacteriologists working now have handled freshly isolated cultures; it has but slight resemblance to A. lignieresii in that it is a non-motile, Gram-negative rod; in metabolism it is quite different and Wetmore, Theil, Herman & Harr (1963) proposed its transfer to Pseudomonas.

An unnamed addition to the genus is a group of organisms isolated from the vaginal exudate of postpartum sows (Ross et al. 1972); the characters are shown in Table 7.7a. Cultures from swine should be incubated in 5–10 % CO_2 to improve the chances of isolating one of this group; one recognizable character is a narrow zone of β-haemolysis on horse blood agar.

Minidefinition: Actinobacillus. Gram-negative rods; non-motile. Aerobic; facul-

tatively anaerobic. Catalase positive; oxidase positive (one exception – a misplaced species). Attack sugars fermentatively without gas production.

7.7.3   Cardiobacterium (Table 7.7a). This organism is said to be pleomorphic and to be Gram negative with Gram-positive areas. Slotnick & Dougherty (1964) found metachromatic granules and sudanophilic bodies but Midgley et al. (1970) were unable to find them. Like Haemophilus, the organisms prefer a high humidity for growth and need it for aerobic growth when first isolated, so that incubation in a jar seems advisable. Carbon dioxide improves growth but is not essential. Growth under strictly anaerobic conditions is good. Hydrogen sulphide cannot be detected in the butt of TSI agar but lead acetate papers are blackened (Tucker et al. 1962). Midgley et al. found H_2S was produced by only one of their strains.

Few strains of this species have been isolated; CDC workers have examined only twenty-four strains (Weaver et al. 1972) and there is an unusual similarity in the characteristics reported, indicating that the same strains have been examined in several laboratories; the agreement between the results is highly satisfactory.

Minidefinition: Cardiobacterium. Gram-negative rods, sometimes with Gram-positive areas. Non-motile. Pleomorphic and may show metachromatic granules. Aerobic (in a moist atmosphere); facultatively anaerobic. Catalase negative; oxidase positive. Sugars are fermented.

7.7.4   Necromonas (Tables 7.7a; 7.8a, b). A genus created by I. W. Smith (1963) for a bacterium that produces furunculosis in fish.

Fish infected by the organism have not been incriminated in food-poisoning, but public health laboratories are sometimes asked to examine fish and this organism may be isolated. It can be identified provisionally (but rapidly) by its inability to grow at 37 °C, by growth at room temperature (in England) and by the production of a characteristic brown pigment that diffuses into the medium on which the organism is growing. The optimal temperature for growth is about 20 °C but it can grow at 5 °C.

Table 7.7b *Dye sensitivity and some biochemical characteristics of* Pasteurella *and* Yersinia *strains* (after Midgley, 1966)

	1	2	3	4	5	6	7	8	9	10	11	12	13	14
Victoria blue 1/10000	+	+	−	±	−	+	−	+	+	±	+	±	+	+
Methylene blue 1/200000	−	−	−	−	±	−	−	±	±	+	+	+	−	+
Thionin 1/25000	−	−	−	−	−	−	−	−	−	±	+	±	−	+
Malachite green 1/50000	−	−	−	−	−	−	−	−	−	+	+	+	−	+
Safranin O 1/25000	−	−	−	−	−	−	−	+	+	+	+	+	−	+
Pyronin 1/100000	−	−	+	+	+	+	−	−	+	+	+	+	+	+
Carbohydrates, acid from:														
arabinose	d	d	−	−	−	−	−	−	−	+	+	+	.	.
lactose	−	+	−	−	−	d	−	d	−	−	−	−	.	.
maltose	−	−	−	+	+	+	+	+	+	+	+	+	.	.
mannitol	+	+	−	+	−	−	+	+	+	+	+	+	.	.
salicin	−	−	−	−	−	−	−	−	+	+	+	−	.	.
sorbitol	+	+	−	+	−	−	−	+	+	+	−	+	.	.
sucrose	+	+	+	+	+	+	+	+	+	−	−	−	.	.
trehalose	d	d	−	+	−	+	−	−	+	+	+	+	.	.
xylose	d	d	−	+	−	+	−	+	−	+	+	(+)	.	.
ONPG	−	+	−	−	−	+	−	d	−	+	+	+	.	.
Indole	+	+	+	+	+	+	−	−	−	−	−	d	.	.
Urease	−	−	−	+	+	+	+	−	−	+	+	+	.	.
Ornithine decarboxylase	+	+	+	−	−	+	−	−	−	+	+	+	.	.

1 **Pasteurella multocida** Midgley's subgroup *a* (human and animal strains)
2 **Pasteurella multocida** subgroup *aa* (human strains)
3 **Pasteurella multocida** subgroup *b* (human strains, all from dog-bites)
4 **Pasteurella multocida** subgroup *c* (human strains)
5 **Pasteurella multocida** subgroup *cc* (human strains)
6 **Pasteurella pneumotropica**
7 **Pasteurella ureae**
8 **Pasteurella haemolytica A**
9 **Pasteurella haemolytica T**
10 **Yersinia pestis**
11 **Yersinia pseudotuberculosis**
12 **Yersinia enterocolitica**
13 **Actinobacillus** spp.
14 **Enterobacteria**
In the first six lines, + = good growth; ± = some growth; − = no growth.

Other symbols used in the table are explained in Tables 5.1 and 5.2 (facing p. 43).

Minidefinition: *Necromonas. Gram-negative rods; non-motile. Aerobic, facultatively anaerobic. Catalase positive; oxidase positive. Attack sugars fermentatively, and may produce gas. On the surface of an agar medium produce a brown diffusible pigment.*

7.7.5   Yersinia (Tables 7.7a, b; 7.9a, b) is an off-shoot of *Pasteurella*; notes on the history of the genus are given in Section 7.9.16. To show the similarities and differences, characters of the species of *Yersinia* are given in Table 7.7a, b.

    Minidefinition: *Yersinia. Gram-negative rods; non-motile at 37 °C (some species motile at 22 °C). Aerobic; facultatively anaerobic. Catalase positive; oxidase nega-tive. Sugars attacked fermentatively; occasionally gas may be produced.*

7.7.6   'Haemophilus' aphrophilus (Tables 7.7a; 7.10b) seems to be X dependent on first isolation (Boyce, Frazer & Zinnemann, 1969) but loses this requirement fairly rapidly. King & Tatum (1962) thought that this species had much in common with *Actinobacillus actinomycetemcomitans* but would not be any better placed in that genus than in *Haemophilus*. A comparison can be made in Table 7.7a and with *Haemophilus* in Table 7.10b.

7.8   The vibrio and vibrio-like group
    (*Vibrio, Beneckea, Aeromonas, Plesiomonas, Necromonas, Chromobacterium violaceum*)

Characters common to members of the group: Gram-negative rods. Aerobic and facultatively anaerobic. Catalase positive; oxidase positive. Attack sugars fermentatively. Nitrates are reduced.

The group is remarkably homogeneous and apart from the pigment produced by *Chromobacterium violaceum* it is easier to draw up a list of common characters than to find ones by which the various genera can be distinguished. This suggests that there are too many genera and that we have become victims of the splitter's plots. *Beneckea* is a recent offshoot of *Vibrio*, and *Plesiomonas* an older one of *Aeromonas*. To redress the balance Hendrie, Shewan & Véron (1971) would abolish *Plesiomonas* and move the C27 organism (*Plesiomonas shigelloides*) to *Vibrio*. The requirement that the genus *Vibrio* should be made up of vibrios (rod-shaped bacteria with a single shallow curve) is a thing of the past; the requirement of a single flagellum is an even more remote connexion with nineteenth-century bacteriology. The combination of *Aeromonas*, *Plesiomonas* and *Beneckea* and their inclusion in *Vibrio* is an engaging thought, and the action is one we would welcome.

The case for the separation of the salmon-disease bacterium from the aeromonads is rather different; this organism is non-motile, grows at 5 °C but not at 37 °C; it is fermentative and produces a little gas from glucose and we agree with Smith (1963) that it is reasonable to separate it from aeromonads.

The inclusion of *Chromobacterium violaceum* in the group introduces a new determining feature, the production of a non-diffusible pigment that may be no more than a species characteristic, though in orthodox classifications it is given generic significance. But, as our grouping is purely for convenience (and *our* convenience), we do not think that this matters very much, though critics may see it as another example of our unorthodoxy and perhaps irresponsibility in drawing attention to convenience as a reason for grouping organisms together.

7.8.1   Vibrio (Table 7.8*a, b*). We characterize *Vibrio cholerae* in our tables and treat *Vibrio eltor* as a biochemical variant or biotype that is VP positive and haemolytic for human red cells (De

et al. 1954). De found that calcium salts were necessary to detect certain haemolysins, but they inhibited others. In culture, true cholera vibrios may acquire haemolytic properties (de Moor, 1949), but this may be delayed in fresh isolates of the el Tor variety. Feeley & Pittman (1963) showed that when the method using sheep cells was standardized, the haemolytic test was reliable for distinguishing between *Vibrio cholerae* and *V. eltor*. Nevertheless, Feeley (1965) recommended that only one species should be recognized and that the differences between the classical cholera vibrio and the el Tor variety should be regarded as of minor importance. Mukerjee (1963) used a group IV cholera phage to pick out cholera-causing vibrios, but Carpenter *et al.* (1968), in commenting on this and other tests (sensitivity to polymyxin and agglutination of chicken red cells), reported that strains giving aberrant results had been found, that adequate controls were necessary, and that the tests were more suitable for a reference laboratory than for a clinical laboratory.

All cholera-like vibrios share a common H antigen but thirty-nine O groups can be distinguished; of these, O group 1 is the true cholera vibrio. Sakazaki, Tamura, Gomez & Sen (1970) support Feeley in recommending that only one species be recognized, and that this species should be subdivided into serotypes, of which type 1 is the cholera vibrio.

Wahba & Takla (1962) devised a chemical flocculation test for distinguishing between the cholera and el Tor vibrios, but the test did not work with rough strains. The so-called non-agglutinable vibrios (NAG) are not, in themselves, important; they are better named non-cholera vibrios (NCV), and although they do not cause epidemic cholera, they may be responsible for sporadic cases of diarrhoea. NCV can be distinguished from the cholera vibrios by serological methods (they are not serotype 1) and strains need to be put up against only one antiserum (type 1) which will agglutinate the true cholera and the el Tor vibrios (Gardner & Venkatraman, 1935). Identification of NCV is unsatisfactory in that it depends on negative serological results and, as every serologist knows, the failure to react may be a product of bad technical methods and independent of the true nature of the antigen. The antigenic variants of the Ogawa, Inaba, and Hikojima types share three somatic antigens in different proportions; Inaba is a loss variant and lacks the b antigen. More than one antigenic variant may be isolated from the stools of a cholera patient, so that these variants cannot be used for tracing infections and do not have any epidemiological significance (Sakazaki & Tamura, 1971). We do not think that any advantage is gained by subdividing vibrios by sugar reactions; the Heiberg (1936) fermentation groups do not correlate with anything and cannot distinguish vibrios from *Aeromonas* species (Sakazaki, Gomez & Sebald, 1967).

A decision to widen the definition of the species *Vibrio cholerae* was made by the International Committee on Systematic Bacteriology Subcommittee on the Taxonomy of Vibrios (Hugh & Feeley, 1972a); in practice, this means that not only true cholera and other vibrios found in faeces, but also those found in water and other situations – which for want of better names have been known as water vibrios, NAG vibrios, NCV, and cholera-like vibrios – are to be placed under the umbrella name *Vibrio cholerae* and further distinguished only by serotype number. We think that this is a most unfortunate decision, a committee decision taken without regard for the consequences in medicine; it is likely to mislead clinicians who, in their naivety, assume that the name attached to an organism and given in the laboratory report, should tell them something. We, as laboratory workers, know that this is not so, and that names can be misleading; but we should not add to the clinician's difficulties by introducing a terminology (it is not nomenclature) that is so misleading that the meaning of the report will be lost. For our part we shall continue to use the common terms for these organisms and reserve the name *Vibrio cholerae* for the classical cholera and el Tor vibrios, and we shall ignore the pontificating recommendations made 'to sharpen the meaning of concepts, convey precise ideas, and expedite international communication' (Hugh & Feeley, 1972a).

The Subcommittee recommended that the micro-aerophilic vibrios should be excluded from the genus *Vibrio* and in this followed the suggestions made by Véron (1965, 1966) for the reorganization of the systematics of *Vibrio* and similar organisms. A misfit among the aerobic vibrios, the organism known as *Vibrio fetus* will, in this edition, be found in Section 7.10.3 under the name *Campylobacter fetus*.

The International Subcommittee (Hugh & Feeley, 1972b) also adopted a minimal characterization for the identification of *Vibrio cholerae* suggested by Hugh & Sakazaki (1972); this was as follows: a Gram-negative, non-sporing rod. Oxidase positive. Glucose fermented without gas production; acid produced from mannitol but not from inositol. H_2S not produced in TSI or Kligler's iron agar. Lysine and ornithine decarboxylated; arginine dihydrolase not produced. Growth in 1% tryptone broth without NaCl. Guanine+cytosine ratio (of DNA) 40–50 mole per cent. The Subcommittee then had a few practical thoughts and rather condescendingly agreed that for routine screening of field strains the decarboxylase and dihydrolase tests and the G+C determinations might be omitted 'where substrates or equipment are not available'. We do not think that G+C ratios will be determinable in routine diagnostic laboratories for some years to come, and not within the useful lifetime of this edition of our *Manual*, so we do not show these values in our diagnostic tables; we hope (and believe) that users will be able to identify vibrios without this item of molecular biological information. However, we recognize that, taxonomically, the G+C of 40–50% for *Vibrio* and 57–60% for *Aeromonas* (Véron, 1966) is the most important character that distinguishes vibrios from aeromonads.

For the isolation of *Vibrio cholerae* and other vibrios both direct plating and enrichment methods should be used. Alkaline peptone water (with subculture from the surface) still has its uses but it should be supplemented by newer media such as salt colistin broth and glucose salt teepol broth. Direct plating of the specimen and also subcultures from the enrichment media are made on selective media such as thiosulphate citrate bile salt sucrose (TCBS) or bromthymol blue salt teepol (BTBST) agars (see Section A2.4.4). After overnight incubation at 37 °C, medium- or large-sized yellow (sucrose-fermenting) colonies are subcultured, checked for purity, and tested against a group 1 antiserum. Biochemical characterization can follow to complete and confirm the identification. Green colonies (sucrose non-fermenting) on TCBS and blue–green colonies on BTBST should be considered as possible strains of *Vibrio parahaemolyticus* (Barrow & Miller, 1972*b*). Normally, *Vibrio cholerae* is a late fermenter of lactose and takes 48 hours to show acid, but in the 1970 cholera season in Calcutta rapid lactose-fermenting strains were isolated (Sanyal, Sakazaki, Prescott & Sinha, 1973).

The species *Vibrio parahaemolyticus* is facultatively halophilic and chitinolytic; it has a world-wide distribution, and travellers infected in one place may become ill on the journey or at their destinations (Peffers *et al.* 1973); medical bacteriologists should, therefore, be aware of it and watching for it. We show its characteristics in Table 7.8*b*. *V. parahaemolyticus* has been isolated from human faeces, sea-water, salt-water fish, and food. Another facultatively halophilic organism, *V. alginolyticus*, is found in sea-water, salt-water fish, and human faeces in descending order of frequency (Sakazaki, Iwanami & Fukumi, 1963; Sakazaki, 1968); this organism swarms on the surface of media without bile salts or one of the Tweens; other characteristics are shown in Table 7.8*b*.

Vibrio parahaemolyticus, like other intestinal pathogens, does not always produce symptoms and its pathogenicity is not easy to prove. Apparently the main reservoir is in salt-water fish and, as the Japanese are great eaters of uncooked fish, it is responsible for more than half of the food-poisoning in Japan (Sakazaki, 1965*a*; Sakazaki, Tamura, Kato, Obara, Yamai & Hobo, 1968). Strains from human faeces differ in haemolytic activity from strains isolated from fish or sea-water, and the human strains show the Kanagawa phenomenon on Wagatsuma agar (the original descriptions are in Japanese but synopses in English are given by Sakazaki *et al.* 1968). A laboratory infection and some feeding tests convinced Sakazaki and his colleagues that strains that produced the Kanagawa phenomenon were potentially pathogenic.

In European waters the organism was thought to be less frequent for only one (a haddock) of 407 samples of fish on sale in Holland yielded *Vibrio parahaemolyticus* (Kampelmacher *et al.* 1970), but Barrow & Miller (1969, 1972*b*) found it

Table 7.8*a* *Second-stage table for* Vibrio, Beneckea, Aeromonas, Plesiomonas, Necromonas *and* Chromobacterium

	1	2	3	4	5	6
Motility	+	+	+	+	−	+
Growth at 37 °C	+	?	+	+	−	D
Growth without NaCl	−a	−	+	+	+	.
Growth in 6% NaCl	D	+	−	−	−	−
Growth in KCN medium	d	.	+	−	−	d
Citrate as C source	+	.	+	−	−	d
Gas from glucose	−	−	d	−	w/−	−
Carbohydrates, acid from:						
inositol	−	−	−	+	−	−
lactose	(+)	−	d	(+)	−	−
sucrose	D	D	+	−	d	d
VP	D	.	d	−	−	−
Starch hydrolysis	+	+	+	−	+	−
Nitrates reduced	+	+	+	+	+	+
Indole	+	D	+	+	−	−
Gelatin hydrolysis	+	D	+	−	+	(+)
Casein hydrolysis	+	D	+	−	.	D
Arginine hydrolysis	−	.	+	d	+	D
Lysine decarboxylase	+	.	−	+	−	−
Ornithine decarboxylase	+	.	−	+	−	.
Lipase	+	.	+	−	+	D
Sensitivity to O/129	+	.	−	−	−	−
Chitin decomposition	d	+	−	.	.	D

1 *Vibrio* spp.
2 *Beneckea* spp.
3 *Aeromonas* sp.
4 *Plesiomonas* sp.
5 *Necromonas* sp.
6 *Chromobacterium* spp.

a Growth in tryptone broth without added NaCl (Hugh & Sakazaki, 1972) but not in peptone water without added NaCl (Sakazaki *et al.* 1963).

in oysters bred in Cornwall. It occurs off both the western and eastern seaboards of the USA (Baross & Liston, 1970; Fishbein *et al.* 1970). Probably many strains have been misidentified; a strain described as a new species, *Aeromonas proteolytica*, by Merkel *et al.* (1964) was probably *Vibrio alginolyticus*. Serological relations between *V. parahaemolyticus* and *V. alginolyticus* were shown

Table 7.8*b* *Third-stage table for* Vibrio, Beneckea, Aeromonas, Plesiomonas, Necromonas *and* Chromobacterium

	1	2	3	4	5	6	7	8	9	10
Motility	+	+	+	+	+	+	+	−	+	+
Swarming surface growth	−	−	−	−	+	−	−	−	−	−
Growth at 37 °C	+	+	+	+	+	+	+	−	+	−
Growth at pH 9	+	+	+	+	.	−	d	−	.	.
Growth without NaCl	−	−	−	−	−	+	+	+	.	.
Growth in 6 % NaCl	−	−	−	+	+	−	−	−	−	.
Growth in KCN medium	d	d	d	+	.	+	−	−	+	d
Citrate as C source	+	+	+	+	+	+	−	−	d	+
Gluconate	d	+	d	−	.	d	−	−	−	−
Glucose, gas from	−	−	−	−	−	d	−	w/−	−	−
Carbohydrates, acid from:										
glucose	+	+	+	+	+	+	+	+	+	−[a]
lactose	(+)	(+)	(+)	−	−	d	(+)	−	−	−
sucrose	+	+	+	−	+	+	−	d	d	−[a]
ONPG	+	+	+	+	+	+	+	+	−	d
VP	−	+	d	−	+	d	−	−	−	−
Indole	+	+	+	+	+	+	+	−	−	−
Gelatin hydrolysis	+	+	+	+	+	+	−	+	+	(+)
Casein hydrolysis	+	+	+	+	.	+		.	+	−
Arginine hydrolysis	−	−	−	−	−	+	d	+	+	−
Chitin hydrolysis	d	d	d	+	+	−	.	.	+	−

1 **Vibrio cholerae**; *V. comma*; cholera vibrio
2 **Vibrio cholerae var. el tor**; *V. eltor*; el Tor vibrio
3 **Vibrio spp.**; NCV (non-cholera vibrio); NAG (non-agglutinating vibrio); water vibrio
4 **Vibrio parahaemolyticus**; *Oceanomonas parahaemolytica*; *Beneckea parahaemolytica*
5 **Vibrio alginolyticus**; *Oceanomonas alginolytica*
6 **Aeromonas hydrophila**; *A. liquefaciens*; *A. punctata*; *A. formicans*
7 **Plesiomonas shigelloides**; C 27; *Aeromonas shigelloides*; *Vibrio shigelloides*; *Fergusonia shigelloides*; *Pseudomonas michigani*
8 **Necromonas salmonicida**; *Aeromonas salmonicida*
9 **Chromobacterium violaceum**
10 **Chromobacterium lividum**

[a] Positive in ASS (Section A 2.6.5).

Symbols used in the table are explained in Tables 5.1 and 5.2 (facing p. 43).

by a common H antigen and some overlapping of the O antigens (Sakazaki, Iwanami & Tamura, 1968).

Vibrio parahaemolyticus may be isolated on media used for the isolation of *Vibrio cholerae* (*sensu stricto*), namely thiosulphate citrate bile salt sucrose (TCBS, obtainable from BBL, Difco, Eiken, and Oxoid; see Appendix H for addresses), or bromthymol blue salt teepol (BTBST) agars (see Section A 2.4.4). Details of isolation techniques are given in English by Sakazaki (1965*a*, *b*; 1969), Barrow & Miller (1972*b*) and Peffers *et al.* (1973). Faeces and small amounts of food may be inoculated into 10 ml volumes of single strength enrich-ment broth (salt colistin, Section A 2.3.1, or glucose salt teepol, Section A 2.3.2). Larger quantities of food should be homogenized in 3 % saline and added to an equal volume of double strength broth. After incubation overnight enrichment media are subcultured heavily to plates of TCBS or BTBST and green or green–blue colonies are subcultured to 3 % NaCl nutrient agar plates for purification. Biochemical tests should be made in media containing 3 % NaCl.

Minidefinition: *Vibrio. Gram-negative rods, motile. Aerobic and facultatively anaerobic. Catalase positive; oxidase positive. Attack sugars by fermentation; gas not produced.*

Lysine and ornithine are decarboxylated; arginine not hydrolysed.

7.8.2   Beneckea (Table 7.8*a*) is a genus of chitin-decomposing bacteria and seems an unlikely candidate for the interest of medical bacteriologists. However one potentially pathogenic vibrio (*Vibrio parahaemolyticus*) is both halophilic and chitino-lytic and Baumann, Baumann & Mandel (1971) would place it in the genus *Beneckea*. The naming of this parahaemolyticus vibrio was discussed at a recent (1973) conference in Japan and on the grounds that the new edition of *Bergey's Manual* (1974) will retain the organism in the genus *Vibrio*, Sakazaki and others argued that the name *Vibrio parahaemolyticus* should be retained, for to change it would cause confusion (personal communication from Dr G. I. Barrow). We accept this recommen-dation, but include a minidefinition of the genus *Beneckea* to indicate the similarity of these organ-isms to those of the genus *Vibrio*.

> **Minidefinition:** *Beneckea. Motile Gram-negative rods. Aerobic and facultatively anaerobic. Catalase positive; oxidase posi-tive. Attack sugars by fermentation; gas not produced. Halophilic; chitinolytic.*

7.8.3   Aeromonas (Table 7.8*a, b*). The subdivision of this genus is not agreed by those who work most closely with the members but it seems likely that only one species is warranted. Eddy (1960, 1962) distinguished the aerogenic, VP-positive, gluconate-positive species (*Aeromonas liquefaciens*) from the anaerogenic, VP-negative, gluconate-negative *A. formicans*; in 1968 *A. formi-cans* was still recognized by Carpenter *et al.* and by Bain & Shewan in their reviews of vibrio-like organisms. On the other hand, Schubert (1967*a, b*) regarded anaerogenic strains as varieties of aero-genic species which he labelled *A. punctata*, *A. hydrophila*, and *A. salmonicida*. Later he (Schubert, 1971) argued that *Aeromonas liquefaciens* was unrecognizable, that the application of the name was doubtful, and that both the taxon and the name should be abandoned; further, that *Aeromonas hydrophila* should be the recognized name of the type species, which he described (and we have taken this description into account in compiling Table

7.8*b*). The main difference between *A. hydrophila* and *A. punctata* (which Schubert had previously favoured as type species) seems to be the production of acetoin (VP positive) by *A. hydrophila*.

We think that Ewing, Hugh & Johnson (1961) were wise to disregard slight strain variations, and to put all strains into one species, *Aeromonas hydro-phila*, and we have followed that course here.

> **Minidefinition:** *Aeromonas. Gram-negative rods; motile. Aerobic and facultatively anaerobic. Catalase positive; oxidase posi-tive. Sugars attacked fermentatively and gas may be produced. Arginine is broken down.*

7.8.4   Plesiomonas (Table 7.8*a, b*). The existence of this genus is almost entirely due to uncertainty about the allocation of its single species, which has been put by different authors into *Aeromonas*, *Vibrio*, and *Pseudomonas*.

The organism is better known by its vernacular designation, C27, than by any of the scientific names that have been applied to it. C 27 (Ferguson & Henderson, 1947) was placed in *Aeromonas* by Ewing & Johnson (1960) and in *Plesiomonas* by Habs & Schubert (1962), supported by Eddy & Carpenter (1964).

The interest that this organism has for medical workers lies in the observation that some strains are agglutinated by phase 1 *Shigella sonnei* antiserum; the organism can readily be distinguished from the shigella by its motility and by its oxidase activity. Its role in human disease is not known but it is not regarded as a pathogen.

> **Minidefinition:** *Plesiomonas. Gram-negative rods; motile. Aerobic and facultatively anaerobic. Catalase positive; oxidase posi-tive. Sugars attacked by fermentation; gas is not produced. Inositol is fermented. Gelatin is not liquefied.*

7.8.5   Necromonas (Tables 7.7*a*; 7.8*a, b*). The single species of this genus is often included in *Aeromonas* as *Aeromonas salmonicida*, and this justifies its place in Table 7.8*a, b*. It does not grow at 37 °C, and although a pathogen for fish it will grow in media without salt.

> **Minidefinition:** *Necromonas. Gram-nega-tive rods; non-motile. Aerobic; facultatively*

anaerobic. Catalase positive; oxidase positive. Attack sugars fermentatively and may produce gas. On the surface of agar media produce a brown diffusible pigment.

7.8.6   Chromobacterium (Tables 7.5; 7.8*a*, *b*) is a genus that encompasses two very different kinds of organism. We dealt with the psychrophilic species, *Chromobacterium lividum*, in Section 7.5.1 and Table 7.5; here we consider *Chromobacterium violaceum*, a mesophilic organism that is more likely to be met in a clinical laboratory. Like *C. lividum*, it produces a violet pigment that is soluble in ethanol, acetone, and amyl alcohol, but it is insoluble in water and does not diffuse through the medium. Pigmentation is encouraged by the presence of mannitol and yeast extract in the medium, but pigment makes the oxidase test difficult to read. Violacein is produced only in the presence of abundant oxygen (Sneath, 1960), and non-pigmented growth from anaerobic cultures might be useful for testing for oxidase.

The older descriptions of *Chromobacterium violaceum* are confusing because the name was given to nearly all cultures that produced a violet pigment. Sneath (1956) applied the name to a mesophil; Leifson (1956) and Eltinge (1956, 1957) to a psychrophil. The nomenclatural problem was referred to the Judicial Commission of the International Committee on Bacteriological Nomenclature which ruled (Opinion 16, 1958) that the mesophilic species should be *Chromobacterium violaceum* and the type species of the genus. Apart from differing in temperature range, *C. lividium* (the psychrophilic species) oxidizes sugars and resembles the oxidative bacteria dealt with in Section 7.5 and Table 7.5; for comparison with the mesophilic species the characters are repeated in Table 7.8*b*.

Chromobacterium violaceum is occasionally pathogenic for man (Sneath *et al.* 1953); a full and useful monograph by Sneath (1960) should be read by those who want to know more of the genus.

Minidefinition: *Chromobacterium violaceum. Gram-negative rods; motile. Aerobic; facultatively anaerobic. Catalase positive; oxidase positive. Attack sugars fermentatively.*

7.9   The enterobacteria
(*Citrobacter, Edwardsiella, Enterobacter, Erwinia, Escherichia, Hafnia, Klebsiella, Morganella, Proteus, Salmonella, Serratia, Shigella, Yersinia*)
***Characters common to members of the group:* Gram-negative rods. Aerobic and facultatively anaerobic. Oxidase negative. Attack sugars fermentatively. Nitrate reduced to nitrite.**

These bacteria are easy to grow on simple media, survive for ten or more years on media in tubes simply sealed with paraffin wax and, being easy and safe to handle, are ideal subjects for students, biochemists, geneticists, and even bacteriologists; laboratory infections do occur but they are rare events. If, as bacteria, they were more exacting in their nutritional requirements or were harder to grow, they would be less popular as bacteriological tools or as 'bags of enzymes', and they would then probably be divided into but a few species in three or four genera. Because some strains are human and animal pathogens and produce intestinal infections and food-poisoning, the group has some epidemiological interest and importance and means have been found to fingerprint the members quite exactly; only a few are pathogenic but these may cause serious infections, so that the importance of the group has become greatly exaggerated. They have been studied exhaustively by large numbers of bacteriologists and have introduced many to taxonomy; they have provided feasts for the splitters and banquets for the geneticists. The result is that they have been divided into a large number of so-called genera and species, and further subdivided into countless serotypes and phage types, but, as Kampelmacher (1959) pointed out, there are no antigenic frontiers in the enterobacteria and there is a great deal of overlapping.

The whole group corresponds to what was *Bacterium* before that genus became the dumping ground for bacteria that could not swiftly and easily be assigned to some other genus. Nowadays it is usual to split the group first into tribes and then into genera, but unless these subdivisions mean something there is little point in making them. As we indicated in a recent review of the group (Cowan in *Bergey's Manual*, 1974), it is conceivable that what are now regarded as tribes may become the genera of the future. In this *Manual* we do not make the division into tribes and our breakdown is simply for convenience, the most pressing reason being the need to fit the table(s) into the book. We have taken genera and species that will be accepted by most (but not by all) bacteriologists and show some characters (not important in themselves) by which they can be distinguished. A second-stage table (7.9*a*) leads on to three third-stage tables (7.9*b*, *d*, *e*) by which an unknown strain of the group can be identified down to species level. The classification of the group is by no means final and the divisions we make do not always correspond to divisions made by others and explains why so many synonyms are necessary. It is only quite recently that the status of Aerobacter has been cleared up by the rejection of this generic name, so that we do not now need to distinguish between Aerobacter and Klebsiella; instead we distinguish Enterobacter from Klebsiella, but this is an advance because Enterobacter is more precisely defined than Aerobacter.

To emphasize that our arrangement is devoid of phylogenetic or hierarchical implications, we have arranged the notes for the subgroups ('genera') in alphabetical order. While our tables are useful in making an identification only down to species level as it is understood in this group, this is well below the level of species in other large groups of bacteria such as corynebacteria and streptococci. We do not proceed to biotypes or to the finer subdivisions made by serological and phage-typing methods since we do not think that many clinical laboratories will have a sufficiently wide range of antisera to carry out this type of work. Fortunately, reference laboratories are available in many countries, and even if their names are national, the services are usually international.

An entirely different method of arriving at an identification of enterobacteria in stages was described by Baer & Washington (1972). In this a score is given to individual characters (acid from mannitol = 5; gas from mannitol = 10; acid from lactose = 20; growth in KCN medium = 320), and the total score is looked up in one or more identification tables. This numerical diagnostic key will be discussed in Chapter 9.

In intestinal infections the enterobacteria may be isolated from the blood stream, intestinal contents (bile or faeces), often from urine, and occasionally from marrow biopsies. When occurring in intestinal contents the enterobacteria are part of a mixed bacterial flora, and isolations are made from enrichment and selective media, from which pure cultures must be obtained by plating on non-inhibitory media.

7.9.1   Aerobacter is a name that has caused much confusion because it has been applied to different organisms. Originally used by Beijerinck (1900) for organisms (motile or non-motile) that had optimal temperatures about 28 °C but would not grow at 37 °C, it was later used by bacteriologists all over the world for organisms that grew at 37 °C or higher, and were usually non-motile. In 1958 Hormaeche & Edwards, who wanted to distinguish klebsiellas from motile bacteria with similar IMViC reactions, used the name for a motile organism that grew at 37 °C; when they realized the difficulties arising from the use of the same name for two different organisms, they changed the name of the group of motile bacteria to Enterobacter (Hormaeche & Edwards, 1960).

Carpenter and many others (1970) asked the Judicial Commission to give an opinion on the use of the name Aerobacter; the Commission issued Opinion 46 (1971) and declared the name rejected.

7.9.2   Bacterium, as a generic name, has been outlawed for a great many years (Opinion 4, revised, 1954) and is now seldom used. The reason for its rejection was the different usage in different countries, although in any one country its use was probably well known and understood.

The English school used it for Gram-negative rods that were essentially the enterobacteria; in the sixth edition of *Bergey's Manual* (1948), which was typical of American practice at that time, the 'genus' *Bacterium* included both Gram-positive and Gram-negative rods.

Most organisms that were formerly *Bacterium this-or-that* in medical laboratories will be found in this *Manual* in Section 7.9 among the enterobacteria. Of the exceptions, *Bacterium anitratum* will be found in Section 7.4.2 under the name *Acinetobacter anitratus*, and not under the strange and tongue-twisting *Acinetobacter calcoaceticus* which purists would inflict on us. *Bacterium typhi flavum*, which for a long time defied our efforts to put it into a suitable genus, has now found a place in *Erwinia* (Section 7.9.6) as *Erwinia herbicola* (Graham & Hodgkiss, 1967).

7.9.3   Citrobacter (Table 7.9*a, b*). The common water and soil forms are rapid lactose fermenters and are *Citrobacter freundii*; a less common variety produces indole and this is one of the intermediate coliforms of water bacteriologists, or *C. freundii* II (see Report, 1956*b*). The Ballerup and Bethesda groups were lactose non-fermenters or late fermenters of the Citrobacter group, and when grown in plate cultures could be recognized by the characteristically foul odour they produced.

Sedlák and his colleagues (1971), in a review of 8000 strains of the genus, think that it is made up of 'conditional' intestinal pathogens, the word conditional, like potential, putative, and opportunistic of other writers, meaning that they can be pathogenic when given the opportunity, that is when conditions are suitable for them to multiply in an unusual situation.

The genus has an unusual history; it was created by Werkman & Gillen (1932) for bacteria that produced trimethylene glycol from glycerol; no one ever used any complicated test for this substance but instead paid attention to the character (utilization of citrate as C source) after which the genus was named. Sedlák *et al.* recognized two species: *Citrobacter freundii*, H_2S positive; indole negative, and malonate positive; and *C. intermedius* with the opposite characters; obviously there are many intergrading forms, which account for the seven species listed by Werkman & Gillen. Of those seven species only *Citrobacter freundii* became established; Ewing & Davis (1972) would revive *C. diversus* for the organism named *C. koseri* by Frederiksen (1970) and *Levinea amalonatica* and *L. malonatica* by Young *et al.* (1971).

Chemical analysis of the lipopolysaccharides of the O antigens indicates that citrobacters are 'closely related to *E. coli*' and that of twenty citrobacter chemotypes identified, eleven were 'identical with

chemotypes occurring in *Salmonella* and *E. coli*' (Keleti *et al.* 1971). Perhaps citrobacters should be considered as a connecting link uniting Escherichia and Salmonella; if that is a fair description of the situation then bacteriologists can be excused for wanting a simple test for differentiating *Citrobacter* from *Salmonella*. Catsaras & Buttiaux (1963) thought that the lysine decarboxylase and KCN tests were useful; citrobacters were lysine negative and KCN positive; salmonellas were lysine positive (with a few exceptions) and KCN negative. Pickett & Goodman (1966) suggested the ONPG test, but this also has its exceptions.

Minidefinition: *Citrobacter. Gram-negative rods; motile. Aerobic and facultatively anaerobic. Catalase positive; oxidase negative. Attack sugars fermentatively; gas is produced. Citrate positive; KCN positive.*

7.9.4   Edwardsiella (Table 7.9*a, b*). Even within the splitters' concepts of the enterobacteria, Edwardsiella seems to be an unnecessary genus. In 1962 it was described (in Japanese) by Sakazaki (1967 in English) as the Asakusa group, but presumably not thought worthy of generic status. It was redescribed by King & Adler (1964) as the Bartholomew group, and elevated to a genus by Ewing *et al.* (1965). The features that distinguish it from Escherichia are mainly quantitative; it produces H_2S in TSI (*Escherichia coli* is negative on TSI but produces H_2S when tested by a more sensitive method). *Edwardsiella tarda* ferments fewer sugars and more slowly (hence the name), and a greater proportion of strains decarboxylate lysine and ornithine. In terms of DNA relatedness, *Edwardsiella tarda* forms a compact group (Brenner, 1973).

Edwardsiella has much in common with some shigellas which, within themselves have differences comparable with those between Escherichia and Edwardsiella. In short, Edwardsiella is a good example of the excessive splitting at 'generic' level that has taken place within the enterobacteria. In our opinion it is better regarded as a biotype of *Escherichia coli*; less satisfactorily as a species, *Escherichia tarda*.

Minidefinition: *Edwardsiella. Gram-negative rods; motile. Aerobic and faculta-*

Table 7.9a *Second-stage table for differentiation of the enterobacteria (majority reactions)*

	1	2	3	4	5	6	7	8	9	10	11	12	13	14
Motility	D	+	D	−	+	+	+	+	+	+	+	+	−	−
Growth in KCN medium	−	−	−	−	D	−	−	+	+	+	+	+	D	+
Citrate as C source	−	−	−	−	+	+	+	−	+	+	+	+	+	d
Gas from glucose	D	+	−	−	+	D	−	+	D	+	d	+	D	D
MR test	+	+	+	+	+	+	−	+	+	−	d	−	D	+
VP test	−	−	−	−	−	−	d	−	d	+	+	+	D	−
Indole	+	+	−	d	D	−	−	+	D	−	−	−	D	−
Gelatin	−	−	−	−	−	D	+	−	D	−	+	(d)	D	−
Urease	−	−	D	−	D	−	−	+	D	−	d	d	+	d
Phenylalanine	−	−	−	−	−	−	+	+	+	−	−	−	−	−
H₂S from TSI	−	+	−	−	D	+	.	−	D	−	−	−	−	−
Lysine decarboxylase	+	+	−	−	−	+	−	−	−	+	d	D	+	d
Ornithine decarboxylase	d	+	D	D	d	D	−	+	D	+	D	+	−	−

Details in Table   7.9b   7.9d   7.9e

1 **Escherichia coli;** A–D group
2 **Edwardsiella tarda;** Asakusa biotype; Bartholomew group
3 **Yersinia** spp.
4 **Shigella** spp.
5 **Citrobacter** spp.; *Levinea* spp.
6 **Salmonella** spp. and serotypes
7 **Erwinia herbicola**
8 **Morganella morganii;** *Proteus morganii*
9 **Proteus** spp. (including Providence group)
10 **Hafnia alvei**
11 **Serratia** spp.
12 **Enterobacter** spp.
13 **Klebsiella aerogenes;** K. atlantae; K. edwardsii; K. oxytoca; K. pneumoniae
14 **Klebsiella ozaenae;** K. rhinoscleromatis

tively anaerobic. Catalase positive; oxidase negative. Attack glucose fermentatively; produce gas. H₂S produced on TSI.

7.9.5   Enterobacter (Table 7.9a, e) was the name proposed by Hormaeche & Edwards (1960) for a group of motile organisms with IMViC reactions − − + +, and *Enterobacter cloacae* (*B. cloacae* Jordan, 1890; *Cloaca cloacae* Castellani & Chalmers, 1919) was designated as the type species. Some strains produce a non-diffusible yellow pigment. Other organisms have been placed in the genus, *Enterobacter aerogenes*, and a psychrophil, *E. liquefaciens*.

The characters of the members of the group are very similar to those of Hafnia and Serratia, and Edwards & Ewing (1972) include *Hafnia alvei* (Section 7.9.8) in *Enterobacter*. We regard Hafnia as a lactose non-fermenting counterpart of Enterobacter and at this revision have not thought it necessary to merge the two groups; our preference is a merger of many more groups but we do not

think that the time is yet ripe for this. On the other hand we think that the psychrophil *E. liquefaciens*, which has much in common with *Serratia marcescens* (Section 7.9.14) should be moved to that group. This leaves *Enterobacter* with two species, *E. cloacae* and *E. aerogenes*. Both these species are only weakly urease positive and so enable Matsen's (1970) ten-minute test for distinguishing between Enterobacter (negative) and Klebsiella (positive) to work, since it depends on the relative inactivity of the *Enterobacter* spp.

> **Minidefinition:** *Enterobacter. Gram-negative rods; motile. Aerobic and facultatively anaerobic. Catalase positive; oxidase negative. Attack sugars fermentatively; gas is produced. VP positive; gluconate positive. Gelatin may be liquefied slowly. Produce ornithine decarboxylase.*

7.9.6   Erwinia (Table 7.9a, d). This genus was named by Winslow *et al.* (1917) after Erwin F. Smith, a plant pathologist who did not agree with

Table 7.9b *Third-stage table for the enterobacteria* (*part* 1)

	1	2	3	4	5	6	7	8	9	10	11	12	13	14	15
Motility	d	−	+	−	+	+	−	−	−	−	−	−	+	+	+
Catalase	+	+	+	+	+	+	−	+	+	+	+	+	+	+	+
Growth in KCN medium	−	−	−	−	−	−	−	−	−	−	−	−	+	−	+
Growth on 4 % selenite	+	+	+	−	+	d	+	+		·	+	+	+	·	·
Citrate as C source	−	−	−	−	−	−	−	−		·	+	+	+	·	·
Malonate	−	−	−	−	−	−	−	−	−	−	−	−	−	+	d
Carbohydrates:															
gas from glucose	+	−	+	−	−	−	−	−	−	d	−	−	+	+	+
acid from:															
adonitol	−	−	−	−	+	−	−	−	−	−	−	−	−	−	−
arabinose	+	+	−	+	+	+	−	d	+	d	+	−	+	+	d
dulcitol	d	d	−	−	−	−	−	−	−	(d)	+	+	+	+	+
lactose	+	d	−	−	−	−	−	−	−	(d)	−	−	(+)	(d)	(d)
maltose	+	+	+	+	+	+	−	d	d	d	d	+	+	+	+
mannitol	+	+	−	+	+	+	−	−	+	+	+	+	+	+	·
rhamnose	d	d	−	(+)	+	−	−	d	−	−	−	d	+	+	+
salicin	d	−	−	+	+	−	−	−	−	−	−	−	d	+	+
sorbitol	d	d	−	−	−	+	−	d	d	d	d	−	+	+	+
sucrose	d	d	−	−	−	+	−	−	−	−	−	(+)	d	d	−
trehalose	+	·	−	+	+	+	+	+	d	(+)	+	+	+	+	−
xylose	d	d	−	+	+	(+)	−	−	−	−	−	−	+	+	·
ONPG	+	d	+	+	+	+	+	d	−	−	−	+	+	+	·
Aesculin hydrolysis	d	·	−	+	+	−	−	−	−	−	−	−	−	−	+
Indole	+	+	+	−	−	d	−	d	d	−	d	−	−	+	+
Urease	−	−	−	−	+	+	−	−	−	−	−	−	−	+	+
H$_2$S from TSI	−	−	+	−	−	−	−	−	−	−	−	−	−	w	+
Arginine dihydrolase	d	d	−	−	−	−	−	−	−	d	d	−	d	d	−
Lysine decarboxylase	+	d	+	−	−	−	−	−	−	−	−	−	−	−	+
Ornithine decarboxylase	d	d	+	−	−	+	−	−	−	−	−	+	d	+	+

1 **Escherichia coli**

2 **A–D group; Alkalescens–dispar group; Escherichia group**

3 **Edwardsiella tarda**; Asakusa group; Bartholomew group

4 **Yersinia pestis**; *Pasteurella pestis*; the plague bacillus

5 **Yersinia pseudotuberculosis**; *Pasteurella pseudotuberculosis*; *P. rodentium*

6 **Yersinia enterocolitica**; Pasteurella X

7 **Shigella dysenteriae (serotype) 1**; *Shigella shigae*; Shiga's bacillus

8 **Shigella dysenteriae 2–10**; (2 = *S. schmitzii*; *S. ambigua*; Schmitz's bacillus); Large–Sach's group

9 **Shigella flexneri (serotypes) 1–5**; Flexner dysentery bacilli

10 **Shigella flexneri 6**; Boyd 88; Newcastle bacillus; Manchester bacillus (see Table 7.9c)

11 **Shigella boydii (serotypes) 1–15**; Boyd's dysentery bacilli

12 **Shigella sonnei**

13 **Citrobacter freundii**; *Escherichia freundii*; *Salmonella coli*; *S. ballerup*; *S. hormaechei*; Bethesda–Ballerup group

14 **Citrobacter koseri**; *C. diversus*

15 **Levinea spp.**

Symbols used in the table are explained in Tables 5.1 and 5.2 (facing p. 43).

the idea of making plant pathogenicity the foundation stone of a new genus, and continually argued against it. The organisms resemble coliforms in their cultural characteristics and Elrod (1942) thought that they were related both to *Citrobacter freundii* and to *Enterobacter cloacae*.

To anticipate the interest of medical bacteriologists in these organisms, we now think that certain bacteria isolated from human and other animal sources are so similar to organisms isolated from plants that they should all be included in the same genus; as the plant organisms are part of a recognized genus, *Erwinia*, and the strains from mammals have never been satisfactorily classified they are all considered as *Erwinia* species. In favour of this treatment is the observation of Lakso & Starr (1970) that about a third of the animal strains they tested were as pathogenic for plants as

Table 7.9c *Unusual biochemical characteristics of*
Shigella flexneri 6 *biotypes* (modified from
Carpenter, Lapage & Steel, 1966)

	1	2	3	4
Glucose (acid)	+	+	+	+
(gas)	−	d	+	−
Mannitol (acid)	+	−	+	+
Dulcitol (acid)	(d)	(d)	(d)	−
Indole	−	−	−	d

1 **Shigella flexneri 6**; Boyd 88 biotype
2 **Shigella flexneri 6**; Newcastle biotype; *S. newcastle*
3 **Shigella flexneri 6**; Manchester biotype; Denton strains
  (Downie *et al.* 1933)
4 **Shigella flexneri** serotypes 1–5

Symbols used in the table are explained in Tables 5.1 and
5.2 (facing p. 43).

some of the species considered to be natural
phytopathogens.

Going back to strains labelled *Bacterium typhi
flavum* (Cruickshank, 1935), which for many years
could not be placed satisfactorily among the usual
'medical' bacteria, these organisms are now considered to be *Erwinia herbicola* (Graham & Hodgkiss, 1967). Similar organisms have been isolated
in many clinical laboratories but the characterizations do not always agree with those of the plant
pathologists. Discrepancies may be due to differences in media and, probably, temperature of
incubation; for example, Ewing & Fife (1972)
found that about a quarter of their strains produced
gas from glucose, and their characterizations made
them allocate their strains to *Enterobacter* as
Enterobacter agglomerans. Other sources we have
consulted report the human and animals strains to be
anaerogenic and these results point less clearly to
Enterobacter. After studying the descriptions our
preference is towards Proteus, but as we have
condoned so much splitting among the enterobacteria we are content to leave them in Erwinia as
Erwinia herbicola.

Although we are not here concerned with the
classification and identification of the phytopathogenic erwinias, we should note that not all is neat
and tidy, and Starr & Mandel (1969) are agnostic
about the genus. Fermentation end-products merely

support the argument that *Erwinia* is a member of
the Enterobacteriaceae (White & Starr, 1971), but
for the phytopathogens do not provide any better
guide to species than they do for the animal strains.

Two characters not shown in our tables are the
yellow pigmentation of the colonies, and the
symplasmata (sausage-shaped aggregates of bacteria) seen in hanging-drop preparations of the
condensation water from slope cultures (Gilardi *et
al.* 1970a).

> **Minidefinition:** *Erwinia. Gram-negative
> rods; motile. Aerobic and facultatively
> anaerobic. Catalase positive; oxidase nega-
> tive. Attack sugars fermentatively, usually
> without producing gas. Urease negative;
> phenylalanine positive. KCN negative.*

7.9.7 Escherichia (Table 7.9a, b), like many
other enterobacteria, is subdivided into numerous
serotypes, some of which seem to cause infections
in man and are especially associated with gastro-
enteritis of infants (Taylor, 1961, 1966). Biochemical
varieties of *Escherichia coli* (e.g. commune,
communior) formed on the basis of differences in
sugar reactions, have gone out of fashion and are
not now regarded as significant; another important
change in approach to Escherichia is the view that
lactose-negative strains are acceptable in the group.
A–D group was a term used for organisms named
B. alkalescens and *B. dispar* by Andrewes (1918),
which were once thought to be shigellas. They
are now considered to be anaerogenic (and non-
motile) biotypes of *Escherichia*, with which there is
antigenic overlapping (Ewing, 1949b). *B. alkalescens*
is lactose negative and *B. dispar* is lactose positive,
and on the basis of the ONPG test Szturm-
Rubinsten & Piéchaud (1962) recognize two biotypes.

Water bacteriologists have a classification of
their own based on indole and gas production from
lactose at 44 °C (Report, 1956b, c).

Many strains of Escherichia are non-motile or
only feebly motile on first isolation, and for that
reason motility is shown as a 'd' character in
Table 7.9b.

> **Minidefinition:** *Escherichia. Gram-negative
> rods; motile. Aerobic and facultatively
> anaerobic. Catalase positive; oxidase*

Table 7.9d *Third-stage table for the enterobacteria (part 2)*

	16	17	18	19	20	21	22	23	24	25	26	27	28	29	30
Motility	+	−	−	+	+	+	+	+	+	+	+	+	+	+	+
Pigment	−	−	−	−	−	−	−	−	+	−	−	−	+	+	+
Growth in KCN medium	−	−	−	−	−	−	−	+	−	+	+	+	+	+	+
Citrate as C source	−	d	d	(+)	+	+	+	+	+	−	d	(+)	+	+	+
Gluconate	.	.	.	.	.	.	.	.	d	−	−	d	+	+	+
Malonate	−	−	−	−	−	+	+	−	d	−	−	d	−	−	−
Carbohydrates:															
gas from glucose	−	+	−	+	+	+	+	+	−	+	+	+	−	+	−
acid from:															
adonitol	−	−	−	−	−	−	−	−	−	−	−	−	−	−	−
arabinose	−	+	+	−	+	+	+	+	+	−	−	−	+	+	−
dulcitol	(d)	−	+	(d)	+	+	+	+	+	−	−	−	−	−	−
glycerol	(w)	−	(+)	−	(d)	.	.	.	d	(d)	(+)	+	(+)	(d)	(+)
inositol	−	−	−	−	d	−	−	.	d	−	−	+	(+)	(d)	(+)
lactose	−	−	−	−	−	−	+/(x)	−	d	−	−	−	+	−	+
maltose	+	(d)	+	+	+	+	+	+	+	−	+	−	−	−	−
mannitol	+	+	+	+	+	+	+	+	+	−	−	−	−	−	−
rhamnose	−	+	(+)	+	+	+	+	+	+	−	−	−	+	−	−
salicin	−	−	−	−	−	−	−	+	d	−	−	−	d	−	−
sucrose	−	−	−	−	−	−	−	+	+	d	(d)	(d)	d	−	(+)
trehalose	+	+	+	−	+	+	+	+	+	d	(+)	(+)	d	(d)	(+)
xylose	d	+	+	+	+	+	+	+	+	−	(+)	+	d	−	d
ONPG	−	−	−	−	−	−/w	+	−	+	−	−	−	−	−	−
VP test	−	−	−	−	−	−	−	−	d	−	−	d^a	−	−	−
Aesculin hydrolysis	.	.	.	−	.	.	.	.	d	−	d	−	d	−	−
Indole	−	−	−	−	−	−	−	−	−	+	d	−	d	−	−
Gelatin hydrolysis	−	−	−	−	−	(+)	(+)	(+)	+	−	+	−	+	+	+
Urease	−	−	−	−	−	−	−	−	+	−	+	+	−	−	−
H₂S from TSI	+	.	.	d	+	+	+	+	.	−	+	+	+	−	−
Arginine dihydrolase	(d)	+	(+)	(+)	(+)	.	−	.	.	−	−	−	−	−	−
Lysine decarboxylase	+	+	+	+	+	+	+	+	−	+	−	−	−	−	−
Ornithine decarboxylase	−	+	−	+	+	+	+	+	−	+	−	+	−	−	−
Phenylalanine	−	−	−	−	−	−	−	−	+	+	+	+	+	+	+

16 **Salmonella typhi**

17 **Salmonella pullorum**

18 **Salmonella gallinarum**

19 **Salmonella choleraesuis**

20 **Salmonella kauffmannii**; *S. enterica*; *S. enteritidis* serotype (bioser) xyz; Salmonella subgenus I

21 **Salmonella salamae**; *S. dar-es-salaam*; Salmonella subgenus II

22 **Salmonella arizonae**; Salmonella subgenus III; *Arizona arizonae*; *A. hinshawii*

23 **Salmonella houtenae**; Salmonella subgenus IV

24 **Erwinia herbicola**; *Bacterium typhi flavum*; *Enterobacter agglomerans*

25 **Morganella morganii**; *Proteus morganii*; Morgan's no. 1 bacillus

26 **Proteus vulgaris**; *Proteus hauseri* (part of)

27 **Proteus mirabilis**; *P. hauseri* (part of)

28 **Proteus rettgeri**; *Rettgerella rettgeri*

29 **Proteus inconstans**; *Proteus providenciae*; *Providencia providenciae*; *Providencia alcalifaciens*; *Proteus inconstans* A

30 **Proteus stuartii**; *Proteus inconstans* B; *Proteus providenciae* B; *Providencia stuartii*

^{a} More strains are positive at 22 °C than at 37 °C.

Table 7.9e *Third-stage table for the enterobacteria (part 3)*

	31	32	33	34	35	36	37	38	39	40	41	42	43	44
Motility	+	+	+	+	+	+	−	−	−	−	−	−	−	−
Pigment	−	d^b	−	d^b	d^c	−	−	−	−	−	−	−	−	−
Growth in KCN medium	+	+	+	+	+	+	+	+	−	+	+	d	+	+
Citrate as C source	+	+	+	d	+	+	+	+	+	+	d	−	d	
Gluconate	+	+	+	+	+	+	+	+	d	d	+	d	−	−
Malonate	d	d	−	d	d	+	+	.	+	−	d	+	−	+
Carbohydrates:														
gas from glucose	+	d	+	d	+	+	+	+	+	+	−	+	d	−
acid from:														
adonitol	−	d	−	+	d	+	+	+	+	.	.	+	+	+
arabinose	+	−	+	+	+	+	+	+	+	.	.	+	+	+
dulcitol	−	−	−	−	d	d	d	+	+	−	−	−	d	−
glycerol	+	+	+	d	d	+	+	+	+	.	.	+	+	+
inositol	−	d	+	d	−	+	+	+	+	.	.	+	+	d
lactose	−	−	d	+	d	+	+	+	+	(+)	(+)	+	(+)	−
maltose	+	+	+	+	+	+	+	+	+	+	+	+	+	+
mannitol	+	+	+	+	+	+	+	+	+	+	+	+	+	+
raffinose	−	−	d	+	+	+	+	+	+	.	.	+	+	+
rhamnose	+	−	−	−	+	+	+	+	+	.	.	+	+	d
salicin	−	+	+	+	+	+	+	+	+	.	.	+	+	+
sorbitol	d	+	d	d	d	+	+	+	+	.	.	+	+	+
sucrose	d	+	+	+	+	+	+	+	+	+	+	+	+	+
trehalose	+	+	+	+	+	+	+	+	+	+	+	+	+	+
xylose	d	(d)	+	+	+	+	+	+	+	+	+	+	+	+
ONPG	+	+	+	+	+	+	+	+	+	+	+	+	+	−
MR test	−	d	d	d	−	−	−	−	+	+	d	d	+	+
VP test^d	+	+	+	+	+	+	+	+	−	d	+	d	−	−
Aesculin hydrolysis	−	d	d	+	−	+	+	.	.	.	.	.	d	+
Indole	−	−	−	−	−	−	−	+	−	−	−	−	−	−
Gelatin hydrolysis	−	+	+	+	(+)	d	(d)	+	−	−	−	−	−	−
Urease	−	w/−	d	d	d	−/w	+	+	+	+	+	−	d	+
H₂S from TSI	−	−	−	−	−	−	−	−	−	−	−	−	−	−
Arginine dihydrolase	−	−	−	−	+	−	−	−	−	−	−	−	−	−
Lysine decarboxylase	+	+	d	d	−	+	+	+	+	+	+	d	d	−
Ornithine decarboxylase	+	+	+	−	+	+	−	−	−	−	−	−	−	−
DNase	−	+	+	+	−	−	−	−	−	−	−	−	−	−

31 **Hafnia alvei;** *Enterobacter alvei*

32 **Serratia marcescens;** *Erythrobacillus prodigiosus; Chromobacterium prodigiosum*

33 **Serratia liquefaciens;** *Enterobacter liquefaciens; Aerobacter liquefaciens*

34 **Serratia rubidaea;** Serratia biotype II (Bascomb *et al.* 1971); ? Phenon B (Grimont *et al.* 1972)

35 **Enterobacter cloacae;** *Cloaca cloacae; Aerobacter cloacae*

36 **Enterobacter aerogenes;** (NOT *Aerobacter aerogenes* Beijerinck)

37 **Klebsiella aerogenes;** *K. pneumoniae* (*sensu lato*); (NOT *Aerobacter aerogenes* Beijerinck)

38 **Klebsiella oxytoca**

39 **Klebsiella pneumoniae** (*sensu stricto*); Friedländer's pneumobacillus

40 **Klebsiella atlantae** n. sp.; *K. edwardsii* var. *atlantae*

41 **Klebsiella edwardsii;** *K. edwardsii* var. *edwardsii*

42 **Unnamed klebsiella** (Bascomb *et al.*)

43 **Klebsiella ozaenae**

44 **Klebsiella rhinoscleromatis**

^b pigment pink or red.   ^c pigment yellow.   ^d at 22–30 °C.

Symbols used in the table are explained in Tables 5.1 and 5.2 (facing p. 43).

negative. Attack sugars fermentatively; gas normally produced. Citrate negative; KCN negative.

7.9.8 Hafnia (Table 7.9a, e). The Hafnia group was described by Stuart & Rustigian (1943a) as their biotype 32011. It is the lactose non-fermenting counterpart of the Enterobacter group, and Sakazaki (1961) and Ewing (1963) have suggested that these groups should be combined. As with Serratia, the biochemical characters are subject to temperature variations, and the most typical results are obtained at 25–30 °C.

The 32011 organism had the misfortune to be named *Paracolobactrum aerogenoides* by Eveland & Faber (1953) but this name, like that of the 'genus' *Colobactrum* (Borman, Stuart & Wheeler, 1944), will be remembered only as a taxonomic *faux pas*.

Priest, Somerville, Cole & Hough (1973) have transferred a common brewery contaminant to the group as *Hafnia protea*.

> **Minidefinition:** *Hafnia. Gram-negative rods; motile. Aerobic and facultatively anaerobic. Catalase positive; oxidase negative. Attack sugars fermentatively and gas is produced. Gelatin is not liquefied; urea is not hydrolysed.*

7.9.9 Klebsiella (Table 7.9a, e). For many years the main problem in identifying Friedländer's bacillus was to distinguish it from *Aerobacter aerogenes* which was considered to be a non-motile organism. Much less difficult is its separation from the motile organism we now know as *Enterobacter aerogenes* (but for a short time known as *Aerobacter aerogenes* Hormaeche & Edwards 1958); Matsen (1970), using a paper strip test for urease, claims to be able to make the distinction in ten minutes. This contrasts with the lengthy but thought-provoking DNA reassociation experiments made by Brenner, Steigerwalt & Fanning (1972) which provide much more convincing (but not routine) evidence (see also Brenner, 1973).

Another naming problem now enters the arena, since *Klebsiella aerogenes* (Report, 1956b) is, by many workers, named *K. pneumoniae*. The classification of klebsiellas used in this *Manual* is based

on that of Cowan, Steel, Shaw & Duguid (1960), but some slight changes have been made. What we regard as *Klebsiella pneumoniae* is a more closely defined taxon than the *K. pneumoniae* of many other workers (e.g. Ørskov in *Bergey's Manual*, 1974; Edwards & Ewing, 1972) and we accept the term used by Bascomb, Lapage, Willcox & Curtis (1971) for our species as *Klebsiella pneumoniae* (*sensu stricto*) because it helps to contrast *K. pneumoniae* (*sensu lato*) of Ørskov and others. The *K. pneumoniae* (*sensu lato*) taxon embraces our *K. aerogenes* and species we now designate as *Klebsiella edwardsii* and *Klebsiella atlantae* n. sp. by raising the variety *K. edwardsii* var. *atlantae* to a species (thereby eliminating the unintentional confusion created by the transpositions of Ślopek & Durlakowa (1967) and Durlakowa *et al.* (1967)). *Klebsiella atlantae* is the only klebsiella to be negative in a new colorimetric test (Mulczyk & Szewczuk, 1970). The correlation between the species and capsule serotypes is: *Klebsiella aerogenes* (*K. pneumoniae, sensu lato*), all types; *K. pneumoniae* (*sensu stricto*), type 3; *K. edwardsii*, types 1 and 2; *K. atlantae*, type 1; *K. rhinoscleromatis*, type 3; *K. ozaenae*, types 3, 4, 5, and 6. *K. pneumoniae*, *K. edwardsii* and *K. atlantae* are associated with acute infections, *K. ozaenae* with chronic lung disease, but *K. aerogenes* is seldom pathogenic (Fallon, 1973).

The classification of the Enterobacteriaceae Subcommittee takes little account of the great range of biochemical characters within the group (Ørskov, 1957). Like most enterobacteria, the reactivity of klebsiella antigens extends beyond the klebsiella group.

Indole-positive forms are said to be not uncommon and strains that produce indole and liquefy gelatin have been named *K. oxytoca*; Lautrop (1956b) and Hugh (1959) think that these strains should be excluded from *Klebsiella*, but Ørskov (1955, 1957) and Ewing (1963) prefer to retain them in the genus. Cowan *et al.* (1960) excluded both motile forms and strains that liquefied gelatin, but we have now joined Ida Ørskov and Ewing and think that they should be retained; if they are not retained, where would we put them? In Table 7.9e *K. oxytoca* is included for the gelatin- and indole-positive forms.

Some strains of *Klebsiella pneumoniae* (*sensu lato*) are able to fix atmospheric nitrogen (Mahl, Wilson, Fife & Ewing, 1965) but this character does not seem to have any taxonomic value and cannot be used in the identification of Klebsiella species.

> **Minidefinition:** *Klebsiella. Gram-negative rods; non-motile. Aerobic and facultatively anaerobic. Catalase positive; oxidase negative. Attack sugars fermentatively, usually with the production of gas. KCN and VP positive (important exceptions). Ornithine decarboxylase not produced. Urea generally hydrolysed. Phenylalanine negative.*

7.9.10 Levinea (Table 7.9a, b). It would be illogical not to mention this 'genus' when we have included Edwardsiella in our notes. Young *et al.* (1971), who described 108 strains of Levinea, admitted that it closely resembled *Citrobacter* and *Enterobacter*, but justified its creation on the grounds that it produced indole and was methyl red positive. These are not very substantial grounds for making a new genus, especially as in making their comparison with Citrobacter they erroneously recorded that organism as MR negative.

We do not think that the minidefinition we have produced for Levinea from the description of Young *et al.* differs in any significant way from that for Citrobacter (Section 7.9.3) and agree with Ewing & Davis (1972a) that strains of this 'genus' would be better included in *Citrobacter diversus*.

> **Minidefinition:** *Levinea. Gram-negative rods; motile. Aerobic and facultatively anaerobic. Catalase positive; oxidase negative. Attack sugars fermentatively; gas is produced. Citrate positive; KCN positive. Indole produced.*

7.9.11 Morganella (Table 7.9a, d). Bacteriologists have been fascinated by Morgan's number 1 bacillus (Morgan, 1906), a quite unimportant organism in spite of Morgan's belief that it was the cause of 'summer diarrhoea' in infants. Thjøtta (1920) thought that it was a 'metacolon' (*Escherichia coli* in today's terms); Jordan *et al.* (1935) doubted whether there was a species well enough characterized to be recognized and preferred to think

of it as a large and variable group. To Rauss (1936) it was a member of the Proteus group, and he showed that on a solid medium of low agar content it would swarm as Proteus species swarmed on ordinary nutrient agar media. Fulton (1943) proposed a separate genus, *Morganella*, for it. Richard (1965) found that it had four to ten times the urease activity of other Proteus species, and he thought that this put it into a category of its own. Meanwhile, Rauss & Vörös (1959) had joined the ranks of the separatists and supported the creation of *Morganella*.

Convincing evidence for a difference between Morgan's bacillus and Proteus species has come from the research laboratories; Dr H. Lautrop tells us that its urease and phenylalanine deaminase are serologically distinct from those of *Proteus* species, and molecular biologists have shown that the G+C content of the DNAs of the organisms are different, 50% for Morgan's no. 1 and 40% for *Proteus* spp.; such a wide difference is unlikely to be found between members of the same genus.

Unfortunately this kind of information is obtained by methods that are not yet available in routine clinical laboratories; we must make our distinctions and identifications on the results of more routine tests and include sufficient tests in our repertoire to show up differences in as convincing a manner as possible.

From a strictly medical angle, it is doubtful if the effort to distinguish these organisms is worthwhile, for neither *Morganella* nor *Proteus* species appears to have been incriminated as a pathogen.

But as laboratory nuisances they both hold high places.

> **Minidefinition:** *Morganella. Gram-negative rods; motile. Aerobic and facultatively anaerobic. Catalase positive; oxidase negative. Glucose is fermented with the production of a small bubble of gas. Phenylalanine positive; urease positive. Citrate negative; gelatin negative.*

7.9.12 Proteus (Table 7.9a, d). The collection of species in the genus *Proteus* and the various proposals to separate them again as distinct genera have the monotonous sounds of so much taxonomic argument; we shall summarize this and give sufficient references for those who would relish the argument.

Rustigian & Stuart (1945) proposed that four species of the genus should be recognized, *Proteus vulgaris*, *P. mirabilis*, *P. morganii*, and *P. rettgeri*; this arrangement gained wide acceptance, though a few preferred to combine the first two species as *Proteus hauseri*. Because the 29911 group of Stuart *et al.* (1946) was phenylalanine positive it was added to *Proteus* by Singer & Bar-Chay (1954), Buttiaux *et al.* (1954) and Shaw & Clarke (1955) as the Providence group or as *Proteus inconstans*.

In the opposite direction, several splittings and new genera were proposed: *Morganella* by Fulton (1943) for Morgan's no. 1 bacillus; Proom & Woiwod (1951) suggested the exclusion of Rettger's bacillus from *Proteus*, and Kauffmann (1953) created a new genus for it (*Rettgerella*). Kauffmann & Edwards (1952) listed a new genus *Providencia*; Ewing (1962) described it and named two species, *P. alcalifaciens* and *P. stuartii*. Rauss & Vörös (1959) and Rauss (1962) supported the proposals for new genera (*Morganella*, *Rettgerella*, and *Providencia*) but Richard (1966) thought that Rettger's bacillus should be included in *Providencia*. Lautrop, writing in *Bergey's Manual* (1974), reviewed the situation as it existed about the beginning of the 1970s and discussed the possible taxonomic treatments. His general conclusion was that Morgan's bacillus, with its $G+C$ content of DNA of 50%, compared with 40% for the other *Proteus* species, seemed the best candidate for separate recognition.

The usual biochemical characterizing tests often show up aberrant strains as, for example, the indole-positive *Proteus mirabilis* strains reported by Matsen *et al.* (1972), and the lactose-fermenting strains of *Proteus rettgeri* (Sutter & Foecking, 1962). Although the estimation of the guanine and cytosine content of DNA is far from being a clinical laboratory test, we cannot turn a blind eye to it and we think that it supports the case for the separation of Morgan's no. 1 bacillus. This is not to give our approval to further splitting of the groups within the enteric bacteria, but a recognition that we should try to arrange our lesser groups as neat and compact taxa that will be useful in the remodelling of the big group (enterobacteria) that is inevitable.

In the medical laboratory *Proteus* species, because of their swarming propensies, are more of a nuisance than a subject for identification. Various tricks have been devised to inhibit swarming, for although the inclusion of bile salts in the medium (as in MacConkey agar) is one of the most successful, it may make the medium unsuitable for the growth of the organisms we want to isolate. Other measures include exposure to ether vapour (Bray, 1945), chloral hydrate (Gillespie, 1948), increased concentration of agar (Hayward & Miles, 1943) and NaCl (Kopper, 1962).

We have not yet mentioned Proteus OX strains, which are strains of *Proteus vulgaris* isolated by Felix from typhus infections. Such strains do not need to be identified among the strains of *P. vulgaris* that are isolated; their importance is in their use as diagnostic agents. Although they are not connected in any way with the infecting agent (*Rickettsia prowazekii* or *R. mooseri*) they are, in the O (non-motile) form, agglutinated by the sera of typhus patients; a titre of 1 in 50 or more suggests rickettsial infection, but should be confirmed by looking for a rising titre during the course of the clinical illness. Proteus OX19 is agglutinated by sera from patients with classical typhus (*R. prowazekii* infection) and Proteus OXK by sera of patients with tsutsugamushi fever (*R. orientalis* infection).

Minidefinition: *Proteus. Gram-negative rods; motile. Aerobic and facultatively anaerobic. Catalase positive; oxidase negative. Attack sugars fermentatively, usually with gas production. Phenylalanine positive; urea often hydrolysed. Utilize citrate as carbon source.*

7.9.13 Salmonella (Table 7.9*a, d*). The identification of a bacterium as a salmonella is not difficult but, with that done, two problems arise. The first is the complex antigenic analysis (and sometimes phage typing) needed to identify strains in sufficient detail to be helpful in tracing a source of infection; the second is how to label (name or number) the strain in the report that must be made to the clinician and to the local health authority. The Salmonella Subcommittee (1934) thought that serology was the ultimate criterion in the classification (and by implication, identification) of the group but did not suggest that it should be based on serology alone. Antigenic analysis and phage typing are not routine procedures for a clinical laboratory, and reference laboratories are available to help in most countries. Simplified diagnostic schemes using a limited number of sera have been suggested (Edwards & Kauffmann, 1952; Spicer, 1956) and their use makes possible the presumptive serotyping of most salmonellas isolated from clinical material. A polyvalent salmonella–arizona phage was found useful for distinguishing salmonellas from other enterobacteria but was not a substitute for classical methods (Talley, 1968).

One serotype, *Salmonella typhi*, is distinct both serologically and biochemically and warrants separate description; it differs from most other salmonellas in being citrate negative and in not producing gas when it breaks down a sugar. *Salmonella gallinarum*, which causes disease in poultry, also does not produce gas. Other serotypes may produce anaerogenic variants and this is particularly common in *S. paratyphi-A* strains isolated in Egypt and Syria, but the normal forms produce gas. *S. paratyphi-A* is atypical in other characters: few strains produce H_2S from TSI; it does not use citrate as C source or produce acid from xylose; it does not decarboxylate lysine.

The type species of the genus, *Salmonella choleraesuis*, is biochemically atypical and does not ferment arabinose or trehalose. The arizona group (*S. arizonae*) strains often ferment lactose, are ONPG positive, liquefy gelatin slowly, and are usually malonate positive (Shaw, 1956). Most other serotypes are biochemical variants on a fairly stable pattern; Borman, Stuart & Wheeler (1944) proposed that they should be named *Salmonella kauffmannii*. For a similar all-embracing species Kauffmann & Edwards (1952) suggested the name *Salmonella enterica*, which would have been unusually meaningful; Ewing (1963) proposed that the name *Salmonella enteritidis* should be followed by the serotype name (when it had one) or number; this system has been tried out in the United States but does not seem to be used elsewhere.

Kauffmann (1963a) divided the Salmonella group into what he called subgenera; these are now accepted (though not as subgenera) and if Salmon-

ella is regarded as a genus, then the subdivisions can conveniently be considered as species: *Salmonella kauffmannii* (subgenus I), *S. salamae* (II), *S. arizonae* (III), and *S. houtenae* (IV) (Le Minor, Rohde & Taylor, 1970).

The typically non-motile salmonellas (*S. pullorum* and *S. gallinarum*) from poultry are often combined, but as one produces gas and the other does not we show them separately in Table 7.9d; the other distinguishing features of these organisms were described by Trabulsi & Edwards (1962), but Costin (1965) could not confirm the differences in the sugar reactions.

Isolation methods do not seem to have changed much since Hobbs & Allison (1945), after comparing several media, found Wilson & Blair to be the most valuable solid medium, with deoxycholate citrate a close second, but recommended that both media should be used as the combination gave more positives than either medium alone. For enrichment, selenite F seemed to give the best results when plated on Wilson & Blair's bismuth sulphite medium. Harvey & Thomson (1953) obtained more positives when cultures were incubated at 43 °C than at 37 °C, but found that temperature regulation had to be accurate as 44 °C was inhibitory for salmonellas. Incubation of selenite F at 43 °C is recommended by Georgala & Boothroyd (1965) and this enrichment is followed by plating on brilliant green agar.

Minidefinition: *Salmonella. Gram-negative rods; motile (a few exceptions). Aerobic and facultatively anaerobic. Catalase positive; oxidase negative. Attack sugars by fermentation with production of gas (important exception does not produce gas and is citrate negative). Citrate usually positive; KCN negative.*

7.9.14 Serratia (Table 7.9a, e). Classically, members of this group produce a bright pink or red pigment but in culture non-pigmented variants are constantly thrown off; non-pigmented strains occur in nature and in a five-month period 92% of strains isolated in a Boston hospital were not pigmented (Wilfert *et al.* 1970); consequently, the bacteriologist must be able to identify the organism in the absence of pigment. However, if pigment is present, the identification is made much easier, and various media have been devised to encourage pigment production. Meat extract seems to inhibit pigment formation but it can be restored by transfer to a medium without meat (Goldsworthy & Still, 1936). Kharasch, Conway & Bloom (1936) thought that glucose was necessary for pigment production by *Serratia marcescens*; on the other hand, Goldsworthy & Still (1936, 1938) found that glucose inhibited and mannitol stimulated pigment production by their strains. Our experience has confirmed all these findings, which indicates that strains vary in the way in which they respond to glucose in the medium. Medium A of King, Ward & Raney (1954) (Section A2.5.3) is one of the most satisfactory media for showing pigment potential; Sedlák and his colleagues (1965) reported good results on Dorset egg (Section A2.1.9) at 22 °C. As with Hafnia, the most characteristic results of biochemical tests are obtained at about 25 °C.

Sometimes serratias are found in human secretions and, by growth in sputum after expectoration, may suggest that the patient has haemoptysis (Robinson & Woolley, 1957). Serratias are suspected of being the cause of infections in man and, with their recognition in the non-pigmented form, reports of their isolation are becoming more frequent. A VP-negative variety, *S. marcescens* var. *kiliensis*, has been isolated from sputum (Bøvre & Tønjum, 1963), but we do not think that a variety need be recognized or named.

Serratia marcescens liquefies gelatin very rapidly, and in this and other characters Pederson & Breed (1928) noticed that it closely resembled the liquefying species of Aerobacter (*Enterobacter liquefaciens* in modern terminology) and thought that non-pigmented strains might be included in *Serratia*. The resemblance extends to deoxyribonuclease activity (DNase) which occurs more frequently and is more active in strains of *Serratia marcescens* and *Enterobacter liquefaciens* than in other enterobacteria (Vörös, 1969). Black, Hodgson & McKechnie (1971) compared methods for carrying out this test in a routine laboratory and preferred that of Jeffries, Holtman & Guse (1957). A rapid and easily read method (combined with the PPA test) was described by Oberhofer & Maddox (1970). We have accepted the suggestion of Pederson & Breed,

which has been repeated by many others, and now include *E. liquefaciens* in *Serratia*.

Traub (1972) compared typing methods based on serology and bacteriocin sensitivity and thought that the latter were the more successful. The significance of the divisions is unknown, but that is not unexpected since we do not know much about the pathogenicity of serratias. The fascinating story of *Serratia marcescens* has been well told by Gaughran (1969).

Another species, *Serratia rubidaea*, described by Breed in *Bergey's Manual* (1948) as having characters much like those of *S. marcescens*, has been revived by Ewing, Davis & Fife (1972); some strains came from human sources but the clinical significance was not indicated and presumably was unknown.

> **Minidefinition:** *Serratia. Gram-negative rods; motile. Aerobic and facultatively anaerobic. Catalase positive; oxidase negative. Attack sugars fermentatively, often with gas production. VP usually positive. Gluconate positive. Produce ornithine decarboxylase; deoxyribonuclease positive. Often produce a red pigment when grown on suitable media.*

7.9.15 Shigella (Table 7.9*a, b, c*). Modern ideas on the classification of this group are largely due to Ewing who built on the foundations laid by Murray (1918), Andrewes & Inman (1919), and by Boyd (1938) whose recognition of group and specific antigens introduced some system into the antigenic analysis of shigellas. Ewing is also responsible for showing that many so-called shigellas are non-motile, anaerogenic members of the Escherichia group. The two groups not only seem to be closely related but may be interfertile, the progeny resembling the A–D group (Luria & Burrows, 1957).

A good case can be made for combining Shigella with Escherichia; the similarity is especially close with *Shigella sonnei* (Cowan, 1956*b*) which, like *Escherichia coli* and the A–D biotypes, is Eijkman positive and reduces trimethylamine (Stuart & Rustigian, 1943*b*; Wood, Baird & Keeping, 1943). Ewing (1953) found that of thirty-three known serotypes, only four were unrelated to the O groups of *E. coli*; unfortunately he did not follow up this pointer to the fusion of the two groups, but by 1972 (Edwards & Ewing, 3rd edition) only two serotypes were not related to the extended O-group range of *E. coli*. One must not put too much weight on antigenic overlaps for they can occur between such culturally dissimilar organisms as pneumococci and klebsiellas, and between *Shigella sonnei* and *Plesiomonas shigelloides* (Ferguson & Henderson, 1947; Martin, Mock & Ewing, 1968), but the relatedness between Escherichia and Shigella (and especially *S. sonnei*) is confirmed by polynucleotide sequences. Brenner *et al.* (1973) think that on the molecular information available, *E. coli* and *Shigella* species should be included in the same genus.

Biochemically the Shigella group is divided into the mannitol fermenters and the mannitol non-fermenters but Ewing (personal communication) has found exceptions in nearly all serotypes. The mannitol-negative subgroup (*Shigella dysenteriae*) differs from all the others in that serotype 1 (Shiga's bacillus) is catalase negative; among other shigellas catalase-negative strains are occasionally found, especially in *S. flexneri* type 4*a* (Carpenter & Lachowicz, 1959) but this is not a constant character of any serotype except *S. dysenteriae* 1. Strains of *S. dysenteriae* 2 (Schmitz's bacillus) always produce indole, a character shared among the mannitol non-fermenters by the rarer serotypes 7 and 8. Among the mannitol fermenters the distinction between *Shigella flexneri* and *S. boydii* is made almost entirely on serological grounds; the only biochemical test of distinguishing value is growth in 0.4 % selenite (Lapage & Bascomb, 1968), and even that test does not give an absolute distinction for a few strains of *S. boydii* fail to grow, and a few of *S. flexneri* will grow in 0.4 % selenite.

Strains of *Shigella flexneri* 6 may differ in some biochemical characters from *S. flexneri* 1 to 5, and Russian workers regard *S. flexneri* 6 as a distinct species (Gekker *et al.* 1965; Timakov *et al.* 1972); the special characteristics of the Newcastle and Manchester varieties (Downie *et al.* 1933) of *S. flexneri* 6 are shown in Table 7.9*c*, which is adapted from a table of Carpenter, Lapage & Steel (1966). Gas is produced by some strains, but see Orr Ewing & Taylor (1945) for the influence of peptone. These aerogenic varieties were originally reported to produce only small bubbles of gas but

Carpenter (personal communication) found that with modern peptones the amount of gas produced was quite large.

The isolation of shigellas is usually made by direct plating of washed mucus (perhaps better described as rinsed mucus) from 'blood and mucus' stools, the loose stool if it does not contain mucus, and in convalescents, from a suspension of the solid stool. Enrichment methods are much less successful with shigellas than with salmonellas (Taylor & Harris, 1965) but a highly selective medium for *Shigella flexneri* (Wilson & Blair, 1941) and a 'new family of media' introduced by Taylor (1965) could make their isolation and recognition easier.

Shigella sonnei produces colicines which, when tested on 'indicator' strains, can be used to sub-divide strains into epidemiologically significant types (Abbot & Shannon, 1958). Typically *S. sonnei* is a late fermenter of lactose and sucrose, but not all strains ferment the sugars and Szturm-Rubinsten (1963) recognized different biotypes. The ONPG test shows up the inherent ability of the late lactose fermenters to ferment the sugar (Le Minor & Ben Hamida, 1962) and tests of other shigellas show that many serotypes are made up of potential lactose fermenters (Szturm-Rubinsten & Piéchaud, 1963).

Minidefinition: *Shigella. Gram-negative rods; non-motile. Aerobic and facultatively anaerobic. Catalase positive (an important exception is negative); oxidase negative. Attack sugars by fermentation without gas production (a few exceptions produce gas). Citrate negative; KCN negative.*

7.9.16 **Yersinia** (Tables 7.7*a, b*; 7.9*a, b*) is a genus originally created for the plague and pseudotuber-culosis organisms by van Loghem (1944–5) who separated them from the pasteurellas. Other organisms have been added since; *Yersinia entero-colitica* (Pasteurella X) from animals and man (Mollaret & Chevalier, 1964); an unnamed variant from hares (Mollaret & Lucas, 1965); and *Y. philomiragia* (Jensen, Owen & Jellison, 1969) from the muskrat and from water.

Many strains with divergent biochemical charac-ters have been included in *Yersinia enterocolitica*, so Knapp & Thal (1973) published a redescription of the species and the characters shown in Table 7.9*a*, *b* agree with the characters recorded in the redescription. It is worth noting that while *Y. enterocolitica* is VP negative at 37 °C, it may be positive at 22–25 °C. Growth temperature seems to be more than usually important in the characterization of yersinias; *Y. pestis* produces a capsule (or envelope) at 37 °C but not at 20 °C (Schütze, 1932*a*); *Y. pseudotuberculosis* is motile at 22 °C but not at 37 °C (Preston & Maitland, 1952), and a similar temperature sensitivity is found in *Y. enterocolitica* (Niléhn, 1967) which produces more or stronger positives at 22 °C than at 37 °C in tests for motility, VP, ONPG, and ornithine decarboxylase. On the other hand, Niléhn found the urease reaction was stronger at 37 °C than at 22 °C.

The variant strains isolated from hares are serologically identical with other strains of *Yersinia enterocolitica* but differ in a few biochemical characters: they are not nitrate reducers, ornithinine is not decarboxylated, the ONPG test is negative and trehalose is not fermented. The staining of the muskrat organism is made difficult by the presence of mucoid material; cultures washed in physiological saline are usually stainable and then resemble the plague bacillus except, perhaps, for their rather smaller size. In culture the organism differs from other yersinias by liquefying gelatin, and like the hare variants, does not reduce nitrate.

The plague bacillus, which needs haematin (Lapage & Zinnemann, 1971), grows slowly in Hugh & Leifson's medium; acid appears first in the open tube and only later in the sealed tube. We think that this should be interpreted as fermentation following an initial oxidation; consequently we describe the organism as fermentative and include it with the enterobacteria, as was indicated by the numerical analysis by Sneath & Cowan (1958), and the antigenic relations shown by Schütze (1928, 1932*b*) between *Pasteurella pseudotuberculosis* and the *Salmonella* group B, and between *P. pseudotuberculosis* and *P. pestis*.

Minidefinition: *Yersinia. Gram-negative rods; motile or non-motile. Aerobic and facultatively anaerobic. Catalase positive; oxidase negative. Sugars attacked fermentatively, occasionally with production of gas. Grow on MacConkey agar.*

7.10   A group of difficult organisms (GDO)
(*Haemophilus, Campylobacter, Eikenella, Streptobacillus*)
Characters common to members of the group: Gram-negative rods. Exacting requirements for isolation and continued growth in subculture.

These organisms have little in common except for the demands they make on the skill and ingenuity of the bacteriologist. If, as in the first edition of this *Manual*, we had a chapter on miscellaneous bacteria and bacteria of uncertain taxonomic position all would have qualified for it, but as we are not overmuch worried by taxonomic position we have collected them into a group we call the GDO (group of difficult organisms). They are difficult in many ways, not least in being fastidious in their nutritional and atmospheric requirements. Neither *Eikenella* nor *Campylobacter* can be isolated from cultures incubated aerobically, and anaerobic cultures are not much more successful – but see below.

Eikenella grows in air+CO_2, while *Campylobacter* prefers air with only 5–10 % oxygen in it. *Haemophilus* species are not so fussy about their atmospheric surroundings but they are demanding in their X- and V-factor requirements. *Streptobacillus* prefers anaerobic conditions and requires a medium much richer in protein than we usually provide; like other members of the group its growth is improved by the addition of carbon dioxide.

7.10.1 Haemophilus (Table 7.10*b*) as we define it, is restricted to bacteria that need one or both of the two factors X (haemin or haematin) and V (co-enzyme I; diphosphopyridine nucleotide) for growth. These species will not grow on the media used in the biochemical tests shown in Tables 7.1 to 7.9, and media supplemented by X and V factors are needed for the indole and carbohydrate tests shown in Table 7.10*b*. Most of the basic fluid and solid media contain traces of X factor, as do some brands and batches of peptone; Zinnemann (1960) recommends Yeastrel agar (Section A2.1.10), used in the examination of water supplies, as a consistently X-free medium for testing the X requirements of *Haemophilus* species.

After isolation the growth requirements may

change as the strains adapt to their new environment; for example, the original cultures of *Haemophilus suis* (Lewis & Shope, 1931), when re-examined by Matthews & Pattison (1961), were found to be no longer dependent on X factor. Biberstein & White (1969) created a new species, *H. parasuis*, for strains that do not need X factor for growth, but as these seem to be culture-collection curiosities rather than wild strains, we do not include them in Table 7.10*b*.

Haemophilus species are not only fastidious in their X and V requirements but also may need some constituent of blood or serum. To obtain consistent results in these tests the use of small inocula (to avoid carry-over) is essential. There is a salt requirement, though the strains are not halophilic in the usual meaning of that term, and this may be associated with an apparent need for carbon dioxide. The mechanism of the 'CO$_2$ effect' has not yet received serious consideration (Boyce, Frazer & Zinnemann, 1969). The need for CO$_2$ may be reduced by incubating cultures in the moist atmosphere of a sealed jar. Under the usual conditions in a bench incubator or incubator room recently isolated strains may grow only feebly or not at all without CO$_2$ (Frazer, Zinnemann & Boyce, 1969); from this it follows that CO$_2$ should figure quite prominently in the development of a routine aimed at isolating *Haemophilus* species.

In-vitro adaptations, by reducing or abolishing specific requirements, may be responsible for conflicting statements in the literature. *Haemophilus aphrophilus* was originally isolated by Khairat (1940) from a blood culture and was so named because it needed X factor and CO$_2$ for growth. King & Tatum (1962) could not confirm the requirement for X factor of the strains sent to them, but they pointed out that these strains had been subcultured an unknown number of times and might have lost their X dependence. They thought that the strains had much in common with strains of *Actinobacillus actinomycetemcomitans*, but had relatively few of the classical characters of either *Haemophilus* or *Actinobacillus*. Boyce *et al.* (1969) discussed the difficulties of classifying strains that adapt quickly to the in-vitro situation, and came to the conclusion that in *H. aphrophilus* the majority of bacterial cells in each culture were

incapable of synthesizing X factor and that the species should be regarded as X dependent. We agree with these conclusions and because we try to show the characteristics of freshly isolated strains, we record this dependence in Table 7.10*b*.

Since carbohydrate breakdown and acid production are much influenced by the medium, the sugar reactions of the haemophils are not sufficiently reliable (or well enough studied) to form a basis for the subdivision of the genus into species; consequently, in Table 7.10*b* we show only the production of acid from glucose, and even this must be read with caution for there are great discrepancies between the results reported by different workers. The mode of carbohydrate breakdown is not known and although the word fermentation is used when discussing this character, we cannot be sure that it is not being used in the loose sense and merely indicates that acid is produced by means that are not known.

The oxidase reaction of all *Haemophilus* species that have been tested is negative (Zinnemann, personal communication). For a review of the genus and its pathogenicity, the reader is referred to Zinnemann (1960). In the fascinating story ('a kind of *Comedy of Errors*') of *Haemophilus influenzae*, Zinnemann (1973) reminds us that although the organism does not cause influenza (whatever that may be), it may be the cause of a meningitis that responds to penicillin therapy.

In addition to the species shown in Table 7.10*b*, Pittman & Davis (1950) distinguished *Haemophilus aegyptius* (the Koch–Weeks bacillus) from *H. influenzae* by differences in acid production from xylose, indole production, and agglutination of human red cells; Orfila & Courden (1961) added differences in the bacteraemia curves after intravenous inoculation, but the modern view seems to be that these differences are not sufficiently great to justify the recognition of *H. aegyptius* as a separate species.

The concept of the genus *Haemophilus* has been blurred, tarnished, and literally stained by a prolonged discussion on the correct classification (i.e. taxonomic position – and this affects the name) of *Haemophilus vaginalis*. At least two different organisms have been given this name; one haemophilic with X and V requirements (Lapage, 1961;

Zinnemann & Turner, 1962), the other a Gram-positive rod which, as cultures aged, became Gram negative, a not unusual sequence for coryneform bacteria. We show the characters of the last organism in Table 6.5b and briefly describe its morphology in Section 6.5.1.

Minidefinition: *Haemophilus. Gram-negative rods; non-motile. Aerobic and facultatively anaerobic. Catalase positive or negative; oxidase negative. Fastidious; do not grow on media unless they contain X and V factors and undefined constituents of blood or serum.*

7.10.2 Eikenella (Table 7.10a) is the name now given to a group of facultatively anaerobic non-sporing rods that will grow aerobically from the first subculture, though anaerobic conditions may be necessary for isolation (Jackson & Goodman, 1972); these organisms form the HB-1 strains of King & Tatum (1962). The genus was named after Eiken who, in 1958, gave the specific epithet to the organism (which he placed in *Bacteroides*). According to Jackson & Goodman two rather different organisms, both of which produced pitting on the surface of the medium, have been named *Bacteroides corrodens*; one is a strict anaerobe (and remains so) and is urease positive; the other (*Eikenella corrodens*) is facultatively anaerobic and urease negative. A few points of difference between these organisms are shown in Table 7.10a. Hill, Snell & Lapage (1970) did not find any of the strictly anaerobic organisms among their strains, which had mostly been isolated in England.

In describing *Eikenella corrodens* Jackson & Goodman (1972) and Prefontaine & Jackson (1972) gave some details of a research laboratory kind which helped to distinguish the facultative from the strictly anaerobic organisms; the G+C content of the DNA was 28–30 % for the strict anaerobe and 57–58 % for *E. corrodens*; the fatty acid compositions of the organisms were different so that they had different 'fingerprints' when these acids were determined by gas chromatography. These are esoteric differences and at the moment only of theoretical importance, but they indicate that we must distinguish (and look for) two similar but different organisms.

Table 7.10a *Second-stage table for* Haemophilus, Eikenella, Campylobacter, Streptobacillus

	1	2	3	4	5	6	7
Motility	−	−	.	+	+	−	−
Growth in air	+	w	−	−	−	+	+
Growth under anaerobic conditions	+	+	+	w	+	+	+
Catalase	D	−	.	+	−	−	−
Oxidase	−*	+	.	+	+	−	−
Swelling of microbial cell	−	−	−	−	−	+	−
Colony adherent to medium	−	+	+	−	−	−	+
Growth at 42 °C	−	w	.	d	−	−	.
Growth favoured by O_2	.	+	−	+	+	+	.
Growth favoured by CO_2	D	+	.	.	.	+ᵃ	.
Growth improved by blood/serum	Dᵇ	+	.	.	.	+	+
Growth improved by moisture (closed jar)	+	+	.	.	.	+ᵃ	.
Carbohydrates [F/O/−]	F	−	.	−	−	F	F/−
Glucose, acid from	+	−	−	−	−	+	+
Starch hydrolysis	.	−	+	.	.	.	+ᶜ
Nitrate reduced	+	+	.	+	+	−	.
Indole	D	−	.	−	−	−	.
Gelatin liquefied	−	−	w	−	−	−	−
Urease	d	−	+	−	−	−	D
H_2S	−	(w)/−	.	d	+	−	D
Arginine dihydrolase	.	−	.	.	.	+	D
Lysine decarboxylase	.	+	.	.	.	.	.
Ornithine decarboxylase	.	+	.	.	.	.	.

1 **Haemophilus** spp.
2 **Eikenella corrodens**; *Bacteroides corrodens*; HB-1
3 **Anaerobic corroding organism** (Jackson & Goodman, 1972)
4 **Campylobacter fetus**; *Vibrio fetus*
5 **Campylobacter sputorum**
6 **Streptobacillus moniliformis**; *Actinobacillus muris*; *Actinomyces muris*
7 **Mycoplasma** spp.; **Acholeplasma** spp.

* Some strains of *H. parainfluenzae* may be oxidase positive (Sneath & Johnson, 1973).
ᵃ Requirement for growth.
ᵇ Blood requirement is for haematin (X factor).
ᶜ False positive due to amylases in serum.

Table 7.10*b* *Third-stage table for* Haemophilus

	1	2	3	4	5	6	7	8	9	10	11	12	13
Catalase	+	+	+	.	+	−	(+)	.	+	+	(+)	−	+
Haemolysis	−	−	+	−	−	−	−	(+)	−	+	−	−	+
Growth on chocolate agar	+	+	+	.	+	+	−[a]	−[a]	+	+	−[a]	.	−[a]
X requirement	+	+	+	+	+	+	+	+	−	−	−	−	−
V requirement	+	+	+	+	−	−	−	−	+	+	+	+	+
CO_2 requirement	−	−	−	+	−	−	+	+	−	−	+	+	+
NaCl requirement (%)	.	.	.	1	0.5	< 2.5	−	.	.	.	.	0.5	0.6
Serum or other enrichment from blood	−	+	−	+	−	−	−	+	−	−	−	+	.
Acid from glucose[b]	+	(w)	.	+	+	+	+	−	+	w	+	+	+
Indole	d	−	d	−	+	−	−	−	−	d	−	−	d

1 Haemophilus influenzae
2 Haemophilus suis
3 Haemophilus haemolyticus
4 Haemophilus gallinarum
5 Haemophilus haemoglobinophilus; *H. canis*
6 Haemophilus influenzaemurium
7 Haemophilus aphrophilus
8 Haemophilus ducreyi
9 Haemophilus parainfluenzae
10 Haemophilus parahaemolyticus; *H. pleuropneumoniae*
11 Haemophilus paraphrophilus
12 Haemophilus paragallinarum
13 Haemophilus paraphrohaemolyticus

[a] Positive in CO_2.
[b] See text, Section 7.10.1, for note on acid production from carbohydrates, and also Sneath & Johnson (1973).

Symbols used in the table are explained in Tables 5.1 and 5.2 (facing p. 43).

Eikenella corrodens has been isolated alone or in mixed culture from pus from various abscesses, pleural fluids, sputum, tonsils, the ear and the nose; Jackson & Goodman regard it as an opportunistic pathogen but Riley, Tatum & Weaver (1973), with histories of 500 strains available to them, thought that it was a normal inhabitant of the alimentary canal.

For isolation, specimens are plated on blood agar and incubated in a closed jar in an atmosphere enriched with 5–10% carbon dioxide. Jackson & Goodman found growth was improved by 0.1% KNO_3, and better with 1% oxygen than under strictly anaerobic conditions. Although anaerobic methods using a closed jar seemed to be essential for isolation, it was not clear whether the anaerobiosis, the moisture, the CO_2, or a combination of these, was the mandatory factor(s). Haematin seems to be essential for growth in air.

The character from which the organism gets its name is the adherent nature of the colony which digs into (corrodes) the surface of agar media; the adherent colonies have wrinkled surfaces. Some colonies are not wrinkled, and these are not adherent; they breed true and have the same biochemical characters as the wrinkled colony form. Biochemically, *E. corrodens* is rather inactive and for that reason has been likened to brucellas and placed in the same family. We draw attention to the similarities to *Campylobacter* (Table 7.10*a*); both grow better in semisolid than in any fluid medium.

Minidefinition: *Eikenella. Gram-negative rods; non-motile. Facultatively anaerobic on first isolation; soon become aerobic. Catalase negative; oxidase positive. Do not attack carbohydrates.*

7.10.3 Campylobacter (Table 7.10*a*) contains the bacterium much better known as *Vibrio fetus* and other 'anaerobic vibrios'. *Campylobacter fetus* had the reputation of being a fairly strict anaerobe but this was both unjustified and inaccurate. In terms of aerobiosis and anaerobiosis the organism does not fit into the usual categories; it grows best in about 5% oxygen; it will not grow on the surface of solid medium when incubated in air, and it will not grow in fluid media containing reducing agent. In sloppy medium containing 0.16% agar *C. fetus* can be incubated aerobically. Slopes should be incubated in a closed jar from which two-thirds of the air has been exhausted, leaving 5–6 % oxygen, or it may be incubated in a jar in which a candle has burnt to extinction (*Anaerobe Laboratory Manual*, 1972). Apart from *C. fetus*, the other species of the genus will tolerate reduced media and more strictly anaerobic conditions; they will grow in 5 % oxygen but not under normal aerobic conditions.

Veterinary workers recognize biotypes of *Campylobacter fetus* (Park *et al.* 1962); although Smibert (1970) confirmed the validity of the biotypes we do not think that the differences in the usual (phenotypical) biochemical characters sufficiently compelling, and in Table 7.10*a* we show *C. fetus* without subdivision. Campylobacters have been isolated from human sources (King, 1962); *C. sputorum*, from the gum area, was described by Loesche *et al.* (1965); this is shown in Table 7.10*a* without breakdown into varieties.

> **Minidefinition:** *Campylobacter. Gram-negative rods; motile. Optimal oxygen concentration for growth is 5%; will not grow in air, under strictly anaerobic conditions, or on reduced media. Catalase positive or negative; oxidase positive. Do not ferment or oxidize sugars. Nitrate reduced to nitrite; do not produce indole.*

7.10.4 Streptobacillus (Table 7.10*a*). An organism that needs a medium enriched by 20 % serum, ascitic fluid or blood, prefers anaerobic conditions for isolation, and for whose growth additional CO_2 is needed; it differs from other members of the GDO in growing more slowly and producing less growth (R. G. Wittler & S. G. Cary, personal communication). Obviously, it is not an organism that will be isolated by our usual routines, and must be specially looked for if its presence is suspected.

Only one species is now listed, but what we know as *Streptobacillus moniliformis* may be only a representative of an almost unknown group of organisms. In morphology the organism is filamentous in young culture but later the filaments break up into shorter sections. Swellings occur in the filaments but these are not caused by spores or metachromatic granules. Biochemical characters may be determined, using media enriched with

serum and yeast extract, by methods that are also suitable for use with L-forms (L-phase variants) of bacteria. A paper by Cohen, Wittler & Faber (1968) describes the methods and gives a table of strains for positive and negative controls.

The organism is pathogenic for mice, which die within a couple of days of intraperitoneal infection; apparently it is avirulent for rats and may be a member of the normal mouth flora of that animal. It is one of the causes of rat-bite fever in man, and has also been isolated from patients with endocarditis.

> **Minidefinition:** *Streptobacillus. Filamentous Gram-negative rods; non-motile. Non-sporing, but filaments may show swellings. Aerobic and facultatively anaerobic. Need enriched medium for growth. Catalase negative; oxidase negative. Attack sugars fermentatively.*

7.10.5 Mycoplasma and **Acholeplasma** (Table 7.10*a*) are considered to be distinct from bacteria and in a class of their own called Mollicutes (Edward & Freundt, 1967). The two genera are distinguished by the requirement (*Mycoplasma*) and lack of need for sterol (*Acholeplasma*) (Edward & Freundt, 1970). They seem quite out of place in a book devoted to bacteria, but they deserve mention because they may be isolated in a bacteriological laboratory from clinical specimens and from tissue cultures. As they are decolorized and take the counterstain (very feebly) when stained by Gram's method, they may be considered Gram negative. Unlike bacteria, they do not have rigid cell walls and in this respect resemble L forms of bacteria, with which they may be confused. Like L forms, they grow in the presence of antibiotics at concentrations inhibitory to normal bacteria; unlike L forms, they do not change, on subculture to antibiotic-free media, into bacteria with normal cell walls.

Mycoplasms (the final 'a' of the generic name should be dropped to form the common name – Andrewes *et al.* 1965) may be found in so-called normal serum and can pass some types of bacterial filter; since they are heat labile serum can be made suitable for use in media by heating at 56 °C for 30 minutes.

Mycoplasms are not easy to characterize and

special methods have been developed for them (Aluotto *et al.* 1970; Williams & Wittler, 1971) which are useful also for *Streptobacillus moniliformis*.

Like *Eikenella corrodens*, colonies not only adhere to the surface but also grow into the medium, and as the growth spreads over the surface the colony resembles a poached egg. While they are not necessarily anaerobic, they grow well in a closed jar, benefiting from the moisture trapped in it.

Serological methods seem to be the most reliable for the identification of species (Lemcke & Leach, 1968). A simple method uses paper disks, each saturated with 0.02 ml antiserum (these can be freeze-dried in open dishes in an Edwards 30P machine), which inhibit growth by the homologous mycoplasm (Dighero, Bradstreet & Andrews, 1970).

7.11 Sources of information for the tables

In revising the tables and developing new ones, a great many papers and monographs were consulted and the sources not in the text are listed in Table 7.11.

Once again there were conflicts of evidence, and when this happened we resorted to two sources which, from familiarity, we regard as most reliable. These bed-rock sources were: (i) E. O. King's tables (1964) and the version brought up to date (1972) by Weaver, Tatum & Hollis, and (ii) the first edition of this *Manual*, in which the tables were based mainly on the results of work in the National Collection of Type Cultures. We admit prejudice, but believe these are two unusually reliable sources of information on the cultural characters of bacteria dealt with in medical laboratories.

We were greatly helped by numerous letters and comments from those working with the Gram-negative organisms described here, and we append a list of those whose influence came under the heading 'personal communications'. These included G. I. Barrow, the late Patricia Carpenter, S. G. Cary, W. H. Ewing, W. Frederiksen, H. Lautrop, S. P. Lapage, L. Le Minor, J. Midgley, J. B. Morgan, F. Ørskov, I. Ørskov, J. E. Phillips, M. J. Pickett, M. Pittman, R. Sakazaki, J. Sedlák, J. M. Shewan, J. E. Smith, P. H. A. Sneath, E. Thal, R. G. Wittler, and K. Zinnemann.

Table 7.11 *Additional sources consulted for Tables 7.1 to 7.10*

Author(s)	Table(s)
Ballard (1968)	7.6
Berger (1962)	7.3
Bergey's Manual of Determinative Bacteriology (1974)	7.2, 7.9, 7.10
Colwell (1970)	7.8
Cook (1948)	7.9
Ewing & Ball (1966)	7.9
Ewing & Davis (1971, 1972b)	7.9
Ewing *et al.* (1971, 1972)	7.9
Fife *et al.* (1965)	7.9
Frederiksen (1964)	7.4, 7.9
Gilardi (1969)	7.4
Gilardi *et al.* (1970b)	7.8
Grimont & Dulong de Rosnay (1972)	7.9
Heyl (1963)	7.7
Hugh & Leifson (1963)	7.6
Hugh & Reese (1968)	7.4
Jones (1964)	7.4
Jonsson (1970)	7.6
Kauffmann (1954)	7.9
King (1964, 1972)	7.4, 7.5, 7.6, 7.7, 7.10
Knapp (1965)	7.7, 7.9
Lysenko (1961)	7.6
Moreira-Jacob (1963)	7.4
Muraschi *et al.* (1965)	7.9
Page & King (1966)	7.7, 7.10
Pickett & Manclark (1970)	7.5
Pittman (1953)	7.10
Pulverer & Ko (1970)	7.7
Ryan (1968)	7.10
Shreeve *et al.* (1970)	7.7
Stanier *et al.* (1966)	7.6
Tunnicliffe (1941)	7.7
Vallée *et al.* (1963)	7.7
Zinnemann *et al.* (1968, 1971)	7.10

8
Identification by cards

Identification is not always an art; it can be mechanized and common diagnostic characters used in a visual sorter (Olds, 1966, 1970) based on the Peek-a-boo system (Wildhack & Stern, 1958; Yourassowsky *et al.* 1965). Hand-sorted punched cards have been used for recording quite varied taxonomic information (Wood, 1957) and in the first edition of this *Manual* we remarked that our 'tables could form the basis of a set of diagnostic punched cards to be used with similar cards on which the characteristics of the unknowns are punched'. Soon after that was written Schneierson & Amsterdam (1964) described a punched card used for identifying bacteria at the Mount Sinai Hospital, New York, but did not give details of the 'authoritative reference' sources from which the characters for the master cards were obtained; and it is the tables of characters that are the meat in this pie. We did not pursue the matter until this edition was being prepared.

A disadvantage of the diagnostic table is that as more detail is included it becomes less easy to use. In the present revision the early drafts of what became Tables 6.1 and 7.1 stretched to more than twenty columns and up to ten lines of characters, and to check them a set of punched cards was made, one (or more) card for each genus. This first check indicated some similar columns, previously unnoticed; these were combined and the tables were re-arranged. The exercise, though laborious, was rewarding by showing how quickly, once characters had been notched on a card, an identification could be made, and seemed to open up a new and perhaps better way of using the tables.

8.1   Minimal-difference Identicards for genera
For the identification of bacterial genera dealt

with in medical and veterinary laboratories, only eleven holes are needed; a spare space (hole) can be used for some character that is a particular favourite of the bacteriologist who intends to use the method. Cards 127×77 mm (5×3 in) are punched as shown in Fig. 8.1; a corner is cut from each card so that all can be faced for notching.

The characters used must include the Gram reaction, which is not shown in our tables; other characters are the ten used in Table 6.1, which also cover the characters in Table 7.1 and many of those mentioned in the minidefinitions given in Chapters 6 and 7.

The name of the genus is written in the middle of each master card, together with any relevant information helpful for isolation (e.g. oxygen requirements of *Campylobacter* or *Eikenella*) or identification.

Sometimes genera need multiple master cards. Examples are *Aerococcus*, in which the catalase test may be read as either weakly positive or as frankly negative; *Clostridium*, in which *C. welchii* is non-motile and is also reluctant to spore; *Gemella*, easily decolorized, has a card for both the Gram-positive and Gram-negative states; *Nocardia* is shown as acid fast and as not acid fast. The enterobacteria are dealt with as one genus (which possibly reflects their value relative to other genera) but three master cards are needed to make possible the identification of shigellas, including Shiga's bacillus, which is unusual in being catalase negative.

The notching of the individual master cards is shown in Table D1*b* (p. 182), which also shows the kind of supplementary information that can be put in the blank central area of the card.

To use the Identicard set no. 1 (for genera), first examine the unknown culture for the characters used on the card. The acid fastness and the sporing

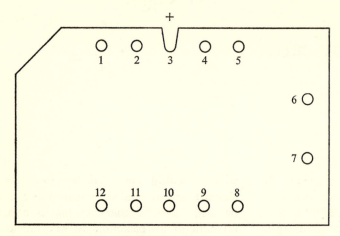

Fig. 8.1. Card punched with a single row of holes. Used for both master cards (characters of known genera) and as cards on which to record the characters of an unknown organism that is to be identified to genus.

Table 8.1 *Aggregations of genera that may occur with Identicard set no.* 1

Aggregation	Genera (species) in aggregation
(i)	*Aerococcus* (catalase read as negative) *Gemella* *Pediococcus* *Streptococcus*
(ii)	*Actinomyces* *Bifidobacterium* *Clostridium welchii* (not sporing) *Eubacterium*
(iii)	*Arachnia* *Erysipelothrix* *Lactobacillus*
(iv)	*Mycobacterium* *Nocardia*
(v)	*Leuconostoc* *Peptostreptococcus*
(vi)	Enterobacteria (*Shigella dysenteriae* 1) *Streptobacillus*
(vii)	*Bordetella* *Brucella* *Moraxella*
(viii)	*Actinobacillus* *Pasteurella* *Necromonas*
(ix)	*Aeromonas* *Beneckea* *Chromobacterium violaceum* *Plesiomonas* *Vibrio*

ability will probably not be determined in all strains, and we should be surprised if every user tested for anaerobic growth unless the culture failed to grow aerobically at the first attempt. Positive characters of the unknown are notched from the appropriate hole of a blank card. Rod-shaped organisms (bacilli, vibrios) are assumed unless hole 5 (coccus) is notched.

8.1.1 Aggregation of cards. In many cases the characters chosen will identify (to genus) bacteria likely to be isolated in medical and veterinary laboratories, but because so few characters are used in marking up (notching) the cards, some sortings will end with more than one card, and the complete identification must be made by studying characters given in the second-stage (or third-stage) tables of Chapters 6 and 7, or from using further sets of Identicards (see Section 8.2). The most surprising aggregation we found was Shiga's bacillus and *Streptobacillus* (Table 8.1, no. vi) but we do not think that anyone would have difficulty in distinguishing them at the bench; the similarity begins and ends with the characters we chose for Table 7.1. The other aggregations are of similar organisms such as *Actinobacillus* and *Pasteurella* (*sensu stricto*) that are difficult to separate even by expert veterinary bacteriologists.

124

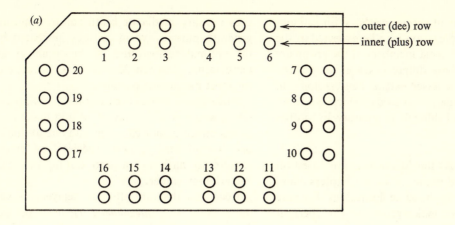

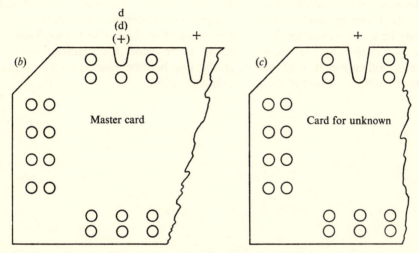

Fig. 8.2. (*a*) Card punched with two rows of holes. Used for master cards (characters of known species) in sets for species identification. May be used as cards for characters of unknowns.

(*b*) Master card, showing method for notching d, (d), (+) and + characters.

(*c*) Card of unknown organism (to be identified) notched for a positive character.

8.2   Identicards for species

The user of Identicard set no. 1 (for genera) will probably find species identification easy by consulting the tables of Chapters 6 and 7, but where the tables are large a further set of Identicards may be helpful. The notching of the master cards for species is complicated by the presence of many 'dee' (d and D) characters and late reactions, recorded in the tables within round brackets. The example of Identicards for species will deal with the enterobacteria, the characters of which are shown in Table 7.9*a*–*e*. The difficulties introduced by the dee characters are overcome by having two rows of holes in the master cards (Fig. 8.2*a*); on them, characters recorded by + signs in the tables are notched to the second (inner or plus) row of holes, and characters shown by d, (d), or (+) (i.e. different or delayed reactions) are notched only to the first (outer or dee) row (see Fig. 8.2*b*). The notching of the master cards for set no. 2 (enterobacteria) is shown in Table D2*b* (p. 184).

Positive characters of the unknown strain (to be identified) are notched to the inner row of holes (Fig. 8.2*c*), or special cards with one row of holes in line with the inner row of the master set may be used.

8.2.1   Aggregates of species cards. With salmonellas in the set, aggregation is to be expected as the differences between most members of the group are serological, and these differences are not entered on the cards. To a lesser extent, aggregation will apply to the shigella-group cards, which Bascomb *et al.* (1973) found difficult to identify by probabilistic methods.

8.2.2   Variants. As the Identicards are based on characters recorded in the tables of Chapters 6 and 7, they are subject to the same limitations. Like the tables, they do not make provision for aberrant strains or the varieties that may occur, sometimes limited to a particular locality – the so-called 'local races'. It should always be borne in mind that a non-motile organism may be a non-motile variant of a motile species, or its non-motility may be a technical failure (however difficult that may be to contemplate) to detect motility. Whether one

uses motility media or broth cultures, motility is generally most active in cultures incubated below the optimal temperature of the organism, and a temperature between 22 and 25 °C is satisfactory for most mesophilic bacteria.

Anaerogenic variants of normally gas-producing salmonella serotypes may occur and make identification difficult; they can even lead one to think that one has isolated a new 'species', an error we confess to have fallen into during our clinical bacteriology career.

Reactions that are slow or delayed, as gelatin liquefaction by *Enterobacter cloacae*, or lactose fermentation by *Shigella sonnei*, are notched to the first (outer) row of the two-row master cards; by so doing and combining it with the probing method recommended in Appendix D (see Table D2c), a reading made before the character has developed (or the test become positive) will not lead to a misidentification.

9
Taxonomy in theory and practice
(but only for those interested)

This chapter is not compulsory reading for users of this *Manual*, neither is it compulsive, for no one will get a kick from it. I cannot pretend that the chapter is a revision, for it did not appear in the first edition, and so I propose to drop the editorial 'we' used in the earlier chapters. This does not imply that my former, and much missed, colleague would have disapproved of what is set down in this chapter, but it would not be seemly to involve his memory in the heresies and unorthodox views that I have been able to express since I gave up office in the International Committee on Bacteriological Nomenclature, now renamed the International Committee on Systematic Bacteriology.

As a subject, taxonomy can be stimulating and exciting; it can also be depressing and uninspiring. Much depends on how one approaches it, and that will be based on what one has read (often deadly dull), been taught (in terrible lectures full of mumbo-jumbo and pseudo-Latin), or been told (or warned) about it. But those who are fortunate and have good teachers will regard all bacteriology as an adventure, and taxonomy as an inspiring probe, not of how bacteria work or what they are made of, but a probe into the differences between them, what those differences mean to the bacteria themselves and how they affect the bacterium's relations with other living things and with the environment. For taxonomy is a search into all these things; it is not just a list of names or collections of species; it is a study of living organisms, potentially beneficial and potentially dangerous, a study that can inspire the humanist and the devout; the only one it cannot (or should not) inspire is the politician (more about him when we deal with nomenclature in Section 9.3). To be a taxonomist and enjoy it, one needs a desire to be tidy, methodical, and orderly, even if one has the most untidy desk and book-

shelves. If you are one of these it is likely that you live, like Alice, in Wonderland and are able to enjoy the absurdities that occur around you.

If you have read Bulloch's (1938) *History of Bacteriology* or Brock's (1961) *Milestones in Microbiology* and enjoyed them you will want to know something of what the early taxonomists did for us and how they approached the subject. Bacteriology developed as an applied science, applied chiefly to diseases of wines, plants, and animals, and not much thought was given to theoretical aspects such as taxonomy. The main lines of investigation were to isolate causes and, if possible, find cures and from them diagnostic bacteriology and preventive medicine were born. To the medical bacteriologist systematics did not matter, but botanists who took an interest in bacteria tried to apply botanical practice to the names. By and large, the medical bacteriologist was content to let names look after themselves; if he isolated what he believed to be the cause of the patient's illness he called it *Bacillus* . . . (a name usually formed from the name of the disease) or . . .*coccus*; other organisms were discarded as contaminants or later as commensals.

Some people do not (or cannot) distinguish between classification and identification; the confusion may arise from the use of dichotomous keys which may look like classifications but are not. In the literature the word taxonomy is often used as a synonym for classification, but in my view this is incorrect, for taxonomy describes what a taxonomist does, and this involves what I once described as the 'Trinity that is Taxonomy', namely classification, nomenclature, and identification.

9.1   Kinds of classification
The early bacteriologists were too busy isolating bacteria to bother about their classification and all

the early systematics on bacteria were made by botanists who introduced their latinized nomenclature; this was followed by a few but ever-increasing number of bacteriologists who needed some sort of name tag so that they could refer to an organism without giving a summarized description of it. While botanists and the few purely academic bacteriologists classified bacteria along the classical lines of orders, families, genera, and species, other practical bacteriologists collected them into groups that meant something to those who practised a particular application of bacteriology. The different forms taken by these classifications can be grouped under a few headings.

9.1.1 Minimal difference classifications are extracts from larger and more comprehensive classifications; they are, in fact, part of minimal difference identification schemes such as are used by bacteriologists concerned with a limit range of bacteria. Water bacteriology probably provides the best example and the classification of coliforms summarizes older classifications based on morphology, sugar reactions, and some biochemical characters. For classifications of this kind Johnston (1895) suggested that a numerical code would be the easiest way to describe (and identify) an organism; he commented that the tests (and so the characters described) were chosen 'more because they happen to form part of laboratory routine than on account of their special value for species differentiation and grouping'. The water bacteriologist's classification that has developed has little in common with modern enterobacteriological classifications, but it still serves a useful purpose by indicating possible pollution of a potable water supply. It is based on a few simple tests and the results of these tests can be expressed by plus and minus signs, using the acronym IMViC (Parr, 1936) for indole, methyl red, Voges–Proskauer, and citrate utilization tests.

9.1.2 Classification by discipline. Because bacteriology started as an applied science, each discipline formed its own classification of bacteria. With pathologists at the head, medical bacteriology classified and identified organisms with the diseases they were thought to produce; other organisms regarded as contaminants were dismissed as unimportant unless they were so similar to a pathogen that the two might be confused; in that event they were given a place in some scheme of labelled bacteria. Similar attitudes were taken in other disciplines, and except between human and veterinary medicine there was little co-operation or exchange of information; thus, medical and plant pathologists might work with similar organisms but, by use of different methods, not realize that they were the same.

Medical bacteriology, with which we are mainly concerned, did not include much systematic work until epidemiological investigations required more and more splitting of the relatively few species so that sources of infection could be pin-pointed and the courses of epidemics traced; this need was satisfied by a development and proliferation of serological typing systems, and these were followed by phage and colicine typing. Until 1929, when the first edition of Topley & Wilson's *Principles of Bacteriology and Immunity* was published, medical bacteriologists in the United Kingdom were content to follow the lead of the pathologists, and only when diseases were clinically similar, as in the enteric fevers, were bacteria considered to be related. This 'relationship' of bacteria and association with a clinical syndrome is perpetuated to this day in the placing of the pertussis and parapertussis organisms in the same genus.

9.1.3 All-purpose classifications. Circumstances and developments were rather different in the United States, where fewer bacteriologists had their initial training in medicine and in pathology departments. There, bacteriologists of all disciplines formed a society, the Society of American Bacteriologists, and to them, inspired no doubt by the young SAB President, R. E. Buchanan, the concept of a hierarchical system presented in the reports of Winslow *et al.* (1917, 1920) did not seem to be so revolutionary as it did to the English and the Scots. But the Winslow Committee's reports did not help those who had to identify cultures, and their needs were no longer met by Chester's (1901) *Manual of Determinative Bacteriology*. The Bergey Committee of the SAB planned and produced the first edition of *Bergey's Manual of Determinative*

Bacteriology in 1923, and this provided both a classification and a scheme intended to help the diagnostician. Since then successive editions of that Manual have been regarded as representing the best of current thought on bacterial classification; indeed, some authors have quoted it as if it had been written in Heaven (which it had not) and its opinions expressed the will of some bacteriological Big Brother (a view not held by any of the editorial boards for the successive editions). The newest edition (1974) abandons any attempt to make a hierarchical classification of the bacteria.

9.1.4 Classifications of convenience.

A commonly held view was expressed by Rahn (1929) when he said that 'It does not matter very much how we divide and which of the many stages of the fluctuating varieties we chose to represent the species, as long as all bacteriologists agree and use the same symbols and names'. But Rahn was a heretic; in 1937 he created the family Enterobacteriaceae with only one genus, and did not characterize it except by lumping together all the co-called genera (*Escherichia, Salmonella, Aerobacter, Klebsiella, Proteus, Erwinia, Eberthella, Shigella* and the gas-formers of *Serratia, Pseudomonas, Flavobacterium* and *Achromobacter*) that he considered should be included in his genus *Enterobacter*, made up of 112 species. (This, of course, is a more inclusive genus than the *Enterobacter* of Hormaeche & Edwards.) Apart from introducing the pseudomonads, Rahn's idea was good and deserved much more serious consideration than it got from the enterobacteriologists of the day.

Hierarchical classifications are mainly of theoretical interest. On the other hand identification is a practical exercise and the diagnostician (using the term in its medical and not its taxonomic sense) is involved with day-to-day identifications and is not concerned with ranks higher than genus or with any supposed phylogeny. For him classification does not have an immediate appeal; it is only the hanger on which he puts his coat, and the groups of convenience used in Chapters 6 and 7 of this *Manual* are such hangers. The characteristics of the members of the different communities described in the tables do not represent anything more permanent than the thinking behind this edition or anything

more than the grouping that must arise when, as in our scheme, certain characters are chosen to form the first signposts to the next set of tables. The groups of convenience do not form part of any classification, but they could form the basis for one; I do not press the point.

9.1.5 Classifications made by statistical methods.

A statistical appraisal of the correlation of characters (as distinct from the expression of characters by numerals) is quite old, as is the principle of attaching equal significance to all characters. Levine (1918) used such a method to classify 333 coliforms, based his subdivisions on 13 variable characters and excluded characters, such as glucose fermentation, that were common to all strains.

It was a long time before further progress was made along these lines; Sneath's (1957a, b) reappraisal, and the development of what became known as numerical taxonomy (Sneath & Sokal, 1962; Sokal & Sneath, 1963) was described succinctly by Sokal (1965) as 'based on observed characters of taxa rather than on phylogenetic speculation', but he also warned that 'Enthusiasm for . . . statistical methods . . . should be tempered by caution against possible abuse'.

A successful approach to numerical taxonomy demands that three points should be satisfied: (i) The characters of a large number of strains should be determined. (ii) Many characters should be examined and, as far as possible, these characters should not be selected. (In practice, ease of determination makes some characters more popular than others.) (iii) All characters should be treated as if they have equal value (i.e. they should be given equal weight) in a classification. It was feared that numerical methods might result in a great splitting and the creation of large numbers of taxa that showed but small differences, but Focht & Lockhart (1965) think they are more likely to clump taxa by showing up spurious differences in orthodox classifications; many of these differences may be due to imperfectly standardized techniques (Lockhart, 1967). Numerical taxonomy is as dependent on good bench work as is intuitive classification, and all efforts to standardize methods are to be encouraged.

One of Focht & Lockhart's (1965) findings should

make all designers of diagnostic tables pause to think: the elimination of all sugar reactions after (or except) glucose does not make any significant difference to a classification made by numerical methods. If this holds true for identification we should be able to make many of our tables smaller without affecting their usefulness. I shirked putting this to the test and leave sugar reactions in the hope that the additional information, although presumably unnecessary, will characterize the organisms more fully.

9.1.6 Classification by computer is a misnomer; this is classification based on statistical principles and is numerical classification under the name of its handmaiden, but what's in a name? Colman (1968), working with streptococci, compared the effect of different computer programmes; with two of them the results agreed well with accepted classifications but the results produced by a third programme seemed unrelated to conventional arrangements. His conclusion, which is indisputable, is that numerical methods will only be successful when the right programme is chosen. The whole subject of computers as taxonomic tools was surveyed by Sneath (1972) and this review should be read by all who propose to use computers for classification.

9.2 Identification

In Section 9.1 the different approaches to classification were traced; here I shall consider the ways by which an identification can be attempted. Whatever method is used, to be satisfactory it must be based on good characterization of the unknown organism; in other words, the data that make up the input must be accurate and reliable. The demand for speed in clinical bacteriology is sometimes made the excuse for poor workmanship in the laboratory or for the application of rapid but crude methods. There cannot be any objection to rapid methods just because they are rapid; as long as they give reliable results they must be accepted; it is only when rapidity leads to shoddy work that they cannot be tolerated. To obtain reliable characterization, by whatever method, the first essential is that the starting point is a pure culture; this rules out any method in which the inoculum of a set of tests is

taken from a colony of the primary plate when that is a selective medium.

Identification has been described as the lowest form of taxonomic work; on the other hand taxonomy has been characterized as 'essentially the technique of identification' (Mayr, 1968). What is indisputable is that identification is the only part of taxonomy for which a bacteriologist will be paid a salary; the intricacies of classification and the complexities of nomenclature are sidelines to be pursued by workers in their spare time.

Sometimes identification is considered as classification in reverse; Skerman (1949) objected to this as a principle and thought that it would lead to the use, or attempted use, of indeterminable characters. Identification consists in characterizing the unknown as thoroughly as one is able, and comparing the characters found with those of known, classified, and named organisms. When the characters can be matched, the unknown will be identified with one of the knowns. If the number of characters compared is small then the perfect match will be common; more often, when many (some would say enough) characters are compared it is seldom possible to make a perfect match (i.e. find true identity) and one must be satisfied with a near match in which the number of divergencies is small. The choice of characters and methods for ascertaining them have been described earlier in this *Manual*; we should now consider the methods for recording the characteristics and comparing them with the unknown.

9.2.1 Identification by tables. Conn (1900) used tables with +, ±, and − signs for characters, and recorded the characters of his unknowns on a slip of paper which he moved over the table in much the same way as we moved a Perspex strip over our tables (Cowan & Steel, 1961). In 1907 Conn and his colleagues commented that 'unless the characteristics of species can be clearly and distinctly *tabulated*, it is almost a hopeless task ... to identify a new culture with one previously described'. Tables of characters, mostly sugar reactions, became popular and formed large and interesting sections of books such as Castellani & Chalmers' (1919) *Manual of Tropical Medicine*. But even simple positive results were often given a symbol more complex than a plus sign, and when attempts were made to combine in one symbol two characters such as acid and gas production the tables became too complicated for use and, in the absence of a standardization of symbols, they fell into disrepute.

Tables began to gain favour again when a simple, standardized arrangement and clear descriptions of characters were introduced in the reports of the Enterobacteriaceae Subcommittee (Report, 1954a, b; 1958); these lists of characters could be combined and we used them in our earlier work on diagnostic tables (Cowan, 1956b; Cowan & Steel, 1961). The tables of the first edition of this *Manual* apparently worked reasonably well in the field; they were used in all parts of the world and their simplicity made them suitable for use in small laboratories. In my view the most remarkable feature of these tables, increasingly evident from Cowan & Steel (1961) to Tables 6.1 and 7.1 of this edition, is the small number of characters (or tests) needed to place the bacteria we deal with in a genus, and this has been confirmed by the use of punched cards in place of tables (see Chapter 8).

9.2.2 **Dichotomous keys** have never been popular with clinical bacteriologists who like to be able to establish a routine that can be followed for most organisms isolated from specimens. The keys in the front of *Bergey's Manual* were not at all helpful to the medical bacteriologist, and it was said that to use *Bergey's Manual* one had to be a good enough bacteriologist to be able to do without the keys and find one's own way to the genus; it was not until Skerman's key was added to the seventh edition that keys were taken seriously in medical bacteriology. Obviously the usefulness of keys varies with the kind of organism to be identified; according to Küster (1972) they are the most useful way of identifying *Streptomyces* species; on the other hand, they are unlikely to be used to identify enterobacteria.

9.2.3 **Mechanical devices**. Bits and pieces of paper, card, plastic, wood and metal have been put together to make gadgets aimed at simplyfying the identification of bacteria. Some years ago Difco Laboratories distributed a 'Microbial Identification Aid' devised by C. D. Graber; this was fascinatingly simple, if not entirely reliable. Our own Determinator (Cowan & Steel, 1960, 1961) fell into this category, and of the two versions described the second was both simpler to make and easier to use; but apart from demonstrating the device we never took it into our normal routine. The tables that we compiled for it were more useful and developed into the tables used in this *Manual*. Olds (1966, 1970) made an ingenious device which, from a limited number of characters, enabled an identification to be made, provided always that the machine had been programmed to identify the organism. There must be many more diagnostic gadgets that never came my way, but while I enjoy trying them out (I was once sent a set from Pandora's box), they do not have a serious future for they cannot allow enough leeway for the exceptions that constantly occur among biological materials. One, recently developed as an extension of the API system for identification of enterobacteria, may be the exception that proves the truth of my generalization.

9.2.4 **Punched card systems**, with or without computer sorting, have been developed for the identification of limited groups of bacteria. The schemes mentioned here are simple, do not involve statistical assessment of associations, and can be used with equipment no more elaborate than a card punch, scissors, and a knitting needle or probe. If one is available, a computer can be used.

Corlett, Lee & Sinnhuber (1965) inoculated strains from foods on to a plate of basal medium (20–40 strains per plate) and by replica plating (Lederberg & Lederberg, 1952) transferred the inocula to ten selective media containing different antibiotics. After incubation growth was recorded on punched cards and to this was added information on pigmentation, morphology, and the Gram reaction. Sorting was by digital computer. With this simple scheme more than 99 % of 408 isolates from fish and minced beef were identified to genus. The lesson to be learnt from this is the usefulness of the replica plating method for characterization; the punched cards and sorting system seem to be incidental.

A more elaborate system was described by Schneierson & Amsterdam (1964) in which details of staining reactions, morphological, and the usual physiological and biochemical characters were recorded on a card measuring 191×165 mm. Information for notching the master cards was from 'authoritative references sources'.

To be practicable card systems must be based on the most useful distinguishing characters in the descriptions of the organisms, and it will be obvious that a punched card system can only be as good as the diagnostic tables (or other information) on which it is based. Like our diagnostic tables, cards are suitable for use in a progressive system of identification, using first a minimal difference set of cards to identify the genus (or main group) and other sets (or packs) to identify the species. If not used in a step-by-step system the card holding the character information must be big and have a great many holes in it; to be sufficiently comprehensive such a card would be too clumsy for routine use. A simple and workable progressive punched card system for identification is described in Chapter 8 and Appendix D.

9.2.5 Arithmetical (summation) systems. Fey (1959) worked out a scheme in which he gave a score to each character (acid from mannitol = 5; gas from glucose = 10; growth in KCN = 320, etc.) and added the scores of all positive characters; from the total he turned to a table from which the identification could be made. Steel (1962a) tested this scheme but had trouble with it; he found that all his strains of *Bordetella bronchiseptica* grew in KCN medium, which gave them 320 too many marks, and they were identified as *Proteus mirabilis*. Baer & Washington (1972) applied the scheme to some enterobacteria (salmonellas and shigellas were excluded) and also found discrepant results with the KCN test. They modified the scheme, introduced confirmatory tests, and with this modification claimed an accuracy of 99%. This degree of accuracy suggests that they had standardized their tests well, and that their media (all commercially produced) gave exceptionally consistent results in the various tests.

9.2.6 Statistical methods (identification by computer). Payne (1963) suggested the use of computers for progressive bacterial identification but the examples he gave, based on information and methods developed by Dybowski & Franklin (1968), were far from convincing. Lapage, Bascomb, Willcox & Curtis (1970, 1973) worked out a scheme that was tested on strains difficult to identify by methods used by competent bacteriologists in well equipped laboratories. Whitby & Blair (1970) described the working of an identification routine in a hospital laboratory in which they used the computer available to the hospital for patients' records. The punch cards of their scheme became the work cards for the specimens, and a great deal of time spent on recording, copying, and punching was eliminated.

Systems such as these meet two main difficulties in the planning and development stages. The first is the standardization of technical methods, but within any one laboratory this is not insuperable. In this connexion, each laboratory should attempt from time to time to estimate its own (intra-laboratory) errors by carrying out replicate tests on the control cultures. Within one laboratory this error should not exceed 5%; if it does, either the test should be abandoned or the whole routine of tests and the media used for them should be overhauled until a better standard is attained (Sneath & Johnson, 1972).

The second difficulty lies in the collection of accurate information about the characters of the different species, using the tests employed in the particular laboratory. A promising method for establishing reference descriptions is to work out the Calculated Mean Organism (CMO of Liston, Wiebe & Colwell, 1963) or the Hypothetical Mean Organism (HMO of Tsukamura & Mizuno, 1968) characterizations of the species most often encountered in medical laboratories. Another method, which also needs access to a computer, is to work out the likelihood or probability that a character will be positive and compare this, again with computer help, with the laboratory findings. The theory of this probabilistic method of making an identification, and an example of its application to fermentative and other Gram-negative rods was described in some detail by Lapage, Bascomb, Willcox & Curtiss (1973), Bascomb *et al.* (1973) and Willcox *et al.* (1973), and these papers should be consulted by anyone who contemplates enlisting the help of a computer to solve his identification problems.

9.3 Nomenclature and numericlature

However good a classification may seem, however easy its units are to identify, its usefulness will be tested by its communicability. To be successful the means of communication must be informative and it should be able to reach and be meaningful to those outside the bacteriological field. Communication is made by some form of label, some are descriptive and others are non-descriptive; some labels consist of words (names, acronyms), others of figures (accession numbers, codes), or letters and figures (codes). We describe the naming process as nomenclature; when numbers or codes form the label we call it numericlature or coding. Names are the most popular form of label but in my view numbers and coded forms are more useful because they can be made informative. Names are often believed to be descriptive (which they need not be) and they can confuse the unwary and the ignorant, as the misled politician who wanted the generic name Salmonella to be suppressed because he thought it affected the sales of fish. Accession numbers (used in culture collections) do not change with the reclassification of organisms, neither do descriptive codes; both these have a permanency that a name could never hope to attain.

9.3.1 Aims of nomenclature and numericlature. It is convenient to consider aims under three subheadings which, in order of importance are: (i) ease of reference and comprehension, (ii) permanence and stability, and (iii) descriptiveness (meaningfulness).

(i) Euphonious words are probably the easiest and briefest form of verbal communication, but words that slip from the tongue of natives of one country may be tongue twisters to their neighbours. Latin is used as an international language and because it is a dead language it does not have national overtones or rouse nationalistic prejudice. But in speech Latin is far from being international and one need only compare the pronunciation of the specific epithet 'coli' by Englishmen and Americans to realize that Latin is not a uniform language. And for the deaf the difference in sound may render a name quite incomprehensible.

My dislike of latinized names explains why I take issue with Hugh & Feeley (1972a) on the use of common names. I maintain, with Wilson (1965), that we write in English and not in Latin; English is understood by all English-speaking people (and many more in scientific circles), whereas Latin is understood by a minority, even of educated Englishmen. Whenever possible I use colloquial names and reserve latinized binominals for the rare occasions on which scientific accuracy is essential, as in a book like this.

(ii) Permanence will apply to bacterial labels only when they are descriptive. When the label is a word that is part of a classification (as Pseudomonadaceae derived from *Pseudomonas*) it may change when there is a change in classification. All bacteriologists know that classifications, like clothes, are changed often, and as with clothes, changes in fashion bring changes in names.

(iii) Descriptive labels do not (or should not) change with the revision of a classification; the organism that causes enteric fever has exactly the same characters whether it is called the typhoid bacillus, *Bacillus typhosus*, *Bacterium typhosum*, *Eberthella typhosa*, or *Salmonella typhi*. But if it can be described by a code, as say 'species 12345', that label could be permanently attached to it. But numerical coding schemes are not popular and are often considered to be the work of eccentrics.

9.3.2 Codes of Bacteriological Nomenclature.

Medical bacteriologists were content with labels easy to remember and for them the names of the disease or the discoverer of the organism were both simple and easily recalled, as the diphtheria bacillus, Koch's bacillus, Pfeiffer's bacillus, Shiga's dysentery bacillus and the like, but this kind of name did not appeal to the bacteriologist trained as a botanist, to whom the differences between tonsillitis and scarlatina might be a mystery. Neither did it lend itself to the formation of hierarchies and the other devices of orthodox taxonomists.

Botanists have had a code of botanical nomenclature since 1867 and it was botanists who first applied latinized names to bacteria. They were not very good at bacteriology; most of Cohn's (1872) *Micrococcus* species were, in fact, rods. The

botanists' names did not please medical bacteriologists who have had more than their share of
nomenclatural troubles with changes in anatomical
terminology (three or four times in my lifetime)
and the instability and variation in names of
diseases from one country to another. A code of
nomenclature for bacteria was suggested at the
first international congress of microbiologists in
1930. The history of the Bacteriological Code is
part of the life stories of three men (the three Bs),
R. E. Buchanan, R. S. Breed, and R. St John-
Brooks (see Obituary, R. E. Buchanan, 1973). The
Code was approved in 1947 and has been amended
repeatedly; a completely revised version was prepared (Lapage *et al.* 1973) for consideration by
members of the nomenclature committee in September 1973. Further details are given in Appendix
G, which also indicates the effect of the proposed
changes in rules on the scientific names used in
this edition.

The Bacteriological Code has been criticized
(Cowan, 1970*a*, 1971) but its principles are sound;
it is aimed at fixity of names but, as pointed out in
Section 9.3.1, names may change because of a
change in classification. It is also aimed at avoiding
confusion, but it sometimes creates it. 'In the
absence of a relevant rule ... established custom
must be followed' (Principle 2; Rule 4 in the
proposed revision).* But custom, like fashion, is a
fickle jade, and differs in different parts of the world.

Principle 3 [2] says that the names of bacteria
should not duplicate those of fungi, algae, protozoa,
or viruses, but they may be the same as those of the
larger plants and animals.

Nomenclature (and the Code) deals with the
names of the different categories (ranks) such as
species, genera, and families, and there are recommendations on the formation of generic names and
specific epithets from the names of individuals
(patronymics). The recommendations in the proposed revision (Lapage *et al.* 1973) differ considerably from those of the 1966 and earlier editions of

* All quotations in this section are from the last
approved version of the *International Code of
Nomenclature of Bacteria* (1966). Numbers in square
brackets are those of the equivalent Principles in the
proposed revision (Lapage *et al.* 1973) of the Code,
which was approved before publication of this
edition of this *Manual*.

the Code; if they are accepted the -*ii* ending of
epithets such as morganii will disappear and be
replaced by the -*i* ending (morganii will become
morgani). But see Section G1, p. 191.

Principle 8 [4] which is often forgotten, gives the
purpose of a name as a means of referring to a
taxon, not to describing it, or giving its history. The
correctness of names is dealt with in Principle 9
[6, 8] and this forms the so-called 'priority rule'.
It is a source of confusion (which it is intended to
prevent) because its application is retroactive (the
proposed revision will make retroactivity unnecessary after 1980 when Approved Lists of Names of
Bacteria will contain the only officially acceptable
names).

Principle 10 [9] urges bacteriologists not to
change the name of a taxon. In this *Manual*
readers will find examples (*Acinetobacter anitratus*
is one) where we have followed Principle 10 and
ignored Principle 9 when its application runs
counter to the greater sense of Principle 10.

Principle 11 [5] is also well-intentioned but
troublesome. It concerns the nomenclatural type,
which is a device for attaching a name to a taxon.
While the designation of types is regulated by rules,
the only essential guiding principle is not one of
them; this should state that the strain chosen to
represent a species (to which the name of that
species is always to be attached) should be characteristic of that species. The requirement seems
obvious to a working bacteriologist, but it was not
in the botanical code and has never been introduced
to the bacteriological code.

The type concept, a favourite of nomenclaturists,
is not popular with all taxonomists; Oldroyd (1966),
an entomologist, wrote of 'The ... evil of the
type concept' and criticized the overriding importance given to names and their correct latinization.
Gordon (1967), an opponent of the designation of a
single strain to represent a species (the type strain),
says that her 'concept of species necessitated the
acceptance of microbial variation as one of the
facts of life'. She believes that a strain should
always belong to the same species, that the identity
of the species should be inherent in the strain itself
and not in its source, history, or someone's note-
book. Gordon's concept of a species is that of a
microbial population and she defines it as 'a group

of freshly isolated strains, of strains maintained *in vitro* for many years and of their variants, that have in common a set of reliable characteristics separating them from other groups of strains'. In her opinion, which I share but know it is not universally accepted, 'The properties of strains persisting after years of cultivation in the test tube . . . [are] useful criteria for defining the species.'

Much of the Bacteriological Code is devoted to the spelling of names but we do not think that the way a name is spelt is half as important as the clarity of the description of the organism; but although this circumscription is not nomenclature, the proposed code intends to improve matters by insisting that names must be accompanied by a description that meets certain minimal standards.

There is, in the Bacteriological Code, a great deal of fuss, in the earlier versions written in a pseudolegalistic jargon brought over from the botanical code, about legitimate and illegitimate names, of effective and of valid publication, and recommendations of doubtful authenticity on the transliteration of words. Such trivialities are irritating, or I find them so and this probably explains my interest in coding schemes to avoid most of the nomenclatural problems.

9.3.3   Descriptive codes. In reviews of coding schemes used in taxonomy these were divided into labelling codes (substitutes for names) and descriptive codes, and outline histories of the two kinds of codes were given (Cowan, 1965*a*, *b*). The application of the Dewey decimal system of classification to bacteria (Harding, 1910) produced numbers of too many digits to be read with ease and accuracy, and one solution suggested was the grouping of characters. Such a solution would necessitate a recasting of diagnostic tables and probably new tables showing the possible (or probable) combinations of grouped characters. The magnitude of the task can be seen from the formula to find the number of possible combinations of characters that can be expressed by + and − signs; this is 2^n, where n is the number of independently variable characters. With a simple code based on the IMViC reactions there are sixteen possible combinations; with more characters the number of possible combinations rises rapidly. In tables in which dee characters, as used in tables of this *Manual*, occur, the characterization of one 'species' would have to extend over many columns if the various dee characters were written out in their + and − forms. Theoretically, it would then be possible to code a strain by the table number followed by the column number which had the same characters as the unknown. But this is much too complicated for everyday use.

A possibility that is being developed is the feeding of information on small groups of characters to a simple mechanical device to give a code number in an easily determined form. Applied to the enterobacteria, the groups of characters can be determined in the Ivan Hall tubes of the API characterizing sets.

APPENDIX A

Preparation of culture media

A1   GENERAL CONSIDERATIONS

The ability of bacteria to grow on media that are inhibitory to other bacteria gives the organisms of the first group special characteristics that may help in their identification; the media themselves, with their selective and differential qualities, have particular interest to diagnosticians and this justifies their inclusion here. In this edition we have added a few notes on the isolation of bacteria and have made passing reference to enrichment and other media used in growing organisms from clinical material, but we have not done justice to these media and methods for this *Manual* is concerned with the organisms that have been isolated and await identification.

In this appendix, media are listed under the following headings and section numbers:

Basic media (A2.1)
Enriched media (A2.2)
Enrichment media (A2.3)
Differential (selective) media (A2.4)
Media for the enhancement of pigmentation (A2.5)
Media for carbohydrate studies (A2.6)

A1.1   Cleaning and sterilization of glassware

Glassware to contain media such as Koser's citrate, in which there is a single source of an element, must be chemically clean to be free from that element. The method recommended by E. A. Dawes (personal communication) is to boil all tubes in 20 % nitric acid for 5–10 minutes and then wash by rinses of glass-distilled water. Tubes are dried in an oven in the inverted position, in baskets lined with filter paper to prevent contact of the mouths of tubes with metal.

Glassware such as Petri dishes and test tubes (metal or cotton stoppered) are sterilized in a hot air oven, preferably with a fan, at 160–170 °C for one hour. The efficiency of the oven and the even distribution of heat should be controlled each day by placing Browne's green spot type III* tubes on each shelf (see Darmady,

* Albert Browne Ltd., Chancery Street, Leicester LE1 5WA.

Hughes & Jones, 1958; Brown & Ridout, 1960). Overheating of cotton-plugged tubes must be avoided; several workers (Wright, 1934*a*; Drea, 1942; Pollock, 1948) have drawn attention to the inhibitory effect of substances volatilized from cotton during dry heat sterilization. Tubes and flasks capped with polypropylene covers (Varney, 1961) and screw-capped bottles (caps loose) are sterilized by autoclaving.

A1.2   Indicators

The pH indicators used in bacteriology are shown in Table A1; some are not readily soluble in water and are dissolved in dilute alkali or ethanol. The preparation of Andrade's indicator and litmus solution are more complex and details are given in Sections A1.2.1 and A1.2.2.

A1.2.1   Andrade's indicator (modified from Andrade, 1906)

Acid fuchsin	5 g
Distilled water	1000 ml
N-NaOH	150–180 ml

Dissolve the acid fuchsin in the distilled water and add 150 ml of alkali solution. Mix and allow the mixture to stand at room temperature with frequent shaking for 24 h; the colour should change from red to brown.

If the dye has not been sufficiently decolorized add a further 10 ml of alkali, mix thoroughly and leave for another 24 h. Subsequent additions of alkali may have to be made. The ultimate colour desired is a straw-yellow and the aim is to attain this with the minimum of alkali.

Test: add 1 % of the indicator to peptone water pH 7.2, mix thoroughly and determine pH; note the rise in pH due to the alkalinity of the indicator and label accordingly. Should the increase in pH be 0.2 all batches of medium to which this indicator is to be added must have an initial pH value 0.2 lower than the desired final reaction.

Table A1 *Indicators and their characteristics*

Indicator	Usual concentration (%)	ml 0.05 N-NaOH per g indicator	Solvent	pH range	Colour change (acid to alkaline)
Methyl red	0.2	—	50% ethanol	4.2–6.3	red–yellow
Chlorphenol red	0.2	47	water or 50% ethanol	4.8–6.4	yellow–purple
Andrade's			water	5–8	pink–yellow
Litmus			40% ethanol	5–8	red–blue
Bromcresol purple	0.2	37 ⎫	water or 50% ethanol	⎰ 5.2–6.8	yellow–purple
Bromthymol blue	0.2	32 ⎭		⎱ 6.0–7.6	yellow–blue
Neutral red	0.1	—	50% ethanol	6.8–8.0	red–yellow
Phenol red	0.2	57 ⎫	water or 50% ethanol	⎧ 6.8–8.4	yellow–red
Cresol red	0.2	53 ⎬		7.2–8.8	yellow–red
Thymol blue	0.2	43 ⎭		⎩ 8.0–9.6	yellow–blue
Phenolphthalein	0.1	—	50% ethanol	8.3–10.0	colourless–red

A1.2.2 Litmus solution (modified from McIntosh, 1920)

Litmus, granular   250 g
Ethanol (40%)   1000 ml

Grind the litmus and place in a flask with 500 ml of the ethanol; boil for 1 min, decant the liquid and add the remainder of the ethanol to the residue; boil for 1 min, decant and add the liquid to the first decoction.

Centrifuge and adjust the volume of the supernatant to 1000 ml with ethanol (40%); add N-HCl drop by drop until the solution becomes purple.

Test for correct reaction: boil 10 ml of distilled water, cool, and add one drop of litmus solution; after mixing the water becomes mauve.

This indicator solution is used at a concentration of about 2.5%.

A1.3 Carbohydrates

'Sugars' used in bacteriology are shown in Table A2, where they are grouped by their chemical structure.

A1.4 Clarification of media

Liquid media may be clarified by filtration through paper, sintered glass, or asbestos fibre (Seitz filtration). To prevent adsorption the use of a filter aid such as kieselguhr or talc is best avoided. Wright (1934b) found that filtration of broth through a thick filtering layer resulted in marked reduction in its growth-promoting capacity.

The grades of material suitable for clarification of media are shown in Table A3.

Agar-containing media must be clarified while in the molten state; paper pulp is often used or a grade of filter paper especially designed for the filtration of agar sols. To prevent solidification during filtration, a steam or hot-water jacketed funnel is used; alternatively, filter rapidly through a Buchner funnel, in which case, a paper of greater wet strength should be used. A method for the filtration of agar-containing media during sterilization in an autoclave was described by Brown (1961).

Gelatin-containing media were in the past clarified with the aid of egg-white or horse serum; gelatin for bacteriological use is now of such quality that this step is unnecessary and gelatin media may be clarified as those containing agar.

A1.5 Sterilization of media

The method of sterilization recommended for each medium is included with the details of preparation.

A1.6 Storage of media

Freshly prepared medium is desirable although with some (e.g. Wilson and Blair's bismuth sulphite agar) maturation is necessary. Many media can be safely kept at room temperature or in a refrigerator for several weeks, or even months, before use. Stability varies with the individual medium and it is not possible to fix a useful storage life. The important point is that moisture should be retained. To prevent evaporation and concentration of the constituents when media are to be stored, they should be kept in screw-capped rather than in cotton-plugged containers. Appreciable evaporation can occur in a refrigerator but this can be prevented by putting tubed media in polythene bags. If nutrient agar

Table A2 *Carbohydrates used in bacteriology*

Class	Carbohydrate	Convenient concentration in water (w/v) at 20 °C
Pentoses	Arabinose (L+)	40
	Xylose	50
Methyl pentose	Rhamnose (isodulcitol)	40
Hexoses	Fructose (laevulose)	50
	Galactose	30
	Glucose (dextrose)	50
	Mannose	50
	Sorbose	40
Disaccharides	Cellobiose	10
	Lactose	15
	Maltose	50
	Melibiose	10
	Sucrose (saccharose)	50
	Trehalose	25
Trisaccharides	Melezitose	10
	Raffinose	10
Polysaccharides	Glycogen	5; dissolves to produce an opalescent solution.
	Inulin	20 at 70 °C; solution may be slightly opalescent.
	Starch, soluble	soluble in hot water
Glycosides	Aesculin (esculin)	0.1; 7.5 on heating
	Amygdalin	7.5
	Arbutin	10
	Salicin	3
Alcohols	Adonitol	40
	Dulcitol	5; readily soluble on heating
	Erythritol	40
	Glycerol	miscible in all proportions
	Mannitol	15
	Sorbitol	50
Non-carbohydrate	Inositol	15

slopes appear to be dry, they should be melted and re-solidified.

Strong light is detrimental to most media and storage in the dark is preferable, especially for those containing dyes or indicators.

Egg media should be kept for a long period before use in order that contaminants that grow only at room temperature have the opportunity to develop into visible colonies.

Cotton-plugged tubes are a potential source of contamination; the moisture absorbed by the cotton is sufficient to permit development of fungi, and hyphae may penetrate a cotton plug.

Media which have been kept in a refrigerator should be allowed to attain room temperature before use. Because the solubility of gases in liquids decreases with

increase in temperature, it is essential to check that gas bubbles do not appear in the Durham's tubes of carbohydrate media as they warm up from storage to room temperature. Fluid media to be used for anaerobic cultivation (particularly those containing thioglycollate) should be heated in a boiling water bath to remove dissolved air and allowed to cool undisturbed before use.

Poured plates may be kept at 4–15 °C, but they should not be put close to the cooling unit of a domestic-type refrigerator. Excess water of condensation can be avoided by allowing the medium to cool before pouring it into Petri dishes. If plates are to be stored in an exposed position they should be stacked with the lid uppermost; in canisters they should be inverted.

Higher forms of life can also be troublesome in a

Table A3 *Materials, and grades, suitable for clarifying media*

	Liquid media	Agar-containing media	
		Simple funnel	Buchner funnel
Papers:			
Green's	798½; 904½	500½; 904½	960; 993
Whatman	1; 30; 52	15	52
Postlip	633E	agar-agar	agar-agar
Schleicher & Schüll	520B½; 598½	520A½; 520B½	520B
Delta	317¾		376
Munktell	5		0
Sintered glass:			
Jena ⎫ Pyrex ⎬	1; 2		
Asbestos pads:			
Seitz	K3; K4; K5		
Sterimats	FCB		
Carlson	K3; K5		

laboratory and we must be on the look-out for insects (beetles) and arachnids (mites). They are potentially dangerous in a medical laboratory, when plates are kept on the bench or incubated at 22 °C, and we have observed the 'footprints' left by mites crossing agar media inoculated with cultures. Dehydrated media are particularly liable to insect attack; the eggs laid by the adult hatching into larvae which can feed upon carbohydrate material.

A1.7 Volumes of Media

The volumes to be put in Petri dishes will vary with the size of the dish. In the United Kingdom there is a British Standard specification (BS 611 : 1952) for glass Petri dishes but none for polystyrene dishes. Recommended volumes are 15–20 ml medium for the 90 mm (3½ in) and 20–25 ml medium for the 100 mm (4 in) dish.

Volumes for media in tubes are shown in Table A4.

A2 FORMULAE OF MEDIA

Two terms need explanation and refer to all formulae.

Agar. In this Appendix the agar concentration relates to Japanese agar; when New Zealand agar is used the amount stated in the formulae should be multiplied by 0.6 to give approximately the same gelling strength. Concentrations for different types of gel are shown in Table A5. Agar is made from seaweed from many parts of the world but the origin is seldom stated on the label of commercial preparations; consequently Table A5 and others like it are not as useful as they appear.

Regard should be paid to the information supplied by the manufacturer and the concentrations advised for different purposes.

Agar is a poor conductor of heat (Bridson & Brecker, 1970) and time must be allowed for heat penetration both in media making and in the safety sterilization of media after cultures have grown on it. The altitude of a laboratory may affect the ease with which agar goes into solution and it may not be practicable to dissolve agar in a steamer; at 2000–3000 feet we had so many soft plates that we resorted to melting agar in the autoclave at about 0.36 kg/cm^2 (5 lb/in^2).

Water. The term water, used in all formulae, implies potable tap water. When distilled water is specified in a formula, de-ionized water may be used.

A2.1 Basic media

A2.1.1 Nutrient broth

Beef extract	10 g
Peptone	10 g
NaCl	5 g
Water	1000 ml

Dissolve the ingredients by heating in the water. Adjust to pH 8.0–8.4 with 10 N-NaOH and boil for 10 min. Filter, adjust to pH 7.2–7.4, and sterilize at 115 °C for 20 min.

Notes. Nutrient agar is nutrient broth gelled by the addition of 2 % agar.

Table A4 *Usual volumes of media (in ml) for tubes of various sizes*

Medium	Tube size			
	75 × 12 mm (3 × ½ in)	100 × 12 mm (4 × ½ in)	125 × 12 mm (5 × ½ in)	150 × 16 mm (6 × ⅝ in)
Liquids	1–2	2–2.5	3	4–5
Slopes (slants)	1	1.5–2	2.5–3	5
Slopes with butts	2.5	2.5	3.5–4	7
Stabs	2.5	2.5	4	7

Table A5 *Concentration (%) of agar in media for different purposes*

Type of medium	Agar			
	Japanese	New Zealand	'Ionagar no 2'[a]	American
Solid (normal)	1.5–2.0	1.0–1.2	1.0	1.5
Solid (to inhibit spreaders)	7	4		
Semisolid	0.1–0.5	0.05–0.3	0.7	0.3–0.4
'Motility media'				0.1–0.4

[a] Ionagar no. 2 was a special purpose agar used only when a defined medium was needed. Now replaced by Purified Agar (Oxoid L28).

Semisolid nutrient agar (Craigie agar, sloppy agar, slush agar) is nutrient broth containing 0.4 % shred agar.

Double-strength nutrient agar follows the same formula as nutrient agar but the volume of water is reduced to 500 ml.

Layered plates consist of two layers of solidified medium; in layered blood agar (Section A2.2.1) the bottom layer consists of blood agar base or peptone water agar (Section A2.1.2) and the top layer is blood agar base + 5 % blood.

The thin top layer may contain other substances under test; some, such as chitin, are insoluble and the suspension is made either in water agar (Section A2.1.12) or saline agar (Section A2.1.11).

A2.1.2   Peptone water

Peptone	10 g
NaCl	5 g
Water	1000 ml

Dissolve the solids by heating in the water. Adjust to pH 8.0–8.4 and boil for 10 min. Filter, adjust to pH 7.2–7.4, and sterilize at 115 °C for 20 min.

Peptone water agar is peptone water gelled by the addition of 2 % agar.

A2.1.3   Robertson's cooked meat medium (modified from Lepper & Martin, 1929)

Minced meat	1000 g
0.05 N-NaOH	1000 ml

Add the minced meat to the alkali solution, mix well and heat to boiling, simmer for 20 min with frequent stirring. Skim off the fat and check pH, which should be about 7.5. Strain through gauze or muslin, squeeze out excess liquor, and dry the meat particles at a temperature below 50 °C. For use, place sufficient dried meat in a screw-capped container to a depth of about 2.5 cm and add sufficient nutrient broth to give a depth of about 5 cm. Sterilize at 115 °C for 20 min; avoid rapid release of pressure in the autoclave after sterilization.

Note. Although called Robertson's cooked meat, the method of preparation differs considerably from the original method (Robertson, 1916).

Cooked meat medium (alternative formula)

Horse meat, fat-free and minced	450 g
Distilled water	1000 ml

Boil the meat in the water for 1 h. Filter through muslin and press the meat dry.

NaCl	5 g
Peptone	10 g

Add the NaCl and peptone to the filtrate, adjust to pH 8.4 with 10 N-NaOH and bring to the boil.

Sodium thioglycollate, 45 % soln   1 ml

Filter and add the thioglycollate soln.

Distribute the dry meat particles to a depth of 2.5 cm into screw-capped bottles, add the broth to a level of 5 cm. Sterilize at 115 °C for 20 min; allow the pressure to fall slowly after sterilization.

A2.1.4 Digest broth (modified from Hartley, 1922, and Pope & Smith, 1932)

Meat, finely minced	600 g
Na$_2$CO$_3$, anhyd.	8 g
Water	1000 ml

Add the alkali and the meat to the water, heat to 80 °C, stir well and cool.

Pancreatic extract, Cole & Onslow's	20 ml
CHCl$_3$	20 ml

Heat the infused mixture to 45–50 °C, add the pancreatic extract (below) and chloroform, and maintain at 45–50 °C for 4–6 h with frequent stirring. Follow the course of digestion by the biuret test (p. 157).

HCl, conc.   16 ml

Add the acid, boil for 30 min and filter. Adjust to pH 8, boil for 30 min and filter. Adjust to pH 7.6, determine the amino acid nitrogen content (Section A3.3.2) and dilute the broth to contain 700–750 mg amino acid N$_2$ per l. Sterilize at 115 °C for 20 min.

Notes. Cole & Onslow's pancreatic extract may be replaced by a commercial trypsin extract or powder.

Pope & Smith recommend the fractional addition of the enzyme during the digestion process.

Digest agar is digest broth gelled by the addition of 2 % agar.

A2.1.5 Pancreatic extract (Cole & Onslow, 1916)

Fresh pig pancreas	250 g
Distilled water	750 ml
Industrial methylated spirit	250 ml

Add the water and spirit to the fat-free and minced pancreas in a 2 l flask and stopper tightly. Shake thoroughly and leave at room temperature for 3 days with frequent shaking. Filter, add 0.1 % conc. HCl to the filtrate and mix well. Store at 4 °C. The cloudy precipitate which settles in a few days may be filtered off. The extract may be expected to retain its activity for several months when stored at 4 °C.

Note. A satisfactory extract should have a tryptic content of at least 50 units per ml (Section A3.1.8).

A2.1.6 Infusion broth (modified from Wright, 1933)

Meat, minced	450 g
Water	1000 ml

Infuse the meat in the water overnight at 4 °C.

Peptone	10 g
NaCl	5 g

Skim the fat from the infused mixture, add the peptone and salt and boil for 30 min. Filter, adjust to pH 8.4 and boil for 20 min. Filter, adjust to pH 7.6, and sterilize at 115 °C for 20 min.

Infusion agar is infusion broth gelled by the addition of 2 % agar.

A2.1.7 CYLG broth (Marshall & Kelsey, 1960)

Casein digest	10 g
Marmite*	5 g
Sodium glycerophosphate	10 g
Potassium lactate, 50 % w/w	10 ml
Glucose	2 g
Inorganic salts soln	5 ml
Distilled water	1000 ml

Dissolve the ingredients by heating, mix, filter, and sterilize at 115 °C for 20 min.

Inorganic salts solution:

10 N-H$_2$SO$_4$	0.1 ml
MgSO$_4$·7H$_2$O	4 g
MnSO$_4$·4H$_2$O	0.4 g
FeSO$_4$·7H$_2$O	0.4 g
Water	100 ml

Add the acid to the water and dissolve the salts without heating.

Note. This basal medium may be supplemented by the addition of blood or serum, gelled by the addition of agar, and can form the basis of many standard media. It is reproducible, does not require pH adjustment, and can be prepared and stored in concentrated form.

A2.1.8 Thioglycollate broth (modified from Brewer, 1940)

Peptone	15 g
Yeast extract	5 g
NaCl	5 g
Agar	1 g
Thioglycollic acid	1 g
Water	1000 ml

* Marmite Ltd, Burton-on-Trent, UK.

Dissolve the solids in the water with the aid of gentle heat. Add the thioglycollic acid and adjust to pH 8.5 with N-NaOH. Autoclave at 115 °C for 10 min. To prevent darkening of the medium screw-caps should be loosened during autoclaving.

Glucose	5 g
Methylene blue, 1 % aq. soln	0.2 ml

Adjust to pH 7.2, add the glucose and dye soln, mix well and sterilize at 115 °C for 10 min.

Notes. This medium should be stored in screw-capped containers in the dark at 4 °C (Cook & Steel, 1959*b*).

If more than 20% of the medium shows a green colour before use, it should be heated in a boiling water bath or steamer for 5–10 min and allowed to cool undisturbed; this treatment must not be repeated.

A2.1.9   Dorset egg medium

Egg yolk and white	800 ml (about 16 hen eggs)
NaCl, 0.9 % sterile aq. soln	200 ml

Wash the eggs in 70% ethanol and lay on a sterile surface. Break the shells with a sterile knife and let the contents fall into a sterile flask; add the saline aseptically. Shake thoroughly to break up the yolks and produce a homogeneous mixture. Distribute 2 ml volumes into sterile 5 ml screw-capped (bijou) bottles or 5 ml volumes into sterile 30 ml screw-capped (1 oz McCartney) bottles. Slope the containers in an inspissator and heat slowly to 75 °C. Maintain at this temperature for 1 h and repeat the process on each of the following two days.

Note. As an alternative to inspissation for egg and serum media, several workers have described methods of autoclaving which result in uniform slopes free from air bubbles. The following procedure may be used: place the tubes in the autoclave in an inclined position and close the door and all valves of the autoclave; allow steam to enter the chamber rapidly until the pressure reaches 1.1 kg/cm².† Maintain this pressure for 10 min; as the air has not been expelled, the temperature will rise slowly, preventing the formation of air bubbles during coagulation. After 10 min, open the air exhaust valve very slowly ensuring that a pressure of 1.1 kg/cm² is maintained until the valve is fully open; rapid pressure changes will cause disruption of the slopes. Maintain the steam pressure for 15 min and then close both the steam supply and air exhaust valves. Allow the autoclave to cool slowly and do not open it until 5 min after the pressure has fallen to atmospheric.

† 15 lb/in².

A2.1.10   Yeastrel agar (Report, 1956*c*)

Yeastrel*	3 g
Peptone	5 g
Agar	15 g
Distilled water	1000 ml

Dissolve the Yeastrel and peptone in distilled water in the steamer; adjust the reaction to pH 7.4. Wash the agar in a muslin bag under running water for 15 min before adding the Yeastrel–peptone mixture. Autoclave at 121 °C for 20 min; filter through paper pulp; do not clear with egg-white. Adjust pH, if necessary, to 7.0. Tube in 10–15 ml volumes and autoclave again at 121 °C for 20 min.

This medium is free from X and V factors (Zinnemann, 1960) and can be used as a base for testing for these growth factors.

A2.1.11   Saline agar

NaCl	8.5 g
Agar	20 g
Water	1000 ml

Dissolve by steaming; sterilize at 115 °C for 20 min.

A2.1.12   Water agar

Agar	20 g
Water	1000 ml

Dissolve by steaming; sterilize at 115 °C for 20 min.

A2.2   Enriched media

A2.2.1   Blood agar

Defibrinated blood	50 ml
Nutrient agar	950 ml

Melt the nutrient agar, cool to 50 °C and add the blood aseptically. Mix and distribute in tubes or plates.

Notes. Haemolysis can be seen better in layered blood agar plates. For such plates, a layer of peptone water agar is poured into the Petri dish, allowed to set, and the blood-containing medium is poured on top. Alternatively, a simple agar solution without nutrients may be used as the lower layer; it must however be made isotonic to prevent haemolysis of the blood in the upper layer.

The inclusion of glucose in the basal medium for blood agar is not recommended as its presence inhibits haemolysin production by streptococci (Fuller & Maxted, 1939).

Blood broth is prepared by the aseptic addition of 5% sterile defibrinated blood to the appropriate volume of nutrient broth.

* Obtainable from Mapleton's Foods Ltd, Moss Street, Garston, Liverpool L19 2NA.

A2.2.2 **Chocolate agar.** Place a blood agar plate (medium down) in a 65 °C incubator for 1–1½ h until the medium assumes a uniform 'chocolate' colour.

Alternatively, melt nutrient agar and cool to 50 °C. Add 5 % sterile blood, mix and heat in a water bath to 80 °C with frequent mixing. Maintain at 80 °C until the medium has a 'chocolate' colour. Distribute.

A2.2.3 **Fildes' peptic digest of blood** (Fildes, 1920)

Defibrinated sheep blood	25 ml
NaCl, 0.9 % sterile aq. soln	75 ml
HCl, conc.	3 ml
Pepsin	0.5 g

Mix the blood and saline in a glass-stoppered bottle and add the pepsin and acid. Shake thoroughly and place in a water bath at 55 °C for 4 h with occasional shaking. Add 6 ml 5 N-NaOH and check that pH is 7.0. Add 0.25 ml $CHCl_3$ as preservative and shake thoroughly. The digest will keep at least 12 months but should be stored at 4 °C. It is better to leave it too acid rather than too alkaline.

Note. Before use the chloroform must be removed by heating gently in a water bath.

A2.2.4 **Fildes' digest agar**

Fildes' peptic digest of blood	50 ml
Nutrient agar	950 ml

Maintain the Fildes' digest at 55 °C for 30 min to volatilize the chloroform. Then aseptically add it to the base, previously melted and cooled to 55 °C. Mix and distribute.

A2.2.5 **Serum agar**

Sterile serum	50 ml
Nutrient agar	950 ml

Melt the nutrient agar, cool to 50–55 °C and aseptically add the serum. Mix and distribute.

Serum broth is prepared by the aseptic addition of 5 % sterile serum to nutrient broth.

A2.2.6 **Serum glucose agar** (Jones & Morgan, 1958)

Peptone	10 g
Beef extract	5 g
NaCl	5 g
Agar	20 g
Water	1000 ml

Prepare the base as for nutrient agar (p. 140) and sterilize.

Sterile horse serum	50 ml
Glucose, 20 % aq. soln	50 ml
Nutrient base	1000 ml

Add the serum and sterile glucose soln to the base, previously melted and cooled to 50–55 °C. Mix and distribute aseptically.

A2.2.7 **Glucose broth**

Glucose, 20 % aq. soln	50 ml
Nutrient broth	950 ml

Sterilize the glucose soln by filtration and add aseptically to the nutrient broth. Mix and distribute aseptically.

A2.2.8 **Glycerol agar**

Glycerol	50 ml
Nutrient agar	1000 ml

Melt the nutrient agar, add the glycerol, mix, and sterilize at 115 °C for 20 min.

Note. Gordon & Smith (1953) use 7 % glycerol in soil extract agar (Section A2.7.28).

A2.2.9 **Tomato juice agar** (modified from Kulp & White, 1932)

Tomatoes	250 g
Distilled water	500 ml

Cut up the tomatoes and steam in the water for an hour or until they are pulped. Clarify through gauze and filter through paper.

Peptone	10 g
Peptonized milk	10 g
Agar	20 g
Tomato juice	400 ml
Distilled water	600 ml

Dissolve the solids in the water by heating. Add the tomato juice, mix, and sterilize at 115 °C for 20 min. The final pH value of the medium should be 6.0–6.2.

A2.3 **Enrichment media**

Isolation procedures often use enrichment media and many have been developed for this purpose. Some have but a brief trial and are then discarded; those that are successful are developed and may be produced commercially. Some media in Section A2.4 could be described and used as enrichment media.

It should be noted that *Salmonella choleraesuis* is inhibited by selenite media, commonly used for isolation of enteric bacteria.

A2.3.1 **Salt colistin broth** (G. I. Barrow)

Yeast extract (Oxoid)	3 g
Tryptone (Oxoid)	10 g
NaCl	20 g
Colistin sulphomethate sodium (Colomycin)	0.5×10^6 i.u.
Sterile distilled water	1000 ml

Dissolve in the cold; adjust the pH to 7.4, then add the Colomycin. Do not heat. Keep at 4 °C and dispense as required.

A2.3.2   Glucose salt teepol broth (Barrow)

Beef extract (Oxoid)	3 g
Tryptone (Oxoid)	10 g
NaCl	30 g
Glucose	5 g
Methyl violet	0.002 g
Teepol 610 (BDH)	4 ml
Distilled water	1000 ml

Dissolve in the cold and adjust the pH to 9.4. Sterilize at 121 °C for 15 min. Dispense aseptically as needed.

A2.4   Differential and selective media

A2.4.1   Bile agar

Ox bile, dehydrated	10 g
Serum, sterile	50 ml
Nutrient agar	1000 ml

Melt the nutrient agar, add the bile (equivalent to 10 % bile), mix and dissolve. Sterilize at 115 °C for 20 min. Cool to about 55 °C and aseptically add the serum. Mix and distribute.

Notes. For 40 % bile agar, use 40 g dehydrated ox bile per litre. Bile agar can be used as whole plates, or ditches in plates of blood or serum agar.

A2.4.2   Blood–tellurite agar

K_2TeO_3, 2 % aq. soln	16 ml
Sterile blood	50 ml
Infusion agar	1000 ml

Melt the agar medium, cool to 50 °C and aseptically add the blood and sterile tellurite soln. The medium must not be heated after addition of the tellurite. Mix and distribute.

Notes. Sterilize the tellurite soln by filtration, not by heat. K_2TeO_3 concentration in this medium is approx. 0.03 % (1/3333).

Several tellurite media have been described; Anderson *et al.* (1931) used a 'chocolate' (heated blood) agar base, and laked blood was used by Wilson (1934) and Hoyle (1941).

A2.4.3   Bordet–Gengou agar (modified from Bordet & Gengou, 1906)

Peptone	10 g
NaCl	5 g
Glycerol	10 ml
Soluble starch	2.5 g
Water	1000 ml
Agar	30 g

Make a smooth paste of the soluble starch with a few ml of the water. Dissolve the peptone, NaCl, and glycerol in the remaining water, heat, and add the starch suspension. Adjust to pH 7.5, add the agar and dissolve by heating. Sterilize at 115 °C for 20 min.

For use, aseptically add 500 ml horse blood (warmed to 45 °C) to 1000 ml of base melted and cooled to 55–60 °C. Mix and distribute.

Notes. Medium in plates should be thick, at least 5 mm in depth, and must not be overdried; it should be bright red in colour (Bailey, 1933); a dark medium indicates old or overheated blood.

Some brands of peptone are markedly inhibitory to the growth of *Bordetella pertussis* and the original formula of Bordet & Gengou did not include peptone. Dawson *et al.* (1951) consider that 30 % blood is the minimum for a satisfactory product; however, haemolysis is not usually seen when the blood concentration exceeds 30 %; the original medium contained 50 %.

A2.4.4   Bromthymol blue salt teepol agar (BTBST) (Barrow)

Beef extract (Oxoid)	3.0 g
Tryptone (Oxoid)	10.0 g
Sucrose	10.0 g
Teepol 610 (BDH)	2.0 ml
NaCl	30.0 g
Bromthymol blue	0.08 g
Agar	15.0 g
Distilled water	1000 ml

Dissolve by steaming; adjust pH to 7.8 and pour as plates for immediate use. Sterilize stock medium at 121 °C for 15 min. For use, melt by steaming.

Note. Plates should not be overdried.

A2.4.5   MacConkey agar (modified from MacConkey, 1908; Report, 1956c)

Peptone	20 g
NaCl	5 g
Sodium taurocholate	5 g
Water	1000 ml

Dissolve the peptone, NaCl and bile salt in the water by heating. Adjust to pH 8.0, boil for 20 min, cool and filter.

Agar	20 g
Lactose	10 g
Neutral red, 1 % aq. soln	10 ml

Add and dissolve the agar by boiling and adjust to pH 7.4. Add the lactose and indicator soln, mix and sterilize at 115 °C for 20 min.

Notes. The exact quantity of indicator depends on the depth of colour preferred.

Sodium taurocholate, sodium tauroglycocholate or other satisfactory bile salt may be used (see Section A3.1.5).

The use of 0.1 % Teepol (an anionic detergent) in place of bile salt in MacConkey agar has been recommended by Jameson & Emberley (1956).

MacConkey broth see Section A2.6.9.

A2.5   Media for enhancing pigment production

A2.5.1   Potato slopes. Take several large potatoes and scrub them thoroughly under running water. Cut cylinders with an 18–20 mm cork borer, rejecting any that are bruised or diseased. Cut each cylinder obliquely into two and place each half in a 30 ml screw-capped bottle or 25 mm diameter tube with the thick end resting on a small plug of absorbent cotton. Fill the containers with water and steam for 30 min. Pour off the water and sterilize at 115 °C for 20 min.

A2.5.2   Mannitol yeast-extract agar

Peptone	2.5 g
NaCl	2.5 g
Agar	20 g
Water	1000 ml

Dissolve the solids by heating in the water. Adjust to pH 8.0, boil for 30 min and filter.

Mannitol	5 g
Yeast extract	2.5 g

Adjust to pH 7.0, add the mannitol and yeast extract. Mix, dissolve, and sterilize at 115 °C for 20 min.

A2.5.3   King, Ward & Raney's media (King *et al.* 1954)
Medium A – for pyocyanin

Peptone	20 g
Glycerol	10 g
K_2SO_4, anhyd.	10 g
$MgCl_2$, anhyd.	1.4 g
Water	1000 ml

Dissolve the constituents by heating in the water. Adjust to pH 7.2 if necessary. Add 20 g agar and dissolve by autoclaving at 115 °C for 10 min. Filter, and sterilize at 115 °C for 10 min.

Medium B – for fluorescin

Proteose peptone	20 g
Glycerol	10 g
K_2HPO_4	1.5 g
$MgSO_4 \cdot 7H_2O$	1.5 g
Water	1000 ml

Proceed as for medium A above.

A2.6   Media for carbohydrate studies

A2.6.1   Hugh and Leifson's OF medium (Hugh & Leifson, 1953)

Peptone	2 g
NaCl	5 g
K_2HPO_4	0.3 g
Agar	3 g
Distilled water	1000 ml
Bromthymol blue, 0.2 % aq. soln	15 ml

Dissolve the solids by heating in the water. Adjust to pH 7.1, filter, and add the indicator. Sterilize at 115 °C for 20 min.

Add a sterile solution of the appropriate carbohydrate aseptically to give a final concentration of 1 %. Mix and distribute aseptically in 10 ml volumes into sterile tubes of not more than 16 mm diameter.

A2.6.2   Peptone water sugars. The method of preparation will depend on the indicator:

Andrade's. Adjust the reaction of 900 ml peptone water to pH 7.1–7.3 so that the addition of 10 ml Andrade's indicator will bring it to pH 7.5. Sterilize at 115 °C for 20 min; this medium is pink when hot but the colour fades on cooling. Dissolve 10 g of the appropriate sugar in 90 ml of water and steam for 30 min or sterilize by filtration. Aseptically add this to the sterile peptone water + indicator and distribute into sterile test tubes with inverted Durham's tubes and steam for 30 min.

Other indicators. To 900 ml peptone water add 10 ml indicator solution (bromcresol purple, bromthymol blue, or phenol red) and sterilize at 115 °C for 20 min. Dissolve 10 g of the appropriate sugar in 90 ml water and steam for 30 min or sterilize by filtration. Add this to the sterile base, distribute into sterile tubes with inverted Durham's tubes and steam for 30 min.

Notes. The addition of some carbohydrates may cause an acid reaction; in these instances add sufficient 0.1 N-NaOH to restore the original colour.

Where the solubility of a carbohydrate is low (Table A2), the required amount of solid material may be added to the base and, when solution is complete, the medium sterilized.

A2.6.3   Broth sugars. This formula is included here because broth-based sugars are used extensively in the USA and are recommended by the international subcommittee on Enterobacteriaceae (Report, 1958).

Peptone	10 g
Meat extract	3 g
NaCl	5 g
Distilled water	1000 ml
Andrade's indicator	10 ml

Dissolve the solids in the water, add the indicator and adjust to pH 7.1–7.2. Sterilize at 115 °C for 20 min. Aseptically add 1 % of the appropriate carbohydrate, mix, distribute into sterile tubes containing inverted Durham's tubes, and steam for 30 min.

A2.6.4 Serum water sugars

Peptone	4 g
Na$_2$HPO$_4$	0.8 g
Distilled water	800 ml
Sterile serum	200 ml
Bromcresol purple, 0.2 % soln	10 ml

Dissolve the peptone and phosphate in the water, steam at 100 °C for 15 min and filter. Add the serum and steam for a further 15 min. Check pH to 7.6–7.8 and add the indicator. Sterilize at 115 °C for 10 min.

Aseptically add 1 % of the appropriate sugar as a sterile solution and distribute into sterile tubes.

Note. It is an advantage to have perfectly clear media. Different batches of serum differ in their coagulability by heat, and occasionally the medium is cloudy when serum in the amount given above is used. It is a good plan to add varying amounts of each batch of serum (e.g. in concentrations of 10–25 %) to tubes of the basal medium, to autoclave them, and to choose the highest concentration that does not show marked cloudiness after sterilization.

A2.6.5 Ammonium salt sugars (ASS) (Smith, Gordon & Clark, 1952)

(NH$_4$)$_2$HPO$_4$	1 g
KCl	0.2 g
MgSO$_4$·7H$_2$O	0.2 g
Yeast extract	0.2 g
Agar	20 g
Distilled water	1000 ml
Bromcresol purple, 0.2 % soln	4 ml

Add the solids to the water and dissolve by steaming. Add the indicator and sterilize at 115 °C for 20 min. Allow the basal medium to cool to about 60 °C and add the appropriate carbohydrate as a sterile solution to give a final concentration of 1 %. Mix and distribute aseptically into sterile tubes which are inclined so that the medium sets as a slope.

A2.6.6 Sugars for neisserias (Thompson & Knudsen, 1958)

Digest broth	1000 ml
Agar	3 g
Phenol red, 0.2 % soln	10 ml
Sterile rabbit serum	50 ml
Sugar, sterile 10 % soln	100 ml

Dissolve the agar in the broth by heating, add the indicator solution and sterilize at 115 °C for 20 min. Cool to about 55 °C and aseptically add the serum and sugar solution. Distribute into sterile tubes.

Notes. The four sugars used to differentiate *Neisseria* spp. are glucose, lactose, maltose, and sucrose.

Wilkinson (1962) recommends a solid medium containing hydrocele fluid for detecting acid production by *Neisseria* spp.

A2.6.7 Sugars for lactobacilli (Man *et al.* 1960)

MRS broth, modified	1000 ml
Carbohydrate	20 g
Chlorphenol red, 0.2 % soln	20 ml

Prepare the basal broth as in Section A2.7.20, omitting the beef extract and glucose; adjust to pH 6.2–6.5, add the indicator, and sterilize at 115 °C for 20 min. Add the carbohydrate (mannose, xylose, and maltose should be Seitz filtered and added aseptically), mix, and distribute; steam for 30 min.

A2.6.8 Lactose (10 %) agar

Peptone	5 g
Beef extract	3 g
Lactose	100 g
Agar	20 g
Distilled water	1000 ml
Bromcresol purple, 0.2 % soln	10 ml

Dissolve the solids in the water by heating, adjust to pH 6.8 with 10 N-NaOH, filter, and add the indicator solution. Sterilize at 115 °C for 20 min and distribute as plates or slopes.

A2.6.9 MacConkey broth (Report, 1956c)

Peptone	20 g
NaCl	5 g
Sodium taurocholate	5 g
Water	1000 ml
Bromcresol purple, 0.2 % soln	5 ml
Lactose	10 g

Dissolve the peptone, NaCl and bile salt in the water by heating. Adjust to pH 8.0 and boil for 20 min. Cool, filter, and adjust to pH 7.4. Add the lactose and indicator solution, mix and distribute into tubes containing inverted Durham's tubes. Sterilize at 115 °C for 15 min.

Note. See MacConkey agar (Section A2.4.5) for remarks on bile salts.

A2.6.10 MR test medium
Glucose–phosphate medium

Peptone	5 g
K$_2$HPO$_4$	5 g
Distilled water	1000 ml

Steam until the solids are dissolved, filter, and adjust to pH 7.5.

Glucose	5 g

Add the glucose, mix and distribute 1.5 ml volumes into tubes. Sterilize at 115 °C for 10 min.

Note. For sterilization, the tubes must be placed in a solid-bottomed container to protect them from contact with steam; if this is neglected, the medium becomes straw-yellow in colour.

Workers in the USA generally use 7 g peptone.

This medium is also used for the VP test; for other media for this test see below.

A2.6.11 VP test media
Glucose–peptone medium (Abd-el-Malek & Gibson, 1948b)

Peptone	10 g
Glucose	5 g
Distilled water	1000 ml

Mix and dissolve by gentle heating. Filter, adjust to pH 7.6, and distribute into tubes. Sterilize at 115 °C for 10 min in a solid-bottomed container.

Glucose–salt medium (Smith, Gordon & Clark, 1946)

Proteose peptone	7 g
NaCl	5 g
Glucose	5 g
Distilled water	1000 ml

Dissolve the solids in the water, tube, and sterilize at 115 °C for 20 min in a solid-bottomed container.

A2.6.12 Media for dextran and levan production
Sucrose agar

Sterile serum	50 ml
Sucrose	50 g
Digest agar	1000 ml

Melt the digest agar, add the sucrose, and steam for 30 min. Cool to 55 °C, aseptically add the serum, and distribute into Petri dishes.

Sucrose broth

Sucrose	50 g
Infusion broth	1000 ml

Dissolve the sucrose in the broth and steam for 1 h.

A2.6.13 Starch agar

Potato starch	10 g
Distilled water	50 ml
Nutrient agar	1000 ml

Triturate the starch with the water to a smooth cream, and add to the molten nutrient agar. Mix, and sterilize at 115 °C for 10 min. Distribute into Petri dishes.

Notes. This medium should not be filtered after adding the starch suspension.

Overheating may hydrolyse the starch.

A2.7 Miscellanous media

A2.7.1 Aesculin broth

Aesculin	1 g
Ferric citrate	0.5 g
Peptone water	1000 ml

Dissolve the aesculin and iron salt in the peptone water, and sterilize at 115 °C for 10 min.

Aesculin agar is aesculin broth gelled by the addition of 2 % agar.

Aesculin bile agar (Williams & Hirch, 1950; Swan, 1954) can be prepared by the addition of aesculin and iron salt to bile agar (Section A2.4.1).

A2.7.2 Arginine media
Arginine broth (Niven *et al.* 1942)

Peptone (tryptone)	5 g
Yeast extract	5 g
K$_2$HPO$_4$	2 g
Glucose	0.5 g
Arginine monohydrochloride	3 g
Distilled water	1000 ml

Dissolve by heating, adjust to pH 7.0, boil, filter, and sterilize at 115 °C for 20 min.

Note. The original formula of Niven *et al.* specified D-arginine monohydrochloride; we use the L-isomer and find it satisfactory.

Arginine agar (Thornley, 1960)

Peptone	1.0 g
NaCl	5.0 g
K$_2$HPO$_4$	0.3 g
Agar	3.0 g
Phenol red	0.01 g
L+ arginine hydrochloride	10.0 g
Distilled water	1000 ml

Adjust to pH 7.2; distribute into screw-capped (6 mm) bottles to a depth of about 16 mm (3.5 ml); sterilize at 121 °C for 15 min.

A2.7.3 Casein agar (milk agar) (modified from Hastings, 1903)

Milk, skim	500 ml
Nutrient agar, double-strength	500 ml

Prepare the skim-milk as in Section A2.7.18 and sterilize by heating at 115 °C for 10 min. Cool to about 50 °C and add to the double-strength nutrient agar (Section A2.1.1) melted and cooled to 50–55 °C. Mix and distribute in Petri dishes or tubes.

Note. As the acid produced by lactose fermentation had an inhibitory effect on the hydrolysis of casein, Eddy (1960) recommended dialysis of milk before adding to the basal medium.

A2.7.4 Citrate media

Christensen's (Christensen, 1949)

Sodium citrate	3 g
Glucose	0.2 g
Yeast extract	0.5 g
Cysteine hydrochloride	0.1 g
Ferric ammonium citrate	0.4 g
KH_2PO_4	1 g
NaCl	5 g
$Na_2S_2O_3$	0.08 g
Agar	20 g
Distilled water	1000 ml
Phenol red, 0.2 % soln	6 ml

Dissolve the solids in the water by heating, filter; adjust to pH 6.8–6.9, add the indicator, and sterilize at 115 °C for 20 min.

Note. This medium is also suitable for demonstrating H_2S production; if it is not to be used for this purpose the cysteine, $Na_2S_2O_3$, and ferric ammonium citrate can be omitted.

Koser's (modified from Koser, 1923; Report, 1956c)

NaCl	5 g
$MgSO_4 \cdot 7H_2O$	0.2 g
$NH_4H_2PO_4$	1 g
K_2HPO_4	1 g
Distilled water	1000 ml

Dissolve the salts in the water.

Citric acid	2 g

Add to the salts solution and adjust to pH 6.8 with N-NaOH. Filter through a sintered-glass funnel. The medium should be colourless. Sterilize at 115 °C for 20 min.

All glassware must be chemically clean and alkali-free (see Section A1.1).

Note. In his original paper, Koser (1923) used 2 g

sodium citrate or 2.77 g of the hydrated salt in place of the citric acid in the formula given above; it is not known which of the three sodium salts of citric acid was used although Koser stated that it had $5\frac{1}{2}$ molecules of water of crystallization.

Simmons' (modified from Simmons, 1926)
This is the modified Koser's citrate (above) incorporating 0.008 % bromthymol blue (i.e. 40 ml 0.2 % soln per litre), and gelled by the addition of 2 % agar.

A2.7.5 Organic acids as carbon sources (Gordon & Mihm, 1957)

NaCl	1 g
$MgSO_4 \cdot 7H_2O$	0.2 g
$(NH_4)_2HPO_4$	1 g
KH_2PO_4	0.5 g
Organic acid (sodium salt)	2 g
Agar	20 g
Distilled water	1000 ml
Phenol red, 0.2 % soln	4 ml

Dissolve the agar by steaming in about 800 ml of the water. Dissolve the salts in the remainder of the water and add to the agar sol. Adjust to pH 6.8 and add the indicator solution. Sterilize at 115 °C for 20 min.

Notes. Organic acids used as their sodium salts include: acetate, benzoate, citrate, lactate, oxalate, propionate, pyruvate, succinate, tartrate; malate is used as its calcium salt, and mucate as the free acid.

This medium resembles the modified Simmons' citrate (above) but contains less NaCl and a different indicator.

A2.7.6 Decarboxylase media

Møller's (Møller, 1955)

Peptone	5 g
Beef extract	5 g
Pyridoxal	5 mg
Glucose	0.5 g
Distilled water	1000 ml
Bromthymol blue, 0.2 % soln	5 ml
Cresol red, 0.2 % soln	2.5 ml

Dissolve the solids in the water by heating. Adjust to pH 6.0. Add the indicators, mix, and distribute into four equal volumes. Sterilize at 115 °C for 20 min.

For use make the following additions:

1. L-arginine hydrochloride   1 %
2. L-lysine hydrochloride   1 %
3. L-ornithine hydrochloride   1 %
4. no addition

re-adjust to pH 6.0 if necessary.

149

Distribute the 4 media in 1–1.5 ml volumes into small tubes (67 × 10 mm or 3 × ⅜ in rimless) containing liquid paraffin to a height of about 5 mm and previously sterilized. After distribution sterilize at 115 °C for 10 min.

Notes. Møller specifies Orthana Special peptone but we use Evans' and find it satisfactory.

When DL-amino acids are used, the concentration should be 2 %. If glutamic acid decarboxylase activity is also to be investigated, the basal medium should be divided into five portions, to the fifth of which 1 % L-glutamic acid is added.

Falkow's (modified from Falkow, 1958)

Peptone	5 g
Yeast extract	3 g
Glucose	1 g
Distilled water	1000 ml
Bromcresol purple, 0.2 % soln	10 ml

Dissolve the solids in the water, adjust to pH 6.7, and add the indicator soln. Sterilize at 115 °C for 20 min. Divide the base into four equal volumes and make the following additions:

1. L-arginine hydrochloride   0.5 %
2. L-lysine hydrochloride   0.5 %
3. L-ornithine hydrochloride   0.5 %
4. no addition

re-adjust to pH 6.7 if necessary. Tube in 2 ml volumes in small tubes and sterilize at 115 °C for 10 min.

A2.7.7   Ferrous chloride gelatin (Report, 1958)

Beef extract	7.5 g
Peptone	25 g
NaCl	5 g
Gelatin	120 g
Distilled water	1000 ml
FeCl₂, 10 % aq. soln	5 ml

Prepare the base as for nutrient gelatin (Section A 2.7.9). After sterilization and before the medium gels, add the freshly prepared $FeCl_2$ soln. Tube into narrow tubes, cool immediately, and seal the tubes with corks which have been soaked in hot paraffin wax.

A2.7.8   Fluorescence–denitrification medium (FN medium of Pickett & Pedersen, 1968)

Proteose peptone	10.0 g
MgSO₄·7H₂O	1.5 g
K₂HPO₄	1.5 g
KNO₃	2.0 g
NaNO₂	0.5 g
Agar	15.0 g
Water	1000 ml

Adjust pH to 7.2; dispense in 4 ml volumes in 12 mm tubes or about 10 ml in 27 ml screw-capped bottles. Sterilize at 121 °C for 10 min. Set at an angle to give a slope and butt of approximately equal length.

For fluorescence, inoculate the surface; for denitrification, stab the butt.

A2.7.9   Gelatin media

Gelatin agar

Gelatin	4 g
Distilled water	50 ml
Nutrient agar	1000 ml

Soak the gelatin in the water and, when throughly softened, add to the melted nutrient agar. Mix, and sterilize at 115 °C for 10 min. Distribute into plates.

Nutrient gelatin

Beef extract	3 g
Peptone	5 g
Gelatin	120 g
Water	1000 ml

Add the gelatin to the water and allow to stand for 15–30 min. Heat to dissolve the gelatin; add and dissolve the other constituents. Adjust to pH 7.0, and sterilize by heating at 115 °C for 20 min.

Note. This medium must not be overheated.

A2.7.10   Gluconate broth (Shaw & Clarke, 1955)

Peptone	1.5 g
Yeast extract	1 g
K₂HPO₄	1 g
Potassium gluconate	40 g
Distilled water	1000 ml

Dissolve in the water by heating. Adjust to pH 7.0. Filter, and sterilize at 115 °C for 20 min.

Note. The potassium gluconate may be replaced by 37.25 g of sodium gluconate.

A2.7.11   Glucose phenolphthalein broth (Clarke, 1953b)

Glycine buffer

Glycine	0.6 g
NaCl	0.35 g
Distilled water, freshly boiled	60 ml
0.1 N-NaOH	40 ml

Dissolve the glycine and NaCl in the water and add the alkali.

1 % Glucose broth (p. 144)	900 ml
Glycine buffer	100 ml
Phenolphthalein, 0.2 % soln	5 ml

Mix and keep overnight in a refrigerator in a stoppered flask. Sterilize by filtration and aseptically distribute into sterile 5 ml screw-capped bottles leaving as little air space as possible. Incubate overnight to check sterility and discard any bottles not showing a definite pink colour.

Note. This medium should be used as soon as possible after preparation.

A2.7.12 Hippurate media

Hippurate agar (modified from Hajna & Damon, 1934; Thirst, 1957*a*)

NaCl	5 g
$MgSO_4 \cdot 7H_2O$	0.2 g
$NH_4H_2PO_4$	1 g
K_2HPO_4	1 g
Sodium hippurate	3 g
Agar	20 g
Distilled water	1000 ml
Phenol red, 0.2 % soln	5 ml

Dissolve the solids in the water by heating, check that the pH is 6.8–7.0, and add the indicator. Sterilize at 115 °C for 20 min.

Hippurate broth (Hare & Colebrook, 1934)

Sodium hippurate	10 g
Infusion broth	1000 ml

Dissolve the hippurate in the broth and sterilize at 115 °C for 20 min.

A2.7.13 KCN broth (modified from Møller, 1954*b*; Rogers & Taylor, 1961)

Peptone	3 g
NaCl	5 g
KH_2PO_4	0.225 g
$Na_2HPO_4 \cdot 2H_2O$	5.64 g
Distilled water	1000 ml

Dissolve the solids in the water, filter through a sintered-glass funnel and distribute in 100 ml volumes in screw-capped containers. Sterilize at 115 °C for 20 min.

For use, add 1.5 ml of a freshly prepared 0.5 % KCN solution in sterile water to 100 ml of base. Mix and aseptically distribute 1 ml amounts into sterile 5 ml screw-capped bottles.

Note. Store at 4 °C and use within 4 weeks of preparation.

A2.7.14 Loeffler serum slopes

Glucose	5 g
Nutrient broth	250 ml
Serum, sterile	750 ml

Dissolve the glucose in the nutrient broth and steam for 10 min. Cool and add aseptically to the filtered serum. Distribute 2.5 ml volumes into sterile tubes and heat at 75 °C for 2 h on each of 3 successive days, keeping the tubes in such a position that a slope is made.

Notes. It is essential that during the first period of heating the temperature is raised slowly, otherwise the surface serum will be coagulated before the dissolved air has been driven off and the finished medium will have an uneven surface.

For an alternative sterilization procedure see Section A2.1.9.

A2.7.15 Lowenstein–Jensen medium (modified from Jensen, 1932)

Mineral salt–starch solution

KH_2PO_4	1.2 g
$MgSO_4 \cdot 7H_2O$	0.12 g
Magnesium citrate	0.3 g
Asparagine	1.8 g
Glycerol	6 ml
Distilled water	300 ml

Dissolve the ingredients in the water with the aid of gentle heat.

Potato starch	15 g

Mix thoroughly with the mineral salt solution, heat in a water bath at 56–60 °C for 15 min and leave in the water bath for 1 h.

Malachite green	0.2 g
Distilled water	10 ml

Mix and incubate at 37 °C for 2 h or place in the water bath at 56–60 °C to dissolve.

Mix the malachite green soln with the mineral salts soln and sterilize by autoclaving at 115 °C for 10 min.

Egg mixture

Thoroughly wash 11–12 hen eggs in 70 % ethanol. Place on a sterile surface and, using a spatula, break the eggs into a 1000 ml wide-mouth stoppered flask. Mix the whites and yolks by shaking vigorously, then strain the mixture through gauze into a 1000 ml measure.

Aseptically add 500 ml of egg mixture to the mineral salt–starch and malachite green soln. Mix thoroughly and distribute in 5–7.5 ml amounts in sterile 30 ml screw-capped bottles. Screw down the caps and lay the bottles almost horizontally in an inspissator (or steamer). Slowly raise the temperature to 75 °C and maintain this temperature for 1 h. Leave the bottles overnight in the inspissator and again heat at 75 °C for 1 h on the following day.

Notes. The spatula, flask, strainer, and measure must be sterile. Too rapid heating on the first day may cause corrugation of the surface of the medium.

Lowenstein–Jensen + TSC

1 % TSC in dimethylformamide	1 ml
Lowenstein–Jensen medium	1000 ml

TSC (thiosemicarbazone, thiacetazone or *p*-acetamido-benzaldehyde thiosemicarbazone) is dissolved in the solvent; the solution is added to the liquid LJ medium before inspissation. After mixing the medium is distributed and inspissated as above. Final TSC concentration = approximately 10 μg/ml.

A2.7.16 Lecithovitellin agar (LV agar) (Macfarlane, Oakley & Anderson, 1941)

Lecithovitellin solution (egg-yolk saline)

Hen eggs	4
NaCl, 0.85 % soln	1000 ml

Separate the yolks from the whites and beat the yolks in the saline to form a homogeneous mixture. Add 25 g kieselguhr (diatomite), mix and clarify by filtration through paper. Sterilize the clarified material by filtration through a bacteria-proof filter.

Notes. If not to be used immediately, distribute the solution aseptically into sterile containers and keep in a refrigerator; it may decrease in sensitivity slightly over a period of 2 weeks or so, but most batches remain unaltered in sensitivity for months; if a precipitate appears, the batch should be discarded.

Yolks vary in size and in order to overcome the variations in egg-yolk saline due to this, McGaughey & Chu (1948) used 5 % w/v egg-yolk.

Billing & Luckhurst (1957) claim that filtration is easier when distilled water is used in place of saline.

Lecithovitellin agar

Lecithovitellin solution	100 ml
Nutrient agar	900 ml

Melt the nutrient agar and cool to about 55 °C. Add the lecithovitellin solution aseptically, mix and pour plates.

A2.7.17 Malonate–phenylalanine medium (Shaw & Clarke, 1955)

$(NH_4)_2SO_4$	2 g
K_2HPO_4	0.6 g
KH_2PO_4	0.4 g
NaCl	2 g
Sodium malonate	3 g
DL-phenylalanine	2 g
Yeast extract	1 g
Distilled water	1000 ml
Bromthymol blue, 0.2 % soln	12.5 ml

Dissolve the solids in the water by heating. Filter, add the indicator solution, and sterilize at 115 °C for 20 min.

Notes. When L-phenylalanine is used, only 1 g is needed. Another medium, phenylalanine agar, for detecting phenylalanine deaminase is described in Section A2.7.25.

A2.7.18 Milk media

Milk, litmus. Stand fresh whole milk in a refrigerator overnight and remove the skim-milk by siphoning, taking care to avoid the cream layer. Steam for 1 h and cool in a refrigerator. Filter and measure the filtrate. Add sufficient litmus solution (Section A1.2.2) to give a bluish-purple colour and sterilize at 115 °C for 10 min *or* by steaming for 30 min on each of 3 successive days. After heating, this medium is colourless but the colour returns on cooling.

Notes. Overheating must be avoided to prevent caramelization.

Homogenized milk is unsuitable.

Milk, purple as above but replace litmus soln with 10 ml 0.2 % bromcresol purple soln per 1000 ml skim-milk.

Milk, Ulrich's (Ulrich, 1944) as litmus milk but use chlorphenol red (0.0015 %) as the pH indicator, and methylene blue (0.0005 %) as a redox potential indicator. To 1000 ml skim-milk, add 7.5 ml 0.2 % chlorphenol red soln and 2.5 ml 0.2 % methylene blue soln.

A2.7.19 Motility medium (Edwards & Bruner, 1942)

Gelatin	80 g
Distilled water	1000 ml
Peptone	10 g
Beef extract	3 g
NaCl	5 g
Agar	4 g

Soak the gelatin in the water for 30 min, add the other ingredients, heat to dissolve, and sterilize at 115 °C for 20 min.

Note. Hajna (1950) modified this formula to permit the simultaneous detection of H_2S production by the addition of 0.2 g cystine and 0.2 g ferrous ammonium sulphate; 2 g sodium citrate was added to clarify the medium and provide an extra nutrient for citrate-utilizing bacteria.

A2.7.20 MRS lactobacillus broth (Man, Rogosa & Sharpe, 1960)

Notes. This medium may be gelled by the addition of 2 % agar.

As a basal medium for carbohydrate studies this formula is modified by the omission of glucose and meat extract (Section A2.6.7).

Peptone	10 g
Beef extract	10 g
Yeast extract	5 g
Glucose	20 g
Polyoxyethylene sorbitan mono-oleate (Tween 80)	1 ml
K_2HPO_4	2 g
$CH_3COONa \cdot 3H_2O$	5 g
Triammonium citrate	2 g
$MgSO_4 \cdot 7H_2O$	0.2 g
$MnSO_4 \cdot 4H_2O$	0.05 g
Distilled water	1000 ml

Dissolve the ingredients in the water, and sterilize at 115 °C for 20 min or at 121 °C for 15 min.

A2.7.21 Nitrate media

Nitrate–blood agar (Cook, 1950)

KNO_3, sterile 20 % aq. soln	5 ml
Horse blood	60 ml
Nutrient agar or digest agar	1000 ml

Melt the nutrient agar, cool to 50–55 °C, add the sterile KNO_3 soln and horse blood aseptically, mix, and distribute into Petri dishes.

Nitrate broth

| KNO_3 | 1 g |
| Nutrient broth | 1000 ml |

Dissolve the KNO_3 in the broth, distribute into tubes containing inverted Durham's tubes, and sterilize at 115 °C for 20 min.

Notes. Nitrite must not be present in this medium (for test see Section A3.3.3).

With a Durham tube to collect gas, this medium can be used to test for denitrification.

A2.7.22 Nitrite broth

| $NaNO_2$ | 0.01 g |
| Nutrient broth | 1000 ml |

Dissolve the $NaNO_2$ in the broth, distribute into tubes, and sterilize at 115 °C for 20 min.

A2.7.23 ONPG broth (Lowe, 1962)

| ONPG | 6 g |
| 0.01 M-Na_2HPO_4 | 1000 ml |

Dissolve at room temperature the ONPG (*o*-nitrophenyl-β-D-galactopyranoside) in the phosphate soln at pH 7.5; sterilize by filtration.

Note. This solution should be stored in a refrigerator and protected from light.

| ONPG soln | 250 ml |
| Peptone water | 750 ml |

Aseptically add the ONPG soln to the peptone water (Section A2.1.2) and distribute in 2.5 ml volumes in sterile tubes.

Note. The medium is stable for a month when stored at 4 °C.

A2.7.24 Phenolphthalein phosphate agar

Phenolphthalein diphosphate, Na salt 1 % aq. soln

Sterilize by filtration and store at 4 °C.

| Phenolphthalein phosphate soln | 10 ml |
| Nutrient agar | 1000 ml |

Melt the nutrient agar and cool to 45–50 °C. Add the phenolphthalein phosphate soln aseptically, mix, and distribute into Petri dishes.

A2.7.25 Phenylalanine agar (Ewing, Davis & Reavis, 1957)

DL-phenylalanine	2 g
Yeast extract	3 g
Na_2HPO_4	1 g
NaCl	5 g
Agar	20 g
Distilled water	1000 ml

Dissolve the ingredients by heating in the water, filter, tube, and sterilize at 115 °C for 20 min. Solidify in a slanting position to give a long slope.

Notes. When L-phenylalanine is used, only 1 g is required.

A combined medium (with malonate) is described in Section A2.7.17.

A2.7.26 Salt broth. Nutrient broth (Section A2.1.1) with the NaCl content increased to 65 g/1000 g, or the amount needed to give the concentration required.

Note. For *Beneckea* spp. and halophilic vibrios increase the salt concentration of all test media to 3 %.

A2.7.27 Selenite broth (Hobbs & Allison, 1945, modified by Lapage & Bascomb, 1968)

Peptone (Evans)	5 g
Mannitol	4 g
$Na_2HPO_4 \cdot 12H_2O$	4.3 g
$NaH_2PO_4 \cdot 2H_2O$	2.8 g
Water	1000 ml

Adjust pH to 7.2; sterilize at 121 °C for 30 min.

Sodium hydrogen selenite, 40 % aq. soln

Sterilize by filtration and store at 4 °C.

On the day of use add 1 ml 40 % selenite soln to

99 ml water; mix, and distribute 4 ml volumes into sterile 150 × 16 mm (6 × ⅝ in) test tubes; use metal closures.

A2.7.28 Soil-extract agar (Gordon & Smith, 1953)
Soil extract

Garden soil, air-dried	1000 g
Water	2400 ml

Sift the air-dried soil through a no. 9 mesh sieve and add to the water. Mix well and heat the suspension in an autoclave at 121 °C for 1 h or at 126 °C for 20–30 min. Stir and filter through paper.

Notes. If the soil is rich in organic matter, 500 g will suffice. If the soil is insufficiently dry the filtrate will be turbid, but may be clarified by the addition of talc, and then refiltered.

Soil-extract agar

Peptone	5 g
Beef extract	3 g
Agar	20 g
Soil extract	1000 ml

Heat to dissolve, adjust to pH 7.0, and sterilize at 115 °C for 20 min.

A2.7.29 Medium for preparation of Streptomyces extract (modified from Maxted, 1948)

NaCl	5 g
K_2HPO_4	2 g
$MgSO_4 \cdot 7H_2O$	1 g
$CaCl_2$	0.04 g
$FeSO_4 \cdot 7H_2O$	0.02 g
$ZnSO_4 \cdot 7H_2O$	0.01 g
Yeast extract	5 g
Agar	20 g
Distilled water	1000 ml

Dissolve the agar by steaming in 750 ml of the water. Dissolve the salts and yeast extract in the remaining water and add to the agar sol. Mix and sterilize at 115 °C for 20 min.

Glucose, 20 % aq. soln	25 ml

For use, melt and cool to about 60 °C, aseptically add sterile glucose solution, and distribute into sterile Roux bottles.

A2.7.30 Todd–Hewitt broth (modified from Todd & Hewitt, 1932)

Meat, minced	450 g
Water	1000 ml

Soak the meat in the water overnight at 4 °C; skim the fat from the infused mixture, heat to 85 °C, and maintain at this temperature for 30 min; filter and adjust the volume if necessary to 1000 ml.

Peptone	20 g
10 N-NaOH	2.7 ml
$NaHCO_3$	2 g
NaCl	2 g
$Na_2HPO_4 \cdot 12H_2O$	1 g
Glucose	2 g

Add the peptone; mix well and add the alkali, followed by the other ingredients; slowly raise to boiling-point and boil for 30 min; adjust to pH 7.8, filter and sterilize at 115 °C for 20 min.

Note. When this medium is to be used for streptococcal type identification, it is essential that the peptone used does not encourage production of the proteinase that destroys the M antigen (Elliott, 1945). Suitable peptones for this medium include Difco Neopeptone and Evans' peptone.

A2.7.31 Triple sugar iron agar (TSI) (Report, 1958)

Beef extract	3 g
Yeast extract	3 g
Peptone	20 g
Glucose	1 g
Lactose	10 g
Sucrose	10 g
$FeSO_4 \cdot 7H_2O$	0.2 g
NaCl	5 g
$Na_2S_2O_3 \cdot 5H_2O$	0.3 g
Agar	20 g
Distilled water	1000 ml
Penol red, 0.2 % soln	12 ml

Heat to dissolve the solids in the water, add the indicator soln, mix and tube. Sterilize at 115 °C for 20 min and cool to form slopes with deep butts.

A2.7.32 Tween 80 medium (Sierra, 1957)

Peptone	10 g
NaCl	5 g
$CaCl_2 \cdot 1H_2O$	0.1 g
Agar	20 g
Distilled water	1000 ml

Dissolve by steaming; adjust the pH to 7.4. Volumes of 500 ml are sterilized in flasks, which are cooled to 40–50 °C.

Tween 80 is sterilized at 121 °C and 5 ml added to each flask to give a final concentration of about 1 %.

A2.7.33 Tyrosine agar (Gordon & Smith, 1955)

Peptone	5 g
Beef extract	3 g
Agar	20 g
Distilled water	1000 ml
L-tyrosine	5 g

Prepare the base as for nutrient agar (Section A2.1.1); add the tyrosine, mix well, and sterilize at 115 °C for 20 min. Distribute into Petri dishes; ensure a uniform suspension of the insoluble tyrosine.

A2.7.34 Urea media

Christensen's (Christensen, 1946)

Peptone	1 g
NaCl	5 g
KH_2PO_4	2 g
Agar	20 g
Distilled water	1000 ml

Dissolve the ingredients by heating, adjust to pH 6.8, filter, and sterilize at 115 °C for 20 min.

Glucose	1 g
Phenol red, 0.2 % soln	6 ml

Add to the molten base, steam for 1 h, and cool to 50–55 °C.

Urea, 20 % aq. soln	100 ml

Sterilize by filtration and add aseptically to the base. Distribute aseptically into sterile containers and allow to cool as slopes or plates.

SSR medium (Stuart, van Stratum & Rustigian, 1945)

KH_2PO_4	9.1 g
Na_2HPO_4	9.5 g
Yeast extract	0.1 g
Urea	20 g
Phenol red, 0.2 % soln	5 ml
Distilled water	1000 ml

Dissolve the solids in the water without heating, check that pH is 6.8, add the indicator, and sterilize by filtration. Aseptically distribute into sterile chemically clean tubes.

Alternatively, the base can be prepared and sterilized by autoclaving and the urea added aseptically as a sterile solution.

A2.7.35 Xanthine agar (Gordon & Mihm, 1957)
Prepared as tyrosine agar (Section A2.7.33), but substituting xanthine (4 g/l) for tyrosine.

A3   MEDIA CONTROL
Standardized media are as important as standardized methods and reagents. Commercially prepared media are tested to show that, within certain limits, they conform to stated formulae but, as many of the media contain peptone and other material of biological origin, the analysis may not be particularly helpful and often does not indicate the suitability of the medium for the task in hand. In many laboratories, media preparation is left to junior or unskilled personnel and the room in which media is prepared is often called a 'media kitchen'. In our laboratory media preparation has been given the status of a department and the work is far removed from cookery. Although media preparation has many features of an art it also has a scientific basis.

Media control consists of quality control and evaluation; quality control is concerned solely with testing whether the product conforms to a predetermined standard, whereas evaluation implies the determination of its efficiency under the conditions of intended usage. The results of both quality control tests and bacteriological evaluation must be correlated and discrepancies or unexpected results investigated. When a sample of glucose–phosphate medium shows a yellow colour (due to overheating) it is likely to give unsatisfactory results in the methyl red test and it must be discarded. The growth of *E. coli*, or other non-utilizer of citrate, in Koser's citrate solution which appears satisfactory on the basis of chemical tests warrants further investigation; a major cause of such phenomena is the use of dirty glassware or the presence of organic matter from cotton plugs. Most laboratories have at some time omitted the lactose or bile salts from MacConkey agar, or used a wrong ingredient in media preparation.

Quality control is a continuous process extending from the raw materials, through manufacture to the final product.

A3.1   Raw materials
Chemicals, reagents, and carbohydrates should be of analytical reagent quality or conform to Pharmacopoeial standards. The bacteriological laboratory is generally not equipped to carry out the necessary examination of these materials (which may involve spectrophotometry, flame-photometry, ion-exchange, chromatography, titration in non-aqueous media, or potentiometric titration, besides the more conventional assay methods) and must rely upon the integrity of the supplier. Materials of biological origin are generally more difficult to standardize and may vary considerably in composition (Report, 1956*a*).

Details of chemical and microbiological assays are outside the scope of this *Manual* and reference must be made to appropriate monographs and textbooks.

A3.1.1   Agar. The concentration necessary to produce a suitable gel varies with the geographical source of the seaweed from which the agar was made (Table A5). A method for estimating the gel strength of agar was described by Jones (1956). A good indication of the source of a sample of agar may be obtained by observation of the diatoms present. These are obtained either by centrifugation of a dilute agar sol or by ashing and extracting the residue with dilute hydrochloric acid; silica skeletons of diatoms, sand particles, and sponge spicules are in the acid-insoluble ash. Examination of granular or powdered agar is less rewarding as undamaged diatoms are seldom found. Forsdike (1950) examined agars from different sources and his paper illustrates many of the types of diatoms. The presence of nitrogenous material may be detected by heating with soda lime, when ammonia is evolved; adulteration with gelatin will be detectable in this way or, alternatively, by the formation of a turbidity or precipitate when a 1 % agar sol is mixed with an equal volume of 1 % aqueous picric acid.

A3.1.2 Peptone. Although some studies on the constituents of different peptones have been published (Report, 1956*a*; Habeeb, 1960*a, b*), much work remains to be done and until more information is available it is not possible to define standards. All peptones should dissolve completely in water to give clear solutions having a pH value between 5 and 7.

Indole production requires a peptone with a high tryptophan content; a gelatin hydrolysate is deficient in tryptophan as is an acid hydrolysate of casein, although an enzymic casein hydrolysate is suitable. Rosenheim's test is of value in detecting tryptophan: to 2 ml 5 % peptone soln add 0.05 ml 1 % formaldehyde soln and 0.05 ml 2 % $FeCl_3$ soln. Cautiously pour conc. H_2SO_4 down the side of the tube. A purple colour develops at the junction of the liquids when tryptophan is present. Peptones for use in media for carbohydrate studies must be tested for fermentable carbohydrate. Soya peptone generally contains carbohydrate and should be avoided in 'sugar' media. The influence of peptone on the methyl red and other carbohydrate reactions will be discussed under Evaluation (p. 159). It is unlikely that modern peptones will be inhibitory because of a high copper content (O'Meara & Macsween, 1936, 1937) but this possibility should be borne in mind.

A3.1.3 Meat extract. In the absence of standards for the product the only simple tests which can be performed are the enumeration of viable organisms (which should be few) and the detection of fermentable carbohydrate (which should be absent).

A3.1.4 Yeast extract, unlike meat extract, has a high carbohydrate content. The moisture content may be high (about 30 %) and considerable quantities of NaCl may be present; samples containing more than about 15 % NaCl should be rejected.

A3.1.5 Bile salts. The complex nature of bile salts makes attempts at standardization difficult. Of the components present, deoxycholic acid (as its sodium salt) is widely used (Leifson, 1935). In the absence of suitable chemical standardization, biological evaluation is necessary and we recommend the method described by Burman (1955), in which a batch of bile salt is standardized against a batch known to be satisfactory; the inhibitory effect of bile salts can be influenced by other constituents of the medium such as NaCl (Leifson, 1935) and phosphates (Allen, Pasley & Pierce, 1952). The evaluation of sodium deoxycholate for use in inhibitory media is discussed by Taylor *et al.* (1964).

A3.1.6 Gelatin comes from many animal sources and undergoes different processes, consequently it is available in several grades. For bacteriology, edible gelatin is generally used, the technical grades being unsatisfactory as they often contain preservatives and may have a high SO_2 and heavy-metal content. Leffmann & La Wall (1911) considered that a standard should be established for SO_2 in gelatin intended for bacteriological use. Some tests for physical properties and extraneous matter of gelatin are detailed in a British Standard (757:1959) to which reference may be made. This standard gives methods for determining moisture content, gel strength, viscosity, melting point, water absorption, solubility, keeping quality, pH, grease, ash, sulphur dioxide, chlorides, arsenic, and heavy metals.

A3.1.7 Carbohydrates and related products. In our laboratory testing is restricted to solubility, clarity and reaction of solution, and simple tests such as absence of reducing sugar in non-reducing sugars, absence of aglycones in glycosides, and absence of monosaccharides in higher saccharides. Some samples of sucrose may contain invert sugar, detectable by measuring the optical rotation of a solution or more simply by testing with Fehling's or Benedict's solution (Section C1.3) for the presence of reducing substances. Soluble starch should be free from reducing sugars and when treated with iodine soln should give a deep blue colour; a reddish or purple colour would indicate dextrin. Some tests for other carbohydrates are mentioned in Section A3.3.3.

A3.1.8 **Cole and Onslow's** or other pancreatic extracts act by their tryptic content which must be estimated as follows:

(i) *Qualitative.* A 1/100 dilution should digest the gelatin from a used photographic plate or film within 30 min at 37 °C.

(ii) *Quantitative* (modified from Douglas, 1922). To 50 ml fresh milk, from which the cream has been removed by centrifugation, add 50 ml 0.2 M-CaCl₂; mix thoroughly and measure 5 ml volumes of the milk into 150×16 mm ($6 \times \frac{5}{8}$ in) tubes. Place the tubes in a water bath at 38–40 °C. Make dilutions of the enzyme from 1/10 to 1/100 and begin the testing using the 1/100 dilution.

Add 1 ml of the diluted enzyme preparation to a tube of calcified milk, shake thoroughly, return to the water bath and note the time. Examine the tube at intervals and note the time at which a precipitate or clotting occurs. Continue to test dilutions of the enzyme until the clotting time is between 1 and 2 minutes.

Calculation. Suppose 1 ml of a 1/60 dilution of the enzyme clots in 80 s, then 1 ml of the original solution contains:

$$\frac{60 \times 100}{80} = 75 \text{ units}$$

A satisfactory batch of Cole and Onslow's extract should have a tryptic content of at least 50 units per ml.

A3.1.9 **Thioglycollic acid** for inclusion in media should be assayed periodically and rejected when its activity falls below 75 % (Report, 1953); the acid should be kept in a tightly stoppered bottle at 4 °C. The stability of thioglycollate solutions has been studied by Cook & Steel (1959*a, b*) and the assay method of Steel (1958) is recommended.

A3.2 **Intermediate control**
During the preparation of digest media (Section A2.1.4) it is important to follow the course of digestion. Samples are taken at the start and at 30–45 minute intervals; the disappearance of undigested protein is most easily shown by the biuret test: heat a 5 ml sample to boiling to stop digestion, cool and add 0.5 ml 10 N-NaOH. Filter and add 0.1 ml 1 % CuSO₄·5H₂O soln to the filtrate. Proteins give a violet colour, proteoses a reddish-pink, and amino acids produce none.

A3.3 **Final product**
The final product should be examined physically and chemically, as well as by bacteriological tests which are considered under Evaluation (Section A3.5); some of

the causes of faulty media are considered later (Section 3.6). Among the physical properties determined are colour, clarity, pH, viscosity, and gel strength of solid media. Determination of specific gravity does not appear to be valuable. For the pH determination of solid media a spear-shaped electrode is useful and avoids the need to melt the medium and compensate for the increased temperature.

Chemical properties tested may include the presence of the correct ingredients (testing for human error), nitrogen estimations, detection of breakdown products of components (especially those of carbohydrates), and freedom from the end-product(s) which will be looked for after the organism has grown.

A3.3.1 **Total nitrogen** is usually estimated by the Kjeldahl method or some modification of it. In this, organic nitrogen is converted to ammonium sulphate by sulphuric acid in the presence of sodium sulphate with copper and selenium as catalysts. The digested reaction mixture is steam-distilled with sodium hydroxide to liberate ammonia. The ammonia is absorbed and estimated colorimetrically with Nessler's reagent or by titration. In all cases a blank determination on the reagents must be made. For details of the technique see an appropriate textbook of analytical chemistry or original papers, for example, Middleton & Stuckey (1951).

Proteose nitrogen is estimated similarly but proteoses are separated by precipitation with saturated zinc sulphate solution, and their nitrogen content determined.

A3.3.2 **Amino nitrogen:** one of two methods may be used but the results given by the two methods may not be identical as they do not estimate exactly the same compounds; formol titration is the simpler method but in dark-coloured solutions the end-point may be difficult to see.

(i) *Sørenson's formol titration:* in this method, formaldehyde reacts with the NH₂- groups of amino acids to form acidic complexes which are titratable with alkali.

Neutralize 40 % formaldehyde soln (formalin) with 0.1 N-NaOH, until just pink to phenolphthalein. To a 5 ml sample of medium add 0.05 ml phenolphthalein soln and 0.1 N-NaOH until just pink. Add 5 ml neutralized formalin and titrate with 0.1 N-NaOH until the pink colour reappears.

1 ml 0.1 N-NaOH ≡ 1.4 mg amino nitrogen

(ii) *Pope & Stevens'* (1939) method: in this, copper phosphate reacts with amino acids to form soluble copper complexes; the amount of copper in solution is estimated iodometrically.

Copper phosphate suspension:

0.16 M-CuCl$_2$	20 ml
0.18 M-Na$_3$PO$_4$	40 ml
0.075 M-borate buffer (pH 8.5)	40 ml

Mix the three solutions. The suspension should be freshly prepared and discarded after three days.

Place a 5 ml sample of medium in a 50 ml volumetric flask and make just alkaline (blue) to thymolphthalein with N-NaOH. Add one drop of *n*-octanol to prevent foaming and 30 ml copper phosphate suspension. Make up to 50 ml with distilled water, mix well and filter. Acidify 10 ml filtrate with 0.5 ml glacial acetic acid, add 2 ml 50 % KI soln and 10 ml 10 % KCNS soln. Titrate with 0.01 N-Na$_2$S$_2$O$_3$ using starch mucilage as indicator. The Na$_2$S$_2$O$_3$ is standardized by the same method against 0.01 N-CuSO$_4$.

$$1 \text{ ml } 0.01 \text{ N-Na}_2\text{S}_2\text{O}_3 \equiv 0.28 \text{ mg amino nitrogen}$$

A satisfactory digest medium should contain about a quarter of its total nitrogen in the form of amino nitrogen. Typical results from our laboratory for the amino acid content of digest broth (Section A2.1.4) and infusion broth (A2.1.6) are in the range 72–91 and 68–84 mg amino nitrogen per 100 ml respectively. To achieve some degree of standardization it is usual to adjust the amino nitrogen content of both these media to 70 mg per 100 ml by blending weak and strong batches. The amino nitrogen content of Todd–Hewitt broth (Section A2.7.30) is found to be of the order of 117–145 mg per 100 ml.

A3.3.3 Other tests. The methods adopted to detect the presence or absence of particular components in culture media are mainly the straightforward techniques of classical chemical analysis, such as chloride estimation by Mohr titration, but the *Extra Pharmacopoeia* (1955) is useful for particular tests. Some of the test methods used have been borrowed from clinical biochemistry, and a brief selection is given below to illustrate their diversity.

Detection of bile salts in MacConkey broth (Hay's test for bile salts in urine): sprinkle powdered sulphur on the surface of the medium in a wide tube or beaker – bile salts lower the surface tension and the particles sink.

Presence of nitrate and absence of nitrite in nitrate broth: to 5 ml medium add 1 ml nitrite reagent A and 1 ml nitrite reagent B (Section C1.13) – a red colour

indicates nitrite and the batch should be discarded; in the absence of a colour change add 20 mg powdered zinc – the development of a red colour indicates the presence of nitrate.

Molisch's test for carbohydrates: to 5 ml medium add 0.1 ml 5 % ethanolic α-naphthol, mix and cautiously pour conc. H$_2$SO$_4$ down the side of the tube – a purple colour at the junction of the liquids indicates the presence of carbohydrate.

Individual carbohydrates may be detected by standard biochemical tests; the distinction of galactose, glucose, lactose and maltose ultimately depends upon the formation of crystalline osazones and their identification by microscopical examination. Several multitests have been proposed by which different carbohydrates can be detected by the same reagent (Barakat & Abd El-Wahab, 1951; Love, 1953); the results of such tests should be confirmed by other methods.

Detection of starch in starch agar; pour an iodine soln (e.g. Lugol's, Section B1.11) over the medium – a blue colour indicates the presence of starch.

Pentoses may be detected by the orcinol reaction: mix equal volumes of test solution and reagent (orcinol, 0.2 g; conc. HCl, 100 ml; 10 % FeCl$_3$, 0.2 ml) and gently heat to boiling – a green or blue–green colour or precipitate indicates the presence of pentoses.

Detection of citrate in Koser's citrate: boil a 5 ml sample with 1 ml mercuric sulphate soln (5 % HgO in 20 % v/v H$_2$SO$_4$), filter, boil, and add 5 drops 1 % KMnO$_4$ soln – decolorization of the reagent and formation of a white precipitate indicates the presence of citrate.

Detection of hippurate in hippurate broth: add 5 % FeCl$_3$ soln – a brownish-pink precipitate soluble in excess reagent indicates hippurate.

Hydrolysis of salicin in 'sugar media' sterilized by heat treatment is shown by the presence of reducing sugar when the medium is boiled with Benedict's reagent, and by a violet colour when FeCl$_3$ soln is added.

Hydrolysis of starch in starch serum water is indicated by a coloured precipitate when a sample of the medium is boiled with Benedict's reagent. Such hydrolysis of starch by the action of amylase may occur when the serum has not been inactivated by heat (Goldsworthy *et al.* 1938).

Many of the tests used are not specific but give a good indication of whether the medium has been correctly prepared. In contrast to the bacteriological control methods described below, chemical tests have the advantage of speed.

Media in cotton plugged tubes may lose water by evaporation and, by concentration of ingredients, will not be suitable for its intended use; the addition of sterile water to rectify the concentration is not satisfactory (Vera, 1971).

A3.4 Control of equipment

Equipment that should be checked at regular intervals includes air-filters, autoclaves, hot-air ovens, incubators, water baths, pH meters, deep-freezes, and refrigerators (Vera, 1971), and to this list we would add thermometers, other temperature recording devices, filters and filtration techniques, anaerobic jars and anaerobic techniques, either orthodox or the reduced media methods of the VPI Anaerobe Laboratory.

A3.5 Evaluation

It is by the behaviour of media in routine use that the reputation of a media department stands or falls. Sterility is obviously of paramount importance and sterility testing will be discussed below. Bacteriological control will depend on the nature of the individual medium. Its purposes are to test: (i) the ability of nutrient media to support growth from small inocula; (ii) biochemical test media for their ability to show the desired reactions; (iii) differential media to ensure that organisms growing on them are characteristic; (iv) selective and enrichment media for growth of the wanted organisms and inhibition of other bacteria.

A3.5.1 Sterility testing.
A sterility test is a limit test and the conventional sterility testing technique will detect only gross contamination. The sterility of a product cannot be proved unless the whole of the product (or batch) is tested. Bryce (1956) has calculated that there is a 50:50 chance of failing to detect contamination when 10 samples are tested from a batch of 500 items, 6.7 % of which are contaminated. In testing bacteriological media for sterility we have the advantage that a contaminant is more likely to develop in a nutrient medium than in a simple aqueous solution, and in many cases it suffices to incubate the medium to check its sterility. Culture media are not necessarily suitable for the growth of all micro-organisms; the pH value of a medium intended for bacteria may not be suitable for the growth of fungi. The incubation of an inhibitory medium may fail to show contamination; such a contaminated medium could be the start of a mixed culture which would reveal itself only on subculture to a non-inhibitory medium. Inhibitory media should be well diluted with sterile nutrient broth before incubation.

Media likely to be incubated for long periods, such as Dorset egg and Lowenstein–Jensen, must be free

from slow-growing contaminants and it is advisable to prepare sufficient stocks to last for several months. Many contaminants grow at room temperature and we should bear in mind the possible development of psychrophils in media stored at low temperatures. In medical bacteriology, the presence of thermophils is unlikely to be a serious problem in media. Theoretically our sterility tests should detect the presence of all living micro-organisms but we test only for bacteria and fungi. It is recommended that all samples of media sterilized by filtration or by heat treatment other than adequate autoclaving, be subjected to the following tests:

Incubation temperature	Incubation time
55–60 °C	7 days in air
37 °C	7 days in air
37 °C	7 days anaerobically
ambient room (15–20 °C)	14 days in air
4 °C	14 days in air

Incubation at 20–25 °C is better than 30–35 °C for showing evidence of inefficient sterilization of materials for injection (Vera, 1971).

A3.5.2 Growth-supporting ability.
The nature of the medium determines the choice of test organisms, for example with 'chocolate' agar strains of *Haemophilus* spp. and of *Neisseria* spp. should be used, whereas with the nutrient agar less exacting organisms, such as staphylococci and coliforms, are tested. Our method is to grow the organisms in a suitable medium overnight and prepare nine 10-fold serial dilutions in sterile water. 0.02 ml of each dilution is placed on the surface of medium contained in a Petri dish (as in the Miles & Misra (1938) surface-viable counting technique) or added to 5 ml volumes of liquid media. After incubation, the highest dilution giving growth is noted. The ability of media to support the growth of anaerobic bacteria is determined in a similar manner. *Clostridium welchii* is not a good test organism for anaerobiosis; more suitable species are *C. chauvoei* (very exacting), *C. oedematiens*, or a non-toxic strain of *C. tetani*, but the film-like growth of *C. tetani* may be difficult to see. Some fastidious anaerobes may be inhibited by oxidized reducing agent or by Liquoid (sodium polyanethol sulphonate) in medium (Holdeman & Moore, 1972). Messer (1947) found an inhibitory agent in a batch of nutrient agar and traced it to formaldehyde used to increase the wet strength of filter paper used during the preparation of the medium.

With MacConkey agar, the test organisms used are *Escherichia coli*, *Salmonella typhimurium*, *Shigella dysenteriae*, and *Shigella sonnei*. In addition to controlling its growth-promoting ability this test also serves to show whether the medium satisfactorily distinguishes between these enteric bacteria. MacConkey broth should be tested for its ability to show acid and gas formation at 44 °C when inoculated with a strain of *E. coli*.

A3.5.3 Biochemical performance. Samples must be tested with organisms known to produce positive and negative reactions. Examples of such control organisms are given under the individual test methods in Appendix C. Because of strain variation within species it is essential that the particular strain used for control purposes possesses the desired characters and in Table E1 we list suitable strains, maintained in the National Collection of Type Cultures, of the organisms required.

The need for biological control was shown by Orr Ewing & Taylor (1945) who found that certain batches of peptone were unsuitable for making carbohydrate media, for only in some of them did the Newcastle and Manchester biotypes of *Shigella flexneri* 6 produce both acid and gas. Peptone may also affect the results of a finely balanced test such as the MR (methyl red) and each batch of peptone should be tried out in the test, with known MR-positive and -negative strains (Jennens, 1954).

A3.5.4 Differentiation. Differential media must be tested to make sure that organisms growing on them exhibit the typical characters by which they are differentiated from other organisms. The testing of MacConkey agar for its ability to distinguish lactose- and lactose-non-fermenting bacteria has been noted above. Tellurite media should be inoculated with each of the three varieties of *Corynebacterium diphtheriae* and after incubation these should be examined for their characteristic colonial appearances.

A3.5.5 Selectivity. A selective or an enrichment medium should be able to support the growth of a particular organism or group of organisms, and at the same time inhibit others. A convenient method of testing this is to mix broth cultures of the organism to be selected with another organism to be inhibited, in varying proportions (e.g. $1:2 \ldots 2^n$). A loopful of each mixture is plated on solid media or inoculated into liquid media. After incubation an estimate of the selectivity of a solid medium may be made by inspection of the growth. The efficiency of a liquid enrichment medium cannot be judged until a subculture to a non-inhibitory solid medium has been made.

A3.6 Causes of faulty media

Major sources of trouble are errors in weighing and measuring, inadvertent use of the wrong ingredients (e.g. hydrated instead of anhydrous salts), and incorrect pH adjustment. Some faults and their possible causes are listed below:

Loss of growth promoting capacity

Over-sterilization; repeated remelting of solid media; burning or charring; contamination with metallic salts; incorrect molarity due to careless pH adjustment.

Decreased gel strength

Over-sterilization; hydrolysis of agar media of low pH; incomplete solution of agar; repeated remelting.

Darkening

Over-sterilization; caramelization of sugars; local superheating due to inadequate mixing.

pH change

Over-sterilization; incomplete mixing; use of alkaline containers; hydrolysis of ingredients; repeated remelting.

Precipitation

Chemical incompatibility; failure to remove phosphates; over-sterilization; prolonged holding of melted agar media at high temperature.

APPENDIX B
Staining: reagents and methods

B1   REAGENTS

All staining reagents should be kept in well-closed glass-stoppered bottles (except Loeffler's methylene blue) and protected from direct sunlight. They should not be stored in close proximity to concentrated acids or ammonia. Distilled water for reagents should be freshly prepared and neutral in reaction.

Formulae of staining reagents are listed in alphabetical order.

B1.1   Acetone–iodine decolorizer

Strong iodine solution

Iodine	10 g	
Potassium iodide	6 g	
Distilled water	10 ml	
Ethanol (90 %)	to 100 ml	

Dissolve the iodine and potassium iodide in the water and adjust to volume with the ethanol.

Acetone–iodine mixture

Strong iodine soln	3.5 ml
Acetone	96.5 ml

Mix.

B1.2   Acid–alcohol

Conc. HCl	3 ml
Ethanol (95 %)	97 ml

Mix.

B1.3   Albert's stain

Malachite green	0.2 g
Toluidine blue	0.15 g
Ethanol (95 %)	2 ml
Glacial acetic acid	1 ml
Distilled water	100 ml

Dissolve the dyes in the ethanol. Mix the acid with the water and add to the dye soln. Allow to stand for 24 h and then filter.

B1.4   Ammoniacal silver nitrate solution

$AgNO_3$	5 g
Distilled water	100 ml

Dissolve; to 90 ml of this soln add strong ammonia soln (sp. gr. 0.880) drop by drop until the precipitate which forms just dissolves; add sufficient $AgNO_3$ soln drop by drop until the reagent remains faintly turbid even after shaking. When protected from light, this reagent is stable for several weeks.

B1.5   Ammonium oxalate – crystal violet

Solution A

Crystal violet	10 g
Ethanol (95 %)	100 ml

Mix and dissolve.

Solution B

Ammonium oxalate	1 % aq. soln

For use mix 20 ml of solution A and 80 ml of solution B.

B1.6   Aqueous solutions

Simple aqueous solutions of the following are used in staining.

Bismarck brown	0.2 %
Chrysoidin	0.4 %
Malachite green	0.5 %
Malachite green	5 %
Safranin	0.5 %

B1.7   Carbol fuchsin, strong

Solution A

Basic fuchsin	10 g
Ethanol (95 %)	100 ml

Mix and dissolve in a stoppered bottle and keep at 37 °C overnight.

Solution B

Phenol	5 g
Distilled water	100 ml

Mix and dissolve.

For use, pour 10 ml of solution A into 100 ml of solution B.

Carbol fuchsin, weak
Dilute one volume of strong carbol fuchsin with 10–20 volumes of distilled water.

B1.8   India ink
A dense, homogeneous India ink free from large particles or clumps of particles is necessary. Duguid's (1951) practice is to mix the ink with a quarter of its volume of grade-12 Ballotini glass beads (0.2 mm) and shake for 1 h in a Mickle tissue disintegrator. Thin ink may be improved by evaporation to concentrate it.

B1.9   Kirkpatrick's fixative

Absolute ethanol	60 ml
Chloroform	30 ml
Formaldehyde (40 %) soln	10 ml

Mix.

B1.10   Loeffler's methylene blue
Saturated solution

Methylene blue	1 g
Ethanol (95 %)	100 ml

Staining solution

KOH 1 % aq. soln	1 ml
Distilled water	99 ml
Ethanolic methylene blue	30 ml

Mix in order; this reagent must be ripened by oxidation, a process taking several months to complete, but ripening can be hastened by aeration. Bottles should be not more than half-full, the stopper replaced by a light cotton plug and the bottle shaken frequently. The stain improves with keeping and we prepare batches sufficiently large to last 5–10 years.
Note. The ripened stain is sometimes called polychrome methylene blue.

B1.11   Lugol's iodine

Iodine	5 g
Potassium iodide	10 g
Distilled water	100 ml

Dissolve the KI and iodine in 10 ml of the water, and adjust to volume with distilled water.
Note. This reagent is Aqueous Iodine Solution of the *British Pharmacopoeia* (1963).
For use dilute 1/5 with distilled water.

B1.12   Muir's mordant

$HgCl_2$, saturated aq. soln (about 7 %)	20 ml
Potash alum, saturated aq. soln (about 12 %)	50 ml
Tannic acid, 20 % aq. soln	20 ml

Mix.

B1.13   Neisser's stain
Solution A

Methylene blue	0.1 g
Ethanol (95 %)	5 ml
Glacial acetic acid	5 ml
Distilled water	100 ml

Dissolve the dye in the water and add the acid and ethanol.

Solution B

Crystal violet	0.33 g
Ethanol (95 %)	3.3 ml
Distilled water	100 ml

Dissolve the dye in the ethanol–water mixture.
For use, mix 20 ml of solution A and 10 ml of solution B.

B1.14   Plimmer's mordant

Tannic acid	20 g
$AlCl_3 \cdot 6H_2O$	36 g
$ZnCl_2$	20 g
Basic fuchsin	3 g
Ethanol (60 %)	80 ml

Grind the solids together in a mortar and add the ethanol; triturate until dissolved.
Before use, add 1 volume of mordant to 3 volumes of distilled water and mix well.

B1.15   Rhodes' mordant

Tannic acid, 10 % aq. soln	60 ml
Potash alum, saturated aq. soln (about 12 %)	30 ml
Aniline, saturated aq. soln (about 3.5 %)	6 ml
$FeCl_3$, 5 % aq. soln	6 ml

Add the alum soln to the tannic acid soln, followed by the aniline soln. Redissolve the curd which forms by shaking. Add the $FeCl_3$ soln and allow the black soln to stand for 10 min before use.

B2   METHODS
In this section we describe a small selection of methods which we have used and found satisfactory; for a more complete coverage, reference must be made to specialist monographs such as those by Conn, Darrow & Emmel (1960), E. Gurr (1956), and G. T. Gurr (1963).
After examination, used slides should be sterilized by autoclaving. It must never be assumed that bacteria will have been killed by the application of the staining reagents. We have seen stained anthrax spores germinate in the immersion oil left on a slide, and Soltys (1948) reported cutaneous anthrax in a veterinary student infected from a stained film.

B2.1 Simple stains

Loeffler's methylene blue is perhaps the most valuable reagent we have for staining bacteria. It is excellent for bacteria of the genus *Corynebacterium* where beading, barring, and granules may be demonstrated, especially when the organism has been grown on Loeffler serum (p. 151). In sporing bacilli stained with this reagent the spores appear as unstained bodies within blue cells.

1. Stain for 1 min.
2. Rinse with water.
3. Drain or blot to dry.

B2.2 Differential stains

B2.2.1 Gram's method.
In the USA the method given is often referred to as Hucker's modification (Hucker & Conn, 1923), and in this country as Lillie's (1928) modification.

1. Apply ammonium oxalate–crystal violet for $\frac{1}{2}$ min.
2. Wash in water.
3. Apply Lugol's iodine soln for $\frac{1}{2}$ min.
4. Tip off iodine but do not wash.
5. Decolorize with a few drops of acetone.
   (Note: acetone decolorizes very quickly and should not be left on the film for more than 2–3 s.)
6. Wash thoroughly in water.
7. Counterstain with 0.5 % safranin for $\frac{1}{2}$ min. (A few Gram-negative organisms are not well stained by safranin, examples are *H. influenzae* and *Y. pestis*. Films of such organisms should be counterstained with weak carbol fuchsin for $\frac{1}{2}$ min.)
8. Wash and stand on end to drain, or blot dry.

Preston & Morrell (1962) modified Lillie's method by retarding decolorization with an acetone–iodine mixture.

1. Ammonium oxalate–crystal violet for $\frac{1}{2}$ min.
2. Wash off thoroughly with Lugol's iodine soln.
3. Apply Lugol's iodine for $\frac{1}{2}$ min.
4. Wash off thoroughly with acetone–iodine.
5. Apply acetone–iodine for $\frac{1}{2}$ min.
6. Wash thoroughly with water.
7. Counterstain with weak carbol fuchsin for $\frac{1}{2}$ min.
8. Wash and drain or blot to dry.

The whole slide must be flooded with each reagent and the previous reagent must be completely removed at each stage. Insufficient reagent may result in uneven staining or decolorization.

Gram-positive organisms are blue or purple, Gram-negative organisms are red.

Some workers prefer to counterstain with Bismarck brown which they claim gives a better contrast.

B2.2.2 Ziehl-Neelsen's method (Acid-fast stain)

1. Flood the slide with strong carbol fuchsin and heat until steam rises (but do not boil).
2. After 3–4 min apply more heat until steam rises again; do not let the stain dry on the slide.
3. About 5–7 min after the first application of heat wash the slide thoroughly under running water.
4. Decolorize in acid–alcohol until all traces of red have disappeared from the film. Decolorization should not be attempted in one stage; there should be intermittent washings in water and re-application of acid–alcohol.
5. Wash well in water when decolorization is complete.
6. Counterstain with Loeffler's methylene blue or 0.5 % malachite green for 1 min.
7. Wash and stand on end to drain; DO NOT BLOT.

Acid-fast organisms are red, other organisms are blue or green.

Dilute sulphuric acid or other reagents may be used for decolorization. Some authors have distinguished between acid fast and acid–alcohol fast; in our opinion such distinction is fallacious; it is perpetuated by plagiarism and it cannot be confirmed by practice.

Various cold-staining methods have been advocated (for example, Aubert, 1950; Hok, 1962) but they have little if any advantage over the conventional Ziehl-Neelsen method when applied to pure cultures.

B2.3 Special stains

B2.3.1 Spore stains
Method modified from Moeller (1891)
This is similar to Ziehl-Neelsen's method but ethanol is used for decolorization.

1. Flood the slide with strong carbol fuchsin and steam.
2. After 5 min wash well in water.
3. Decolorize with ethanol until all traces of red have been removed. Decolorization of the vegetative bacilli can best be controlled by examining the wet film under low power (after the bottom of the slide has been wiped dry).
4. Wash thoroughly in water.
5. Counterstain with Loeffler's methylene blue for 1–2 min.
6. Wash and drain or blot to dry.

Bacterial bodies stain blue, spores red.

Schaeffer & Fulton's (1933) method
1. Flood the slide with 5 % aq. malachite green and steam for 1 min.
2. Wash under running water.

3. Counterstain with 0.5 % aq. safranin for 15 s.

4. Rinse with water and drain or blot to dry.

Bacterial bodies stain red, spores green.

This method can be used as a cold stain by allowing the malachite green to act for 10 min.

B2.3.2 Capsule stains

Muir's method

1. Flood with strong carbol fuchsin and heat gently for 1 min.

2. Rinse rapidly with ethanol, then wash well in water.

3. Flood with Muir's mordant for 30 s.

4. Wash off with water, and wash with ethanol for 30 s or until the film is pale red.

5. Wash well with water.

6. Counterstain with Loeffler's methylene blue for 30 s.

7. Wash and drain or blot to dry.

Bacteria stain red, capsules blue.

India ink wet-film method (Duguid, 1951)

This is a 'negative' stain, which is not a stain in the true sense of the word but a means of colouring the background so that the cells are shown in relief as clear objects.

1. Place a large loopful of undiluted India ink on a slide.

2. Mix into this a small portion of the bacterial colony or a small loopful of the deposit from a centrifuged liquid culture.

3. Place a coverslip on top and press down under a pad of blotting-paper. Ideally, the film should be of the same thickness as the capsulate organisms. If the coverslip is not pressed down sufficiently, the organisms will tend to drift in the ink and may be obscured by overlying ink; if pressed down too much, the capsules may be distorted.

The capsule appears as a clear light zone between the refractile cell outline and the dark background.

For demonstrating slime production by enteric organisms, Duguid grows them on excess sugar agar, a medium containing maltose, phosphate, mineral salts, and a low concentration of peptone.

B2.3.3 Stains for metachromatic (volutin) granules

For metachromatic granules make a smear from a culture on Loeffler serum (p. 151).

Albert's stain, modified (Albert, 1921; Laybourn, 1924)

1. Stain with Albert's stain for 3–5 min.

2. Wash with water and blot to dry.

3. Stain with Lugol's iodine soln for 1 min.

4. Wash with water and drain or blot to dry.

Cytoplasm appears light green, granules blue–black.

Neisser's stain

1. Stain with Neisser's stain for 10 s.

2. Rinse rapidly with water.

3. Stain with 0.2 % Bismarck brown or 0.4 % chrysoidin for 30 s.

4. Wash rapidly in water, drain or blot dry.

Cytoplasm appears light brown, granules blue–black.

B2.3.4 Flagella stains.
The arrangement of flagella on the bacterial cell has long been used as a taxonomic criterion. Unfortunately it is not one which is easily or unequivocally determined. The most satisfactory method of determining the mode of bacterial flagellation is by electron microscopy but, since a two-dimensional picture of a three-dimensional object is obtained, the electron micrographs must be interpreted with caution.

Flagella staining should not be undertaken lightly, but reasonably satisfactory results can be obtained when care is taken in the preparation of the culture, the film, and the reagents. The interpretation of flagella stains has been discussed briefly by Hodgkiss (1960). For workers who wish to undertake flagella staining two methods are given below. In the USA Leifson's (1951) method is widely used, but as we have only had limited experience of it, we have omitted it from this section.

It is essential to use known peritrichous and polar flagellate organisms as controls.

Bacterial suspension. Inoculate the organism on the surface of nutrient agar slopes (or other suitable media) and incubate at 22–30 °C for 18–24 h. After incubation, carefully pipette 2–3 ml of sterile distilled water into the tubes and allow the bacteria to diffuse off the agar surface into the water. When the suspension is turbid, transfer by pipette into a clean tube containing 2 ml of 1 % formalin (0.4 % formaldehyde). On holding up to the light, the suspension should appear faintly opalescent. If it is turbid, more formalin must be added. The suspension may be washed by light centrifugation and resuspended in 1 % formalin solution.

Leifson (1961) has noted that the addition of formaldehyde to suspensions before flagella staining may cause a change in the shape of the flagella, and this must be borne in mind when examining stained films or comparing them with published illustrations (see for example Leifson, 1960).

Preparation of films. Clean slides with hot nitric acid (see Section A1.1), thoroughly wash to remove all traces of acid and allow to drain; store in a closed container.

Place a loopful of the bacterial suspension near one end of the dry slide which is immediately tipped to a vertical position so that the drop runs down, leaving a thin film with parallel sides. The drop reaches the bottom in a few seconds if the slide is really clean, and is then dried in the air at room temperature. Keep the slide in the vertical position to prevent dust settling on the film. If the liquid does not run down the slide smoothly, a good result is unlikely and it is advisable to make a fresh film.

Cesares-Gill's method, modified (Plimmer & Paine, 1921)

1. Treat with Kirkpatrick's fixative for 5 min.
2. Wash off the fixative thoroughly.
3. Filter the diluted Plimmer's mordant onto the slide and allow to act for 5 min.

4. Wash off with water.
5. Stain for 2 min with weak carbol fuchsin.
6. Wash and allow to dry in air.

Rhodes' (1958) method

This is a modification of Fontana's method of staining spirochaetes.

1. Apply iron tannate mordant for 3–5 min.
2. Thoroughly wash with water.
3. Heat the ammoniacal silver nitrate soln nearly to boiling and apply to the film.
4. Leave to act for 3–5 min.
5. Wash well with water.
6. Drain or blot to dry.

Unless a permanent preparation is made, the stained film disintegrates after about a week on exposure to air.

APPENDIX C

Characterization tests

C1 REAGENTS

Formulae of, and notes on the reagents are shown below. Standard acids and alkalis, and simple aqueous solutions are not listed.

C1.1 Acid ferric chloride

$FeCl_3 \cdot 6H_2O$	12 g
Conc. HCl	2.5 ml
Distilled water	to 100 ml

Dilute the acid with 75 ml of the water, dissolve the ferric chloride by warming gently, and adjust to volume with water.

C1.2 Acid mercuric chloride (Frazier, 1926)

Mercuric chloride	12 g
Distilled water	80 ml
Conc. HCl	16 ml

Mix the $HgCl_2$ with the water, add the acid, and shake well until solution is complete.

C1.3 Benedict's qualitative solution

Sodium citrate	17.3 g
Na_2CO_3, anhyd.	10 g
$CuSO_4 \cdot 5H_2O$	1.73 g
Distilled water	to 100 ml

Dissolve the sodium citrate and carbonate in 60 ml of the water. Dissolve the copper sulphate in 20 ml of the water and add, with constant stirring, to the first solution. Adjust to volume with water.

Note. The solution is liable to crystallize in cold weather and should be stored in a warm place.

C1.4 Creatine solution

1 % creatine in 0.1 N-HCl

This solution avoids the rather vague 'knife-point of creatine' and is relatively stable; a solution of creatine in alkali is often recommended, but is unstable (Levine, Epstein & Vaughn, 1934).

EHC disks (synonym: Optochin disks), see Section C1.16.

C1.5 Ehrlich's reagent

p-dimethylaminobenzaldehyde	1 g
Absolute ethanol	95 ml
Conc. HCl	20 ml

Dissolve the aldehyde in the ethanol and add the acid. Protect from light.

C1.6 Hydrogen peroxide

H_2O_2, 3 % aq. soln ('10 volume')

Protect from light and store in a cool place. Keep in a bottle closed with a glass stopper, paraffined cork or plastic screw-cap.

C1.7 Kovács' (1928) reagent for indole

p-dimethylaminobenzaldehyde	5 g
Amyl alcohol	75 ml
Conc. HCl	25 ml

Dissolve the aldehyde in the alcohol by gently warming in a water bath (about 50–55 °C). Cool and add the acid. Protect from light and store at 4 °C.

Note. The reagent should be light yellow to light brown in colour; some samples of amyl alcohol are unsatisfactory, and give a dark colour with the aldehyde.

For micromethods this reagent is prepared with *iso*-amyl alcohol.

Lugol's iodine solution see p. 162.

C1.8 Lytic enzyme for streptococcal grouping

(Maxted, 1948). *Streptomyces griseus* NCTC 7807, originally stated by Maxted to be *Streptomyces albus*, is grown on a suitable medium (Section A2.7.29) in Roux bottles for 4 to 5 days at 37 °C. After growth, the agar gel is destroyed by freezing in solid CO_2. The fluid which exudes on thawing contains the lytic principle and can be sterilized by filtration but this is not essential; the pH is not adjusted, nor is a preservative added. Store in a refrigerator.

166

C1.9 Methyl red solution

Methyl red	0.04 g
Ethanol	40 ml
Distilled water	to 100 ml

Dissolve the methyl red in the ethanol and dilute to volume with the water.

C1.10 α-naphthol solution

5 % α-naphthol in ethanol
(not 95 % ethanol)

The soln should not be darker than straw colour; if necessary the α-naphthol should be redistilled (Fulton, Halkias & Yarashus, 1960).

C1.11 Nessler's reagent

Dissolve 5 g potassium iodide in 5 ml freshly distilled water. Add cold saturated mercuric chloride solution until a slight precipitate remains permanently after thorough shaking. Add 40 ml 9 N-NaOH. Dilute to 100 ml with distilled water. Allow to stand for 24 h.

Alternative formula: dissolve 8 g potassium iodide and 11.5 g mercuric iodide in 20 ml water and adjust to 50 ml. Add 50 ml 6 N-NaOH. Mix and allow to stand for 24 h.

Notes. The water used in its preparation must be ammonia-free. Allow the reagent to settle before use. Protect from light.

C1.12 Niacin test reagents

(i) 4 % aniline in 95 % ethanol
or 1.5 % o-tolidine in 95 % ethanol
(ii) 10 % aq. cyanogen bromide

Store at 4 °C for up to 2 weeks. Cyanogen bromide soln is toxic and must be treated with an equal volume of ammonia soln (sp. gr. 0.880) or 10 N-NaOH before disposal.

C1.13 Nitrite test reagents

Solution A

0.8 % sulphanilic acid in 5 N-acetic acid

Dissolve by gentle heating.

Solution B

0.6 % dimethyl-α-naphthylamine in 5 N-acetic acid
or
0.5 % α-naphthylamine in 5 N-acetic acid

Dissolve by gentle heating.

Zinc dust *or* 10 % zinc dust suspended in 1 % methyl-cellulose soln (Steel & Fisher, 1961)

CAUTION. α-naphthylamine is carcinogenic and should be handled with care.

C1.14 Oxidase test reagents

Solution 1

1 % tetramethyl-*p*-phenylenediamine dihydro-chloride aq. soln

The reagent should be colourless and be stored in a glass-stoppered bottle, protected from light, at 4 °C. The solution should not be used if it becomes deep blue. The autoxidation of the reagent may be retarded by the addition of 1 % ascorbic acid (Steel, 1962b).

Solution 2

1 % α-naphthol in 95 % ethanol

Solution 3

1 % *p*-aminodimethylaniline oxalate aq. soln
(also known as dimethyl-*p*-phenylenediamine oxalate)

As with solution 1 autoxidation may occur; if ascorbic acid is not used to delay the process the solution should be freshly prepared each week.

C1.15 Test papers (detecting)

Cut filter paper strips 5–10 mm wide and 50–60 mm long, and impregnate with the appropriate solution; dry at 50 to 60 °C. Store in screw-capped containers.

For the detection of H_2S (Clarke, 1953a)

hot saturated aq. lead acetate soln

Note: for the NCTC micromethod the papers should be 4 to 5 mm wide.

For the detection of indole (Holman & Gonzales, 1923)

hot saturated oxalic acid aq. soln

For the detection of indole (Gillies' solution, 1956)

p-dimethylaminobenzaldehyde	10 g
o-phosphoric acid	20 ml
methanol	100 ml

Dissolve the aldehyde in the methanol and add the phosphoric acid.

For the detection of phenylpyruvic acid (PPA) (Goldin & Glenn, 1962)

0.5 % phenylalanine in phosphate buffer
(pH 7.4)

Dry at room temperature.

C1.16 Test papers (sensitivity)

Sterile filter paper disks (6 to 8 mm diam.) are soaked in the appropriate solution, drained, and dried at 37 °C. Dried disks can be stored in small screw-capped bottles and should be kept at 4 °C.

For sensitivity to O/129 (Bain & Shewan, 1968)

2,4-diamino-6,7-di-*iso*propyl	
pteridine phosphate*	0.1 g
acetone	100 ml

For sensitivity to optochin

0.05 % ethylhydrocuprein hydrochloride aq. soln

C1.17   Tween 80-peroxide mixture (Kubica, 1973)

10 % Tween 80 made by adding 10 ml Tween to 90 ml distilled water. Sterilize at 121 °C for 10 min. If the Tween separates, rotate the flask to ensure mixing.

Before use mix equal volumes of 10 % Tween 80 and 30 % H_2O_2.

C1.18   X- and V-factors (Marshall & Kelsey, 1960)

X-factor. Centrifuge the red cells from 40 ml blood and add to them with shaking 100 ml acetone containing 1.2 ml conc. HCl; filter and add 100 to 120 ml water to the filtrate to precipitate the haemin. Collect by filtration and wash with water. Dissolve the crude haemin in 25 ml 0.1 M-Na_2HPO_4 and sterilize at 115 °C for 10 min.

V-factor. Suspend 50 g yeast in 100 ml 0.2 M-KH_2PO_4 and heat at 80 °C for 20 min. Clarify by centrifugation and sterilize the supernatant by filtration. Store in a refrigerator or deep-freeze.

X-, V-, and X+V-factor disks. Cut filter paper (such as Whatman no. 3 or other suitable absorbent paper) into disks about 10 mm in diameter. Soak the disks with X-, V-, or a mixture of X- and V-factor solution. Drain and dry at 37 °C, or freeze-dry. Store in a refrigerator in a closed container.

C2   BUFFER SOLUTIONS

C2.1   McIlvaine's buffer
Solution A

0.1 M-citric acid
($C_6H_8O_7 \cdot H_2O$, mol. wt = 210.15)

Solution B

0.2 M-disodium phosphate
(Na_2HPO_4, mol. wt = 141.97)

	soln A	soln B
pH 4.0	61.45 ml	+ 38.55 ml
pH 6.0	36.85 ml	+ 63.15 ml

* Obtainable from BDH Chemicals Ltd, Poole, Dorset (Cat. no. 44169).

C2.2   Phthalate buffer, 0.0125 M, pH 5.0
Solution A

0.05 M-potassium hydrogen phthalate
(C_6H_4 (COOH) COOK, mol. wt = 204.23)

Solution B

0.05 N-NaOH (carbonate-free)

	soln A	soln B
pH 5.0	50 ml	+ 23.85 ml
		dilute to 200 ml with distilled water.

In the micromethod for decarboxylases, 5 ml 1 % ethanolic bromcresol purple is added to 200 ml buffer.

C2.3   Phosphate buffer, 0.025 M
Solution A

0.025 M-Na_2HPO_4
(Na_2HPO_4, mol. wt = 141.97;
$Na_2HPO_4 \cdot 12H_2O$, mol. wt = 358.16)

Solution B

0.025 M-KH_2PO_4 (mol. wt = 136.09)

	soln A	soln B
pH 6.0	12 ml	+ 88 ml
pH 6.8	50 ml	+ 50 ml

For the malonate and urease micromethods, 5 ml 0.1 % ethanolic phenol red is added to 100 ml buffer.

C2.4   Sørensen's citrate buffer, 0.01 M, pH 5.6
Solution A

0.1 M-citric acid
($C_6H_8O_7 \cdot H_2O$, mol. wt = 210.15)

Solution B

0.1 M-*tri*-sodium citrate
($Na_3C_6H_5O_7 \cdot 2H_2O$, mol. wt = 294.11)

	soln A	soln B
pH 5.6	13.7 ml	+ 36.3 ml
		dilute to 500 ml with distilled water.

All buffer solutions should be stored in well-closed bottles made of alkali-free glass; they should not be used later than 3 months after preparation.

C3   CHARACTERIZATION TEST METHODS

Unless otherwise indicated, cultures are incubated at 37 °C or at their optimum temperature.

Recommended control organisms are listed in Table E1.

C3.1 Acetylmethylcarbinol production; the Voges–Proskauer reaction

Method 1 (Barritt, 1936). After completion of the methyl red test (Section C3.32) add 0.6 ml 5 % α-naphthol soln (Section C1.10) and 0.2 ml 40 % KOH aq. soln; shake, slope the tube (to increase the size of the air/liquid interface), and examine after 15 min and 1 h. A positive reaction is indicated by a strong red colour.

Method 2 (O'Meara, 1931). Add 2 drops (about 0.05 ml) creatine soln (Section C1.4) and 1 ml 40 % KOH aq. soln; shake, slope, and examine after 1 and 4 h. A positive reaction is indicated by an eosin-pink colour.

Method 3 (modified from Barrow). Inoculate by stabbing semisolid (0.3 % agar) nutrient agar containing 1 % glucose; incubate overnight. Drop on to the surface 1 drop creatine soln (Section C1.4) and about 0.5 ml freshly prepared mixture of 3 parts 5 % α-naphthol (Section C1.10) and 1 part 40 % KOH; shake gently, and read after 1 h. A positive reaction gives a red colour.

Method 4 (NCTC micromethod; Clarke & Cowan, 1952). Grow the culture overnight on 1 % glucose agar; wash off with water or saline; spin and resuspend deposit in water or saline so that the density corresponds approximately to 10^9 *Escherichia coli* per ml. Test: using capillary pipettes that deliver 50 drops/ml, pipette into small tubes (we use 65 × 10 mm) as follows:

10 % glucose	1 drop	0.02 ml
0.2 % creatine	1 drop	0.02 ml
0.025 M-phosphate buffer, pH 6.8	2 drops	0.04 ml
Suspension from glucose agar	2 drops	0.04 ml

Incubate in water bath at 37 °C. Test after 2 h. Add 3 drops (0.06 ml) 5 % α-naphthol in ethanol (Section C1.10); shake well to mix; then add 2 drops (0.04 ml) 40 % KOH, shake, leave on bench and after 10 min read the result.

Red colour = positive.

Controls: positive – *Enterobacter cloacae*
negative – *Escherichia coli*

Acid production from sugars: see Carbohydrate breakdown (C3.7.1).

C3.2 Aesculin hydrolysis

Inoculate aesculin broth and examine daily up to 7 days for blackening, this indicates hydrolysis of the aesculin. Alternatively, inoculate aesculin agar and look for blackening in and around the bacterial growth.

Controls: positive – *Streptococcus faecalis*
negative – *S. agalactiae*

C3.3 Arginine hydrolysis

Method 1. Inoculate 5 ml arginine broth and after incubation for 24 h add 0.25 ml Nessler's reagent (Section C1.11). Arginine hydrolysis is indicated by the development of a brown colour.

Method 2 (Thornley, 1960). Make a stab inoculation into arginine agar; pipette on to the surface a 5 mm layer of molten sterile petrolatum. Incubate at an appropriate temperature (pseudomonads at 30 °C, streptococci at 37 °C); a positive reaction is shown by a colour change (to red) after incubation for 3 to 7 days.

Controls: positive – *Streptococcus faecalis*
negative – *S. salivarius*

C3.4 Bile solubility

Method 1. To 5 ml of an 18-hour culture of the test organism in serum, digest, or infusion broth add 0.5 ml 10 % sodium deoxycholate soln and incubate at 37 °C. Pneumococci are lysed within 15 min of adding the bile salt.

Note. A glucose-containing medium is unsatisfactory for this test as the reaction should be not more acid than pH 6.8.

Method 2. Grow the organism in serum broth or Todd–Hewitt broth for 24 h. Centrifuge and discard the supernatant. Resuspend the organisms in 0.5 ml isotonic saline adjusted to pH 7.0 or in buffer solution at pH 7.0. Add 0.5 ml 10 % sodium deoxycholate soln and incubate at 37 °C for 15–30 min. Under these conditions, a rapid clearing of the suspension occurs with pneumococci; when clearing has not taken place in 30 min the organisms are not pneumococci.

Method 3 (Hawn & Beebe, 1965). For a rapid presumptive test on the primary plate touch a suspected colony with a loop charged with 2 % sodium deoxycholate (pH 7.0) soln. Incubate the plate for 30 min at 37 °C. Colonies of pneumococcus disappear and, on blood agar, leave an area of α-haemolysis.

Controls: positive – *Streptococcus pneumoniae*
negative – *S. faecalis*

C3.5 Bile tolerance

Inoculate onto 10 % and 40 % bile agar plates and incubate at 37 °C for 24–48 h. Growth indicates resistance to bile. Alternatively, 'ditch' plates comprising blood agar on one side and bile agar on the other may be used; strains should not be regarded as bile tolerant unless they grow right across the bile agar half.

Controls: positive (10 % and 40 %) – *Streptococcus faecalis*
positive (10 % only) – *Streptococcus salivarius*
negative – *Streptococcus dysgalactiae*

C3.6 The **CAMP test** (Christie, Atkins & Munch-Petersen, 1944)

Prepare a plate by covering a layer of Oxoid blood agar base no. 2 with a layer of the same base + 10 % (v/v) sheep blood. Inoculate the test culture to obtain discrete colonies. After incubation overnight, and in the incubator room to avoid chilling the plate, drop 0.02–0.04 ml (1 or 2 drops) of staphylococcal β-toxin (10 units/ml) on the area of discrete colonies. Continue incubation for a further 2 h before examining the plate. A clear zone of the medium around colonies covered by β-toxin is a positive CAMP test.

Controls: positive – *Streptococcus agalactiae*
negative – *Streptococcus faecalis*

C3.7 **Carbohydrate breakdown**
Acetylmethylcarbinol production: see Section C3.1

C3.7.1 **Acid from carbohydrates**

Method 1. Peptone water and nutrient broth sugars. Inoculate and examine daily for 7 days for acid or acid and gas production. Reversion to alkalinity should also be noted. Negative tests should be examined at regular intervals up to 30 days.

With some organisms the ability to produce visible gas depends on the temperature of incubation, and if equivocal or suspect results are obtained the tests should be repeated at a lower temperature. As some anaerobes can produce gas from proteins, gas production is not reliable as an indicator of fermentation.

When incubated anaerobically, some indicators may be 'bleached' (reduced to a colourless state); in such cases, test for acid production by the addition of fresh indicator soln.

Method 2. Serum water sugars.
Inoculate and examine for acid production or acid and clot formation.
Method 3. Media for neisserias and lactobacilli.
Inoculate and examine for growth and acid production.
Method 4. Ammonium salt sugars and 10 % lactose agar.
Inoculate the surface of the slopes and examine for growth and acid production.

β-**galactosidase**: see ONPG test (Section C3.39)

C3.7.2 **Oxidation or fermentation of glucose** (Hugh & Leifson, 1953)
Some workers steam the OF medium, to remove dissolved air, and quickly cool immediately before use.

Inoculate duplicate tubes by stabbing with a straight wire. To one of the tubes add a layer of melted soft paraffin (petrolatum) to a depth of about 1 cm. Incubate and examine daily for up to 14 days.

Results:	open tube	sealed tube
Oxidation	yellow	green
Fermentation	yellow	yellow
No action on carbohydrate	blue or green	green

Note. This medium can also be used for detecting gas production and motility.

Controls: oxidation – *Acinetobacter anitratus*
fermentation – *Escherichia coli*
no action – *Alcaligenes faecalis*

C3.8 **Carbon source utilization (CSU) tests**
Apart from the citrate utilization tests (Section C3.8.1) and tests for use of organic acids (Section C3.8.2), other CSU tests are not yet well enough developed for use in identification. Those interested in their use in classification should consult Stanier, Palleroni & Doudoroff (1966) where the methods are described.

C3.8.1 **Citrate utilization**
Make a light suspension of the organisms in sterile water or saline; inoculate citrate media with a straight wire. Incubate at 30 °C (enterobacteria) or optimum temperature (other organisms).

Method 1. Inoculate Koser's citrate and examine daily up to 7 days for turbidity. Confirm positives by subculture to Koser's citrate.

Turbidity = citrate utilized
No turbidity = citrate not utilized

Method 2. Inoculate by making a single streak over the surface of a slope of Simmons' citrate. Examine daily up to 7 days for growth and colour change. Confirm positives by subculture to Simmons' or Koser's citrate.

blue colour and streak of growth = citrate utilized
original green colour = citrate not utilized

Controls: positive – *Klebsiella aerogenes*
negative – *Escherichia coli*

Method 3. Inoculate Christensen's citrate by stabbing the butt and then drawing the wire over the surface of the slope. Examine for up to 7 days for colour change.

magenta colour = citrate utilized
yellow colour = citrate not utilized

Note. An organism positive in Koser's or Simmons' test will be positive in Christensen's, but an organism positive in Christensen's test may or may not be positive in Koser's or Simmons'.
Controls: positive – *Klebsiella aerogenes*
negative – *Shigella sonnei*

C3.8.2 Utilization of other organic acids as carbon sources

Inoculate the appropriate media and examine at intervals up to 1 month; use of the carbon compound is indicated by alkali production, shown by the colour change of the indicator from yellow to red.

Controls:

	Positive	Negative
benzoate } mucate } oxalate }	*Mycobacterium smegmatis*	*M. phlei*

C3.9 Catalase activity

Method 1. Grow the organism on a slope of nutrient agar or other suitable medium. Run 1 ml 3 % H_2O_2 down the slope and examine immediately and after 5 min for evolution of gas, which indicates catalase activity.

Method 2. Grown the organism in nutrient broth; after incubation overnight add 1 ml 3 % H_2O_2 and examine immediately and after 5 min.

Notes. Blood agar and other blood-containing media are unsuitable for the test.

The addition of 1 % glucose will avoid confusing reactions from pseudocatalase (Whittenbury, 1964).

False positives can be produced by dirty glassware; all tubes must be chemically clean (see Section A1.1).

Anaerobically incubated cultures should be exposed to air for at least 30 min before adding the H_2O_2 (Holdeman & Moore, 1972).

Controls: positive – *Staphylococcus epidermidis*
negative – *Streptococcus faecalis*

Method 3 (for mycobacteria) (Kubica, 1973). Deeps (US = butts) of Lowenstein–Jensen medium are seeded with 0.1 ml 7-day culture in Middlebrook 7H-9 broth (BBL or Difco powder + ADC (albumin–glucose–catalase) enrichment); incubate with caps loose for 2 weeks at 37 °C. Include with each batch of tests controls of a strong (*Mycobacterium kansasii*) and a weak (*M. avium*) catalase producer.

Add 1 ml Tween 80-peroxide mixture (Section C1.17) to each culture and after 5 min measure the height of the column of bubbles above the surface of the medium.

Results: negative – no froth (usually isoniazid-resistant strain of *Mycobacterium tuberculosis* or *M. bovis*)
positive – froth < 45 mm
hyperactive – froth > 45 mm

C3.10 Chitin hydrolysis (Holding & Collee, 1971)

Purified chitin (Lingappa & Lockwood, 1961) is made by treating crude chitin alternately with N-NaOH and N-HCl several times, and then with ethanol until foreign material is removed. Dissolve the purified chitin in cold conc. HCl, filter through glass wool, precipitate in distilled water, and wash until neutral. Add to melted water agar or salt agar at a concentration of about 0.25 % (the medium should be slightly opaque) and pour as a thin layer on top of nutrient agar.

Inoculate the test organism(s) as a streak(s) on the surface and incubate at the optimal temperature of the organism or at 22, 30, and 37 °C. Chitin hydrolysis is shown by a clear zone around the growth.

Note. For halophilic organisms such as *Vibrio parahaemolyticus* the chitin should be suspended in salt agar, and the NaCl concentration of the basal medium increased to 3 % or more.

Controls: positive – *Vibrio parahaemolyticus*
negative – *Escherichia coli*

[N.B. *Vibrio parahaemolyticus* should be treated with respect; it has produced at least one laboratory infection (Sanyal, Sil & Sakazaki, 1973).]

C3.11 Coagulase test

In tube tests, a positive result is indicated by definite clot formation; granular or ropy growth is regarded as doubtful and the organism should be retested.

Method 1 (Cowan, 1938b). Mix 0.5 ml undiluted plasma with an equal volume of an 18–24-hour broth culture and incubate at 37 °C for 4 h. Examine after 1 and 4 h for a coagulum. Negative tubes should be left at room temperature overnight and then re-examined.

Method 2 (Gillespie, 1943). To 0.5 ml of 1/10 dilution of plasma in saline add 0.1 ml of an 18–24-hour broth culture of the organism. Incubate at 37 °C and examine after 1, 3, and 6 h for a coagulum. Negative tubes should be left at room temperature overnight and then re-examined.

Method 3 (Cadness-Graves *et al.* 1943; Williams & Harper, 1946). With the minimum of spreading, emulsify a colony in a drop of water on a microscope slide to produce a thick suspension. Stir the bacterial suspension with a straight wire which has been dipped into plasma. A positive result is indicated by macroscopic clumping within 5 s. Delayed clumping does not constitute a positive reaction.

Method 4 (Subcommittee on taxonomy of staphylococci and micrococci, 1965). A single colony from a 24 h blood agar plate is rubbed up in 1 ml fresh citrated rabbit plasma diluted 1 in 6 with physiological saline. Incubate in a water bath at 37 °C and read after 1, 2, 4, 8, and 14 h. If possible, include among the controls a weakly positive strain (as NCTC 6571). This method detects free coagulase.

Notes. If the plasma has been stored in a refrigerator it may be sufficiently cold to delay coagulation, especially in the slide test; it is advisable to allow the plasma to come to room temperature before use.

The slide test is a valuable presumptive test but as it only detects bound coagulase, negative results should be confirmed in a tube test which will also detect free coagulase.

Known positive and negative strains should always be tested in parallel and, with the tube tests, an uninoculated control should also be set up.

Controls: positive – *Staphylococcus aureus*
negative – *S. epidermidis*

C3.12 Decarboxylase reactions

Method 1 (Møller, 1955). From a plate culture heavily inoculate, with a straight wire, tubes of the four media (arginine, lysine, ornithine, and control) through the paraffin layer. Incubate and examine daily for up to 4 days. The media first become yellow due to acid production from the glucose; later if decarboxylation occurs, the medium becomes violet. The control should remain yellow.

Note. In the diagnostic tables, plus signs indicate only the production of a violet colour in the medium. When a positive reaction is obtained with arginine, the medium may be tested with Nessler's reagent (Section C1.11) for the presence of NH_3; in the absence of urease, the formation of NH_3 indicates that the arginine dihydrolase system has been involved in the reaction (Møller, 1955).

Method 2 (Falkow, 1958). Inoculate tubes of the four media with a straight wire. Incubate and examine daily for up to 4 days. Decarboxylation is indicated by a purple colour, whereas the control and negative tubes are yellow. Falkow's method is not satisfactory with the genera *Enterobacter* and *Klebsiella*.

Method 3 NCTC micromethod (Shaw & Clarke, 1955). Suspension: grow culture overnight on nutrient

agar or other suitable medium, wash off in water, spin resuspend in a small volume of water so that the density is at least equal to 10^9 *E. coli*/ml.

Test: 0.03 M-amino acid (pH 5.0)   0.04 ml
0.0125 M-phthalate buffer, pH 5.0
+ bromcresol purple   0.04 ml
Suspension   0.04 ml

Place tubes in 37 °C water bath. When decarboxylation takes place a colour change is seen. Readings are taken after 2, 4, and 24 h. Each set of tests should include a suspension control without amino acid; when this control is alkaline (blue) buffer is added to all tubes until the control becomes yellow.

This method is not suitable for decarboxylation of glutamic acid.

Controls:

Arginine	Lysine	Ornithine	
−	−	−	*Proteus vulgaris*
+	−	−	*Aeromonas hydrophila*
−	+	−	*Klebsiella aerogenes*
−	−	+	*Morganella morganii*
+	+	−	*Salmonella typhi*
+	−	+	*Enterobacter cloacae*
−	+	+	*Enterobacter aerogenes*
+	+	+	*Salmonella typhimurium*

C3.13 Decomposition of tyrosine or xanthine

Inoculate plates of the appropriate media (Sections A2.7.33, A2.7.35) and examine at intervals up to a month for dissolution of crystals under and around the bacterial growth.

Controls: Tyrosine   Xanthine
positive *Nocardia brasiliensis*   *Nocardia caviae*
negative *Mycobacterium phlei*   *Mycobacterium phlei*

C3.14 Digestion of casein

Inoculate plates of casein agar and at intervals examine for up to 14 days for clearing of the medium around the bacterial growth.

Note. In a few instances clearing may be due to solution of the milk proteins by acid or alkaline metabolic products (see Hastings, 1904); this may be distinguished from true proteolysis by the addition of acid mercuric chloride (Section C1.2), when a decrease in the cleared area shows that the casein has not been digested.

Controls: positive – *Bacillus subtilis*
negative – *Mycobacterium phlei*

C3.15 Digestion of egg

Inoculate a slope of Dorset egg and examine at intervals for up to 14 days for liquefaction.

C3.16 Digestion of meat

Inoculate cooked meat medium and on the container mark the level of the meat. Incubate and examine at intervals for up to 14 days for diminution in the volume of the meat, disintegration, or softening of the meat particles. Blackening or reddening of the meat and/or production of small white feathery crystals of tyrosine may also occur.

C3.17 Digestion of insipissated serum

Inoculate a slope of Loeffler serum and examine after incubation for liquefaction of the medium. With anaerobes, inoculate and examine after incubation in a jar.

C3.18 DNase activity (Jeffries, Holtman & Guse, 1957)

Dissolve DNA in distilled water; prepare sufficient to produce a concentration of 2 mg/ml in the final medium. Add the DNA solution to nutrient agar (or other) base immediately before autoclaving and pour the plates as soon as the medium cools to 50 °C.

Prepare replicate plates; inoculate test culture(s) as lines on the surface. Incubate at several temperatures; 25, 30, and 37 °C are suggested.

After incubation for 36 h flood the plates with N-HCl; a positive result shows as a clear zone around the growth; the surrounding medium – and a negative result of the test – is opaque.

Controls: positive – *Serratia marcescens*
negative – *Enterobacter aerogenes*

β-galactosidase: see ONPG test (Section C3.39)

C3.19 Eijkman test, modified (44 °C fermentation test of Report, 1956c)

Inoculate MacConkey broth (Section A2.6.9), warmed to 37 °C and incubate in a water bath at 44 ± 0.1 °C for 48 h. Production of both acid and gas is a positive result of this test.

Note. Many alternatives to MacConkey broth have been suggested.

Controls: positive – *Escherichia coli*
negative – *Enterobacter cloacae*

C3.20 Ethylhydrocuprein (EHC) sensitivity

Place a disk impregnated with EHC (optochin, Section C1.16) or a tablet containing 0.05 mg optochin on the surface of a blood agar plate inoculated with the organism. Incubate and examine after 18–24 h. Sensi-

tivity to the compound is shown by inhibition of bacterial growth around the disk for a distance of at least 5 mm; resistant organisms will grow up to the disk or may show a small inhibition zone of not more than 1–2 mm.

Controls: sensitive – *Streptococcus pneumoniae*
insensitive – *S. faecalis*

C3.21 Gelatin hydrolysis (or liquefaction)

Method 1. Inoculate nutrient gelatin with a straight wire and incubate at 22 °C; observe daily up to 30 days for growth and presence of liquefaction.

Method 2. Inoculate nutrient gelatin and incubate at 37 °C for up to 14 days; every 2–3 days, cool in a refrigerator for 2 h and then examine for liquefaction. Set up a control tube of uninoculated medium in parallel.

Method 3 (Frazier, 1926). Inoculate a slope or plate of gelatin agar and incubate for 3 days. Flood the surface with 5–10 ml acid mercuric chloride soln (Section C1.2); clear zones indicate areas of gelatin hydrolysis.

When glass Petri dishes are used, metal tops should be avoided; plastic disposable dishes prevent contamination of glassware with mercuric ions.

30 % trichloracetic acid can be substituted for the acid mercuric chloride in Frazier's method (Pitt & Dey, 1970).

Method 4. Ferrous chloride gelatin medium may be used for the determination of both gelatin liquefaction and H_2S production (Section C3.27, method 2).

Method 5. Green & Larks (1955) adapted Kohn's (1953) gelatin disks to a micromethod, with a consequent increase in speed. Formalized gelatin disks are washed in water, sterilized by steaming for 30 min and are stored in a refrigerator. Disks are added to 1 ml volumes of 1 % peptone water, placed in a 37 °C water bath and heavily inoculated with culture from an agar slope. With positive cultures the disks disintegrate in 2–6 h.

Controls: positive – *Aeromonas hydrophila*
negative – *Escherichia coli*

C3.22 Gluconate oxidation

Inoculate gluconate broth and incubate for two days.

Method 1. To 5 ml culture add 1 ml Benedict's qualitative soln (Section C1.3), mix, and boil for 10 min. The formation of a brown, orange, or tan precipitate constitutes a positive reaction.

Method 2 (Carpenter, 1961). Add one Clinitest tablet (Ames & Co.) in place of the Benedict's reagent and look for the formation of a coloured precipitate as in method 1.

Controls: positive – *Klebsiella aerogenes*
negative – *Escherichia coli*

C3.23 Growth on individual media
The ability to grow on a particular medium occurs in
several tables. Media are inoculated and incubated for
a suitable period in accordance with the growth rate of
the bacteria. Growth should not be scored as absent
until adequate time has elapsed for it to have occurred.

The media on which this character is recorded in the
tables are:

	Tables
Bile agar (10 and 40 %)	6.3*b*
Dye-containing media	7.4*b*; 7.7*b*
MacConkey agar	7.5; 7.6*a*; 7.7*a*
Media without salt	7.8*a*
Media with increased salt	6.3*b*; 6.9; 7.8*a,b*
Nutrient agar	7.3; 7.4*a*
Selenite agar	7.9*b*
SS agar	7.5
Tellurite (1/4000) agar	6.3*b,c*

C3.24 Growth at pH 9.6
Inoculate a bottle of glucose phenolphthalein broth
and incubate at 37 °C for 24 h. Tolerance of pH 9.6
is indicated by heavy growth and decolorization of the
indicator.
Controls: positive – *Streptococcus faecalis*
negative – *S. dysgalactiae*

C3.25 Growth in media with increased NaCl concentration
Inoculate broth of the required salt concentration with
the organism to be tested and incubate at the optimal
temperature for growth. Many salt-tolerant organisms
(and most halophils) have optimal temperatures below
37 °C.

C3.26 Hippurate hydrolysis
Method 1 (Hare & Colebrook, 1934). Grow the
organism in hippurate broth for 4 days. Set up a
control tube of uninoculated medium in parallel.
Hydrolysis of hippurate to benzoate is detected by the
addition of acid ferric chloride soln (Section C1.1).

To 1 ml volumes of the control medium, add varying
amounts of acid ferric chloride soln (0.2, 0.3, 0.4, 0.5
ml) rapidly, and shake immediately. With the smaller
amounts a precipitate usually appears, soluble in
excess, with the larger a clear solution is obtained; the
smallest amount of acid ferric chloride soln giving such
a clear solution is then added to 1 ml volumes of clear
supernatant fluids from the broth cultures. A heavy

precipitate is taken as evidence of hydrolysis of sodium
hippurate by the organisms.
Controls: positive – *Streptococcus agalactiae*
negative – *S. salivarius*

Method 2 (Thirst, 1957*a*). Lightly inoculate slopes of
hippurate agar and examine daily for up to 7 days.
Hydrolysis of hippurate is indicated by growth and a
pink colour due to alkali production.
Controls: positive – *Klebsiella aerogenes* (not all strains)
negative – *Enterobacter cloacae*

C3.27 Hydrogen sulphide production
Method 1. Inoculate a tube of triple sugar iron agar
by stabbing the butt and steaking the slope; observe
daily for up to 7 days for blackening due to H_2S
production.
Method 2. Inoculate as a stab a tube of ferrous
chloride gelatin and incubate at 22 °C. Read daily for
7 days for blackening due to H_2S. Gelatin liquefaction
may also be observed in this medium; for this incubation is continued up to 30 days.
Method 3. Grow the organism in nutrient broth or
peptone water, and insert a lead acetate paper (Section
C1.15) between the cap or plug and the tube. Examine
daily for 7 days for blackening of the paper.
Method 4, for *Brucella* sp. Inoculate a serum glucose
agar slope and insert a lead acetate paper strip as in
method 3. Examine and change the paper daily for
7 days.
Method 5 Morse & Weaver (1950). Medium: 2 %
thiopeptone in distilled water, pH 6.8; dispense in 0.8
ml volumes in 75 × 10 mm tubes; heat to 37 °C before
heavy inoculation by means of a swab from a 6-hour
culture on a solid medium. A 5 mm wide strip of lead
acetate paper (Section C1.15) is folded 1 cm from the
end and inserted into the mouth of the tube. Incubation
at 37 °C is continued in a water bath and readings are
made after 15, 30, 45 and 60 min. Morse & Weaver say
that the method is more sensitive than macrotests and
that the 45 min reading gives the best correlation.
Method 6 (Clarke, 1953*a*). Suspension are made from
growth on nutrient agar (see Decarboxylases, Section
C3.12).

0.1 % cysteine hydrochloride, pH 7.4	0.04 ml
0.025 M-phosphate buffer, pH 6.8	0.04 ml
Suspension	0.04 ml

Place a small lead acetate paper (Section C1.15) in
mouth of tube and keep it in position by a loose cotton
plug. Do not allow paper to touch suspension–reagent
mixture. Incubate at 37 °C; read at intervals of 15 min
for 1 h.

Controls: positive – *Proteus vulgaris*
negative – *Shigella sonnei*

C3.28 Indole production
Method 1. Inoculate peptone water or nutrient broth, place an oxalic acid paper (Section C1.15) between the plug or cap and the tube. Incubate and examine daily for up to 7 days. Indole production is shown by the development of a pale pink colour at the lower end of the test paper.

Method 2. Inoculate peptone water or nutrient broth and incubate for 48 h. Add 0.5 ml Kovács' reagent for indole (Section C1.7), shake well, and examine after about 1 min. A red colour in the reagent layer indicates indole.

Method 3. To a 48-hour culture in peptone water or nutrient broth add about 1 ml ether or xylol; shake; run 0.5 ml Ehrlich's reagent (Section C1.5) down the side of the tube. A pink or red colour in the solvent indicates indole.

Method 4 (Arnold & Weaver, 1948). Medium 1: Tryptone, 1 %; beef extract, 0.3 %, in distilled water. Medium 2: tryptophan, 0.03 %; peptone, 0.1 %; K_2HPO_4, 0.5 %, in distilled water. Both media adjusted to pH 7.4.

Inoculate medium heavily from a culture in the logarithmic phase; incubate in a 37 °C water bath. Test by adding 4 drops of Kovács' reagent (Section C1.7, use *iso*-amyl alcohol as solvent). Medium 2 gives positive results more quickly than medium 1 (but with both media the tests should be complete within 2 h).

Method 5 NCTC micromethod (Clarke & Cowan, 1952). Suspensions are made from growth on nutrient agar (see Decarboxylases, Section C3.12).

0.1 % tryptophan	0.06 ml
0.025 M-phosphate buffer, pH 6.8	0.04 ml
Suspension	0.04 ml

Incubate in water bath at 37 °C and test at 1 h by adding 0.06 ml Kovács' reagent (Section C1.7, prepared with *iso*-amyl alcohol); shake. Read immediately; red colour indicates indole.

Controls: positive – *Escherichia coli*
negative – *Enterobacter cloacae*

C3.29 KCN test
Inoculate KCN broth with one loopful of an overnight or 24-hour broth culture. Tightly screw down the cap of the bottle and incubate for up to 48 h. Examine after 24 and 48 h for turbidity indicating growth, which constitutes a positive reaction.

After use, care should be exercised in the disposal of cyanide-containing media; add a crystal of $FeSO_4$ and 0.1 ml 40 % KOH before sterilization.

Controls: positive – *Klebsiella aerogenes*
negative – *Escherichia coli*

C3.30 LV reaction
Inoculate LV agar and after incubation examine for (i) growth, (ii) opalescence within the medium, (iii) 'pearly layer' formation over and around the colonies. (ii) and (iii) constitute positive reactions.

Flood the plate with saturated aq. $CuSO_4$ soln, remove excess reagent and allow the plate to dry in an incubator for 20 min. An insoluble bright greenish-blue copper soap is formed in those areas containing free fatty acid.

Controls: opalescence – *Clostridium welchii*
pearly layer – *C. sporogenes*
no reaction – *Bacillus subtilis*

C3.31 Malonate utilization
Method 1. Inoculate malonate–phenylalanine medium and incubate for 24 h. Examine for colour change and keep the culture for the phenylalanine test (Section C3.41). A positive malonate reaction is indicated by a deep blue colour; a negative reaction by the unchanged greenish colour of the medium (with some negative strains a yellow colour appears).

Method 2. NCTC micromethod (Shaw & Clarke, 1955). Suspensions are made from growth on nutrient agar (see Decarboxylases, Section C3.12).

1 % Na malonate	0.04 ml
0.025 M-phosphate buffer, pH 6.0 (phenol red)	0.04 ml
Suspension	0.04 ml

Incubate in water bath at 37 °C; read at intervals up to 24 h. Red colour indicates a positive test.

Controls: positive – *Klebsiella aerogenes*
negative – *Proteus vulgaris*

C3.32 Methyl red (MR) reaction
Inoculate glucose phosphate (MR) medium (Section A2.6.10) and incubate at 30 °C for 5 days (some workers prefer 37 °C for 2 days). Add 2 drops of methyl red soln (Section C1.9), shake and examine.

Red colour = + ; orange = ± ; yellow = −.

(After reading the MR reaction the same culture can be used for the VP test (Section C3.1).)

Controls: positive – *Escherichia coli*
negative – *Enterobacter cloacae*

175

C3.33 Milk, growth in

Inoculate the appropriate medium (Section A2.7.18) and examine daily for 14 days for colour change and clotting. The following reactions may be seen:

Litmus milk:

acid production indicated by pink colour,

alkali production indicated by blue colour,

reduction of the indicator shown by colourless (white) medium,

acid clot shown by a firm pink clot which does not retract and which is soluble in alkali,

rennet clot shown by a soft clot which retracts and expresses a clear greyish fluid (whey), the clot is insoluble in alkali; peptonization or digestion of the clot may follow,

'stormy fermentation' in which the acid clot is broken up by gas production.

Purple milk:

as above, but acid production is shown by a yellow colour.

Reduction of the indicator is not seen.

Ulrich milk:

the colour changes may be interpreted as follows:

bluish grey – unchanged,

pale yellow green to yellowish orange – acid,

pale bluish purple to reddish purple – alkaline,

bluish green – oxidation,

white – reduction,

acidity or alkalinity are best observed in the lower (reduced) portion of the medium.

Controls:

acid – *Escherichia coli*

alkaline – *Alcaligenes faecalis*

stormy fermentation – *Clostridium welchii*

no change – *Proteus vulgaris*

C3.34 Motility

Method 1. Young broth cultures of the organism, incubated at or below the optimum temperature (e.g. 37 °C and 22 °C), should be examined in 'hanging drop' preparations, using a high-power dry objective and reduced illumination.

Method 2. Inoculate tubes of motility medium by stabbing the medium to a depth of about 5 mm. Incubate at the optimum temperature and below.

Motile organisms migrate through the medium which becomes turbid; growth of non-motile organisms is confined to the stab.

Method 3 (for anaerobes). Take up some of the liquid from a young culture in cooked meat medium into the capillary of a Pasteur pipette; cut the capillary and seal both ends. A fine oxygen flame is needed to give a narrow zone of intense heat which melts the glass quickly.

Examine the sealed capillary under the high-power dry objective.

Notes. OF medium (Section A2.6.1) may be used to test motility but it cannot be relied upon to the exclusion of the methods described above.

For the enhancement of motility inoculate Craigie tubes (Craigie, 1931) or U-tubes containing semisolid nutrient agar; serial passages may be necessary.

C3.35 Niacin test

Method 1 (Marks & Trollope, 1960). Heavily inoculate the surface of Dorset egg medium contained in a bijou bottle; add 0.4 ml sterile water and incubate with the cap loose for 2 weeks at 37 °C; a moist atmosphere must be maintained. Transfer the aqueous extract to a test tube and add 0.6 ml 4 % ethanolic aniline followed by 0.6 ml 10 % aq. cyanogen bromide (Section C1.12). The presence of niacin is indicated by a yellow colour.

Method 2 (Gutiérrez-Vázquez, 1960; modified by Collins & Massey, 1963). Add 0.3 ml sterile water to a 30-day culture on Lowenstein–Jensen medium; autoclave at 115 °C for 15 min. When cool, remove 2 drops of liquor and place on a white tile. Add 2 drops 1.5 % ethanolic *o*-tolidine and 2 drops 10 % aq. cyanogen bromide. A positive result is shown by a pink to orange colour; negatives remain blue–grey.

Note. Cyanogen bromide is toxic; the test must be carried out in a fume cupboard and, after completion, alkali should be added to decompose the reagent before sterilization.

C3.36 Nitrate reduction

Method 1. Inoculate nitrate broth and incubate for up to 5 days. Note any gas formation in the Durham's tube. Add 1 ml nitrite reagent A followed by 1 ml reagent B (Section C1.13).

Red colour shows presence of nitrite and indicates that nitrate has been reduced.

To tubes not showing a red colour within 5 min add powdered zinc (up to 5 mg/ml of culture) and allow to stand. Red colour = nitrate present in the medium (i.e. not reduced by the organism). Absence of red colour = nitrate absent in the medium (i.e. reduced by the organism to nitrite, which in turn was reduced).

Note. Incubation for 5 days is unnecessary with many organisms and Daubner (1962) reported that with the exception of two *Erwinia* spp., all members of the Enterobacteriaceae reduced nitrate to nitrite in 8 h; it is convenient to test a sample of the inoculated medium daily and re-incubate if nitrate has not been reduced.

Method 2. Brough (1950) used small volumes (1 ml in 75 × 10 mm tubes) of medium (0.1 % KNO₃ in nutrient broth) heated at 37 °C before inoculation with a heavy suspension and a rapid return to a 37 °C water bath. Test after 15 min with 3 drops each of sulphanilic acid and α-naphthylamine reagents (Section C1.13).

Method 3 Bachmann & Weaver (1951). Medium: peptone, 1 %; beef extract, 0.3 %; KNO₃, 0.1 % in distilled water; sterilize and store in flasks. Dispense in 1.0 ml volumes into clean, non-sterile 75 × 10 mm tubes. Heat tubes in 37 °C water bath and then inoculate with two 3 mm loopsful of 6-hour culture (inoculum should not be broken up but allowed to settle). After 15 min add 1 drop each of sulphanilic acid and dimethyl-α-naphthylamine reagents (Section C1.13). When nitrite is present a pink colour develops in 5 min.

Method 4 NCTC micromethod (Clarke & Cowan, 1952). Suspensions are made from growth on nutrient agar (see Decarboxylases, Section C3.12).

0.05 % NaNO₃	0.04 ml
0.025 M-phosphate buffer, pH 6.8	0.04 ml
Suspension	0.04 ml

Incubate in water bath at 37 °C and test after 1 h. Add 0.06 ml nitrite test solution A and 0.06 ml test solution B (dimethyl-α-naphthylamine) (Section C1.13). Shake and read after 1–2 min. A pink colour is indicative of nitrite. In each series of tests a blank without suspension should be made to exclude the presence of nitrite in the substrate.

Controls: reduced – *Escherichia coli*
not reduced – *Acinetobacter anitratus*

C3.37 Nitrite reduction

Inoculate nitrite broth (Section A2.7.22) and incubate for 7–14 days. Add nitrite reagents (Section C1.13) as for the nitrate reduction test.

Red colour = nitrite present. Absence of red colour = nitrite absent, i.e. reduced by the organism.

Controls: reduced – *Escherichia coli*
not reduced – *Acinetobacter anitratus*

C3.38 0/129 sensitivity

Method 1 (Davis & Park, 1962). Place a few crystals of the pteridine compound (2,4-diamino-6,7-di-*iso*-propyl pteridine)* on the surface of a plate previously inoculated with the test culture. Incubate the plate overnight and examine for inhibition of growth around the crystals.

Method 2 (Bain & Shewan, 1968). Place an O/129

* Obtainable from BDH Chemicals Ltd, Poole, Dorset.

disk (Section C1.16) on the surface of a nutrient agar plate sown with the test organism. Incubate the plate overnight and look for a clear zone around the disk.

Controls: positive – *Vibrio parahaemolyticus*
negative – *Escherichia coli*

C3.39 ONPG test (Lowe, 1962)

Inoculate a tube of ONPG broth and incubate for 24 h. β-galactosidase activity is indicated by the appearance of a yellow colour due to *o*-nitrophenol.

Controls: positive – *Escherichia coli*
negative – *Morganella morganii*

C3.40 Oxidase (cytochrome c oxidase) activity

Method 1 (Kovács, 1956). On a piece of filter paper (7 cm diam.) in a Petri dish, place 2 to 3 drops of 1 % tetramethyl-*p*-phenylenediamine dihydrochloride (Section C1.14, soln 1); do not allow the drops to dry on the paper. The test organism (grown on a medium free from glucose and nitrate) is removed with a platinum (not nichrome) wire or glass rod and smeared across the surface of the impregnated paper. A positive reaction is shown by the development of a dark purple colour within 10 s.

Method 2 (Gaby & Hadley, 1957). Add 0.2 ml α-naphthol (Section C1.14, soln 2) and 0.3 ml 1 % dimethyl-*p*-phenylenediamine oxalate (Section C1.14, soln 3) to an overnight broth culture. Shake vigorously. A blue colour appearing within 10 to 30 s indicates a positive result; weak reactions occurring between 2 and 5 min should be ignored. For plate cultures mix equal volumes of the two reagents (Section C1.14, solns 2 and 3) and run a few drops over the surfaces of colonies on the plate (Ewing & Johnson, 1960); colour changes and times are similar to the test in broth.

Note. Method 2 is slightly less sensitive than method 1.

Controls: positive – *Pseudomonas aeruginosa*
negative – *Escherichia coli*

C3.41 Phenylalanine deamination

Method 1 (Shaw & Clarke, 1955). After recording the result of the malonate test (Section C3.31) acidify with 0.1–0.2 ml 0.1 N-HCl and add 0.2 ml 10 % FeCl₃ aq. soln; shake and observe any colour change. Watch immediately; a positive reaction is indicated by a green colour which quickly fades.

Note. This method is not suitable for showing phenylalanine deaminase in *Moraxella phenylpyruvica* (Snell & Davey, 1971).

Method 2 (Report, 1958). Inoculate heavily a phenylalanine agar slope. Incubate overnight and run 0.2 ml 10 % FeCl₃ aq. soln over the growth. A positive result gives a green colour on the slope and in the free liquid at the base.

Method 3 (Goldin & Glenn, 1962). Make a suspension of the test organism in a small tube. Place a phenylalanine test strip (Section C1.15) in the tube and let the tip of the paper touch the suspension. Place the tube in a water bath at 37 °C for 1 h, then add 1 drop of 8 % $FeCl_3$ to the strip. A positive test produces a green colour. *Moraxella phenylpyruvica* is not likely to be positive in under 4 h of incubation.

Method 4 Henriksen (1950). Make a heavy suspension of the organism by suspending the growth from one agar slope in 0.5 ml saline. Add 0.2 ml suspension to 0.2 ml 0.2 % DL-phenylalanine in saline. Shake and place the tube in an almost horizontal position in an incubator. After 4 h acidify the mixture by adding 10 % H_2SO_4 using phenol red as indicator. Next add 4–5 drops half-saturated $FeSO_4 \cdot (NH_4)_2SO_4 \cdot 6H_2O$, shake the tube and watch for a green colour (= positive) within a minute; the colour quickly fades.

Method 5 NCTC micromethod (Shaw & Clarke, 1955). Suspensions are made from growth on nutrient agar (see Decarboxylases, Section C3.12).

0.03 M-phenylalanine	0.04 ml
0.025 M-phosphate buffer, pH 6.8	0.04 ml
Suspension	0.04 ml

Incubate at 37 °C in a water bath. Test after 2 h by adding 0.04 ml 2 % ferric chloride; shake. Read a minute later; a green colour indicates the presence of phenylpyruvic acid.

Controls: positive – *Proteus vulgaris*
negative – *Klebsiella aerogenes*

C3.42   Phosphatase test

Method 1. Lightly inoculate phenolphthalein phosphate agar to obtain discrete colonies, and incubate for 18 h. Place 0.1 ml ammonia soln (sp. gr. 0.880) in the lid of the Petri dish and invert the medium above it. Alternatively the medium may be exposed to ammonia vapour by holding above an open bottle. Free phenolphthalein liberated by phosphatase reacts with the ammonia and phosphatase-positive colonies become bright pink.

Note. Baird-Parker (1963) recommends incubation of cultures at 30 °C for 3–5 days before applying the test, and thereby obtains more positives than in cultures incubated at 37 °C for 18 h.

Method 2 White & Pickett (1953). Substrate: dissolve 30 mg phenol-free phenyl disodium phosphate in 100 ml 0.01 M-Sørensen's citrate–NaOH buffer at pH 5.6 (keeps for 3 months at 4 °C in a stoppered bottle).

Indicator: dissolve 50 mg 2:6-dibromo-*N*-chloro-*p*-quinone imine in 10 ml methanol (stable for 2 months at 4 °C in a dark, stoppered bottle).

Test: pipette 0.5 ml substrate into 100×13 mm tube. In this make a heavy suspension (10^{10}/ml) of the organism under test; incubate the tube at 37 °C for 4 h. Add 4 drops indicator solution; shake and stand the tube at room temperature for 15 min. Add 0.3 ml *n*-butanol; shake, stand for 5 min. A purple or blue colour in the butanol layer indicates a positive result.

Controls: positive – *Staphylococcus aureus*
negative – *S. epidermidis*

C3.43   Pigment production

For *Chromobacterium* spp. use mannitol yeast extract agar. Incubate at 22–30 °C.

The production of pigment and the influence of light are important characteristics of *Mycobacterium* spp. For incubation in continuous light, Marks & Richards (1962) recommend that a 37 °C incubator should be fitted with a 25 W lamp; cultures on Lowenstein–Jensen slopes should be placed at 30–60 cm from the lamp.

For most *Pseudomonas* spp. use King, Ward & Raney media. Incubate medium A at 37 °C for 24–96 h and medium B at 37 °C for 24 h followed by 22 °C (or room temperature) for 72 h. Kligler's iron agar (KIA) and TSI show up the pigmentation of *Pseudomonas cepacia*.

Serratia marcescens strains vary in their media requirements for pigment production; try nutrient agar, mannitol yeast extract agar, or King, Ward & Raney medium A at 22 °C or 30 °C.

Note. Non-pigmented strains are not uncommon and a suitable medium for inducing pigment production by all recalcitrant strains has not yet been produced. Micrococci produce pigment well on potato, but staphylococci do not seem to grow well enough on it to show any pigment. In general staphylococci produce pigment best in diffuse daylight.

C3.44   Poly-β-hydroxybutyric acid accumulation

Accumulation of poly-β-hydroxybutyrate (PHB) can be seen by phase microscopy and confirmed by staining with Sudan black (Stanier, Palleroni & Doudoroff, 1966), or dilute carbol fuchsin; it may be confirmed by chemical extraction (Williamson & Wilkinson, 1958). The methods are hardly routine in clinical laboratories, but if the information can be obtained it will be found useful in identifying pseudomonads.

C3.45 Polysaccharide formation on sucrose media

Inoculate sucrose broth and incubate. Much dextran formation is shown by an increased viscosity of the culture and the dextran may be flocculated by the addition of ethanol. The dextran is best recognized by a precipitin test in which the broth culture is set up against an antiserum to *Streptococcus pneumoniae* type 2.

Inoculate a plate of sucrose agar and incubate. Levan-producing organisms grow as large mucoid colonies; dextran-producing organisms (e.g. *Streptococcus sanguis*) may form small glassy colonies on this medium.

Controls: dextran produced – *Streptococcus sanguis*
         levan produced – *S. salivarius*
         dextran and levan negative – *S. faecalis*

C3.46 Starch hydrolysis

Inoculate starch agar and incubate plates at 30 °C for 5 days.

Method 1. Flood the plate with Lugol's iodine solution (Section B1.11); the medium turns blue where starch has not been hydrolysed, while hydrolysis is indicated by clear colourless zones.

Method 2 (Kellerman & McBeth, 1912). Flood the plate with 95 % ethanol; milky-white areas indicate unhydrolysed starch, whereas hydrolysis is indicated by clear zones. This reaction is not instantaneous and is best observed 30 min after addition of the ethanol.

Note. Some strains of *Bacillus* spp. produce only restricted zones of hydrolysis that may not be obvious until the bacterial growth has been scraped away.

Controls: positive – *Bacillus subtilis*
         negative – *Escherichia coli*

C3.47 Streptococcal grouping

Preparation of the extract

1. Acid extraction (modified from Lancefield, 1933). Mix the growth from a quarter of a blood agar plate or the centrifuged deposit from 10 ml of a culture in Todd–Hewitt broth with 0.4 ml 0.2 N-HCl and place in a boiling water bath for 10 min. Cool and neutralize the supernatant with 0.2 N-NaOH, using phenol red as the indicator. Centrifuge and use the supernatant.

2. Formamide extraction (Fuller, 1938). Mix the growth from a quarter of a blood agar plate or the centrifuged deposit from 5 ml of a culture in Todd–Hewitt broth with 0.1 ml formamide and heat in an oil bath at 160 °C for 15 min or until the growth is almost completely dissolved. Add 0.25 ml 95 % ethanol containing 0.5 % HCl, shake and centrifuge. Discard the precipitate and add 0.5 ml acetone to the supernatant. Shake, centrifuge, and discard the supernatant.

Dissolve the precipitate in 0.4 ml saline, and neutralize with 0.2 N-NaOH using phenol red as the indicator.

3. Enzymic extraction (Maxted, 1948). Suspend a loopful of growth from a blood agar plate in 0.25 ml enzyme solution (Section C1.8) and heat in a water bath at 50 °C until clear (about 1½ h).

The test method

Prepare 'grouping pipettes' from 5 mm diam. glass tubing by drawing out one end into a capillary. Cut to a total length of about 3 cm and stand vertically by placing the capillary end in a block of Plasticine (modelling clay). Place a drop of antiserum in the pipette and layer the extract on top. The formation of a precipitate at the interface of the two layers within 2–3 min indicates a positive reaction.

Notes. While strains of groups A, B, C, and G are the ones most often investigated in medical laboratories, the grouping test should be made against all available group antisera. By Lancefield's method, some strains are better extracted with 0.07 N-HCl, and others, particularly group B strains, produce better extracts at 50 °C for 2 h (Williams, 1958).

Cross-reactions may occur when the extract prepared by the formamide method is too alkaline. This method tends to destroy the group O antigens.

Maxted's enzyme method is suitable for streptococci of groups A, C and G but strains of other groups (especially D) are less easily lysed by the enzyme.

Group D strains do not always give good reactions and, when suspected, should be grown in broth containing 0.5 % glucose.

C3.48 Tellurite tolerance

Inoculate blood tellurite agar plates and incubate at 37 °C for 24 h. Tellurite-resistant organisms show a heavy growth of jet-black colonies; tellurite-sensitive organisms fail to grow or show a very light growth, the colonies being visible only with a hand lens.

Controls: positive – *Streptococcus faecalis*
         negative – *S. agalactiae*

C3.49 Temperature range for growth

The general principle of this type of test is that a suitable medium is lightly inoculated with the organism under test and incubated at different temperatures. For temperatures above 37 °C, a thermostatically controlled (± 0.5 °C) water bath is preferable to an incubator.

With aerobic spore-forming bacilli, mycobacteria, and actinomycetes a solid medium (as a slope) is preferable; with other organisms liquid media are used.

For streptococci, Abd-el-Malek & Gibson (1948a) recommend litmus milk; for organisms showing little activity in plain milk they add 0.25 % each of glucose and yeast extract.

At 22 °C and above examine cultures for growth daily for up to 7 days; at lower temperatures after 7 and 14 days. The exact length of incubation will obviously depend upon the normal growth rate of the organism. The ability of an organism to grow at a particular temperature should be confirmed by growth at that temperature after subculture.

C3.50   Temperature tolerance

60 °C for 30 min (streptococci and similar organisms). Place 1 ml of a 24-hour broth or serum broth culture in a small test tube, and place in a water bath at 60 °C for 30 min. Cool under a cold tap and incubate at 37 °C for 24 h. Subculture to a serum agar slope and incubate for 24 h. Examine for growth which indicates the ability of the organism to survive the conditions.

C3.51   Tween 80 hydrolysis

Method 1 (Sierra, 1957). Make a stroke inoculation of the test culture on the surface of Tween 80 nutrient agar (Section A2.7.32); incubate at the optimal temperature of the organism. Look at the plate each day; an opaque halo around the growth indicates hydrolysis of the Tween.

Controls: positive – *Pseudomonas aeruginosa*
　　　　　negative – *Alcaligenes bronchisepticus*

Method 2 (Kubica & Dye, 1967). 0.5 % Tween 80 soln in phosphate buffer, pH 7.0, with neutral red as indicator, is tubed in 4 ml volumes in screw-capped containers, and autoclaved. The final colour should be amber. Store at 4 °C and use within a fortnight.

Inoculate with a large loopful of growth from a solid medium, incubate at 37 °C and read each day for three weeks. In a positive result the indicator changes from amber to pink.

Controls: positive – *Mycobacterium kansasii*
　　　　　negative – (i) uninoculated tube of medium
　　　　　　　　　　(ii) *M. fortuitum*

C3.52   Urease activity

Method 1. Inoculate heavily a slope of Christensen's urea medium; examine after 4 h incubation and daily for 5 days. Red colour = positive.

Method 2. Inoculate fairly heavily a tube of SSR urea medium; incubate and examine daily for 7 days. Red colour = urea hydrolysed.

Method 3 Stuart, van Stratum & Rustigian (1945). Medium for rapid test: to 380 ml distilled water add KH_2PO_4, 364 mg; Na_2HPO_4, 380 mg; urea, 8 g; yeast

extract, 40 mg; 0.02 % phenol red, 20 ml. The pH is 6.8. Filter to sterilize.

Test: pipette 1.5 ml volumes into small tubes and inoculate heavily with 3 loopsful of culture from a solid medium. Incubate at 37 °C in a water bath. *Proteus* spp. produce a red colour in 5–60 min.

Method 4 Hormaeche & Munilla (1957). Test solution: to 100 ml 2 % urea solution add 2 ml 0.04 % cresol red. Distribute in 1 ml volumes into small tubes; sterilization is not necessary when the test is to be made on the same day. Inoculate tubes with 2 loopsful of growth from 24-hour agar culture (old cultures are too alkaline). Place tubes in water bath at 45–50 °C for 2 h. Urease-positive cultures produce a violet red colour.

Method 5. NCTC micromethod. Suspensions are made from growth on either nutrient or glucose agar; the latter usually give stronger reactions.

2 % urea soln	0.06 ml
0.025 M-phosphate buffer, pH 6.0	
(phenol red)	0.06 ml
Suspension	0.04 ml

Place in 37 °C water bath and observe at intervals of 15 min for the first hour; leave negatives for a final reading at 4 h. Positive tests show a red colour.

This is better than the test given in Clarke & Cowan (1952).

Controls: positive – *Proteus vulgaris*
　　　　　negative – *Escherichia coli*

Voges–Proskauer (VP) reaction: see Section C3.1.

C3.53   'X' and 'V' requirements

Method 1. Inoculate a blood agar plate and a nutrient agar plate with the organism and spot inoculate a strain of *Staphylococcus aureus* on each plate. Observe each plate for growth and for 'satellitism'.

Growth on blood agar plate only	– requires X factor
Growth shows 'satellitism' on blood agar	– requires X and V factors
Shows 'satellitism' on both media	– requires V factor
Growth on both media but not showing 'satellitism'	– neither X nor V factor required.

Method 2. Inoculate a nutrient agar plate and lay an X-factor and a V-factor disk (Section C1.18) on the surface at a distance of about 2 cm from each other. Examine for growth in the vicinity of one or both disks.

APPENDIX D

Identicards

D1 IDENTICARD SET FOR GENERA

Use a card with a single row of holes (Fig. 8.1).

The plan for notching the master cards (set no. 1 for genera) is shown in Table D 1b, and the key to the numbered holes in Table D 1a. All positive characters are notched from the hole to the edge of the card. For certain genera two or more cards may be needed to make provision for different reactions (dee characters) or differences in reading a test (catalase in *Aerococcus*). A guide card with the holes numbered will be found useful for the probing (sorting) operation.

Notching the unknown. Positive characters of the strain under test are notched from the appropriate hole (Table D 1a) to the edge of the card.

Probing. When the notching of the unknown's card is completed put it at the front of the pack of master cards, correctly faced, and test each hole in turn with a probe or knitting needle.

A probe through the hole of a positive character (of the unknown) will, when lifted, remove cards that are negative for that character and these can be discarded. The unknown's card and master cards of genera in which that character is positive will drop out of the pack; these cards are collected and tested again for another character.

When unnotched holes (negative characters) of the unknown are probed, the cards that are lifted with the probe are retained for further testing, and the drop outs are discarded (Table D 1c).

The identity of the unknown (as far as it can be determined by this set of cards) will correspond with that of the master card that has similar notchings.

D2 IDENTICARD SET FOR SPECIES

Use cards with two rows of holes (Fig. 8.2a).

In the *master cards* the outer row of holes is notched for characters recorded as d, (d) and (+) in the tables in Chapters 6 and 7. Characters shown as + in the

Table D 1a *Key for numbered holes, Identicard set no. 1 (card with single row of holes)*

Hole no.	Character represented
1	Gram reaction
2	Motility
3	Acid fastness
4	Spore formation
5	Coccus (bacillus is not notched)
6	Growth anaerobically
7	Growth in air
8	Oxidase
9	Catalase
10	
11	Oxidative attack on sugars
12	Fermentative attack on sugars

tables are notched to the inner row of holes (Fig. 8.2b). The notching plan for the enterobacteria is given in Table D 2a, b.

Notching the unknown. Positive characters of the unknown organism are notched to the second (inner) row of holes in the two-row cards (Fig. 8.2c).

Probing. The completed card(s) is placed in front of the pack of master cards, correctly faced, and the probe inserted through the appropriate holes. In species identification the probing procedure is different from that for genus identification (see Table D 2c).

Positive characters of the unknown are probed in the first (outer) hole, the probe lifted to remove master cards in which that character is negative. The cards that drop out are retained for testing other characters on the card.

Negative characters are probed through the second (inner row) hole, and the cards that are retained on the probe are kept for further tests.

As with the cards for generic identification, the probing is continued until only one master card remains or all the holes have been probed.

Table D 1*b* *Notching of master cards for Identicard set no.* 1

		1	2	3	4	5	6	7	8	9	10	11	12	Notes for centre of card
1a	*Aerococcus*	V				V	V	V					V	Catalase = −
1b	*Aerococcus*	V				V	V	V		V			V	Catalase = w
2	*Aeromonas*		V				V	V	V	V			V	
3a	*Acinetobacter*					V		V		V		V		Coccobacillus – coccus card
3b	*Acinetobacter*							V		V		V		Coccobacillus – bacillus card
4	*Actinobacillus*						V	V	V	V			V	Gas not produced
5	*Actinomyces*	V					V						V	May branch
6	*Alcaligenes*		V					V	V	V				
7	*Arachinia*	V					V	V					V	(Also *Actinomyces odontolyticus*) Branched, filamentous
11a	*Bacillus*	V	V		V			V		V		V	V	⎧ Oxidase variable, ? inconstant
11b	*Bacillus*	V			V		V	V	V	V		V	V	⎪ Some spp. facultative [Ø]
11c	*Bacillus*	V	V		V		V	V	V	V		V	V	⎨ Carbohydrates: some spp. F
														some spp. O
														some spp. −
														⎪ One sp. (*B. anthracis*) non-
														⎩ motile
12a	*Bacteroides*						V						V	⎧ Catalase variable
12b	*Bacteroides*						V			V				⎨ Most spp. non-motile
12c	*Bacteroides*		V				V						V	⎩ One sp. motile
13	*Beneckea*		V				V	V	V	V			V	Halophilic; chitinolytic
14	*Bifidobacterium*	V					V						V	Tendency to branch
15	*Bordetella*							V	V	V				Does not grow on simple media
16	*Branhamella*					V		V	V	V				
17	*Brucella*							V	V	V				Carboxyphilic; urease +
21a	*Campylobacter*		V						V	V				⎰ Will not grow under strict [Ø];
21b	*Campylobacter*		V						V					⎱ opt. = 5 % O₂. Catalase = D
22	*Cardiobacterium*						V	V	V				V	Pleomorphic; metachromatic granules?
23	*Chromobacterium lividum*		V					V	V	V		V		Psychrophilic (37 = no growth) ⎫ Violet
24	*Chromobacterium violaceum*		V				V	V	V	V			V	Mesophilic (37 = growth) ⎬ pigment
25a	*Clostridium*	V	V		V		V						V	
25b	*Clostridium* (asporogenous)	V					V						V	*C. welchii*; non-motile; seldom spores
26	*Corynebacterium*	V					V	V		V			V	Pleomorphic
31a	*Eikenella*						V	V	V					⎧ Needs CO₂ at isolation; soon [O]
31b	*Eikenella*						V		V					⎨ Probably cannot grow [Ø];
														⎩ ? a second, anaerobic species
32a	Enterobacteria		V				V	V		V			V	Most produce gas; NO₃ reduced
32b	Enterobacteria						V	V		V			V	Non-motile spp.
32c	Enterobacteria						V	V					V	*Shigella dysenteriae* 1 (Shiga's bacillus)
33	*Erysipelothrix*	V					V	V					V	
34	*Eubacterium*	V					V						V	
36	*Flavobacterium*							V	V	V		V		Yellow pigment
38a	*Gemella*	V				V	V	V					V	⎰ Easily decolorized; usually
38b	*Gemella*					V	V	V					V	⎱ regarded as Gram negative
40a	*Haemophilus*						V	V		V				⎰ Fastidious; needs X and/or V
40b	*Haemophilus*						V	V						⎱ factor; catalase variable
42	*Kurthia*	V	V				V			V				
44	*Lactobacillus*	V					V	V						Grows best at about pH 6
45	*Leuconostoc*	V				V	V						V	
46	*Listeria*	V	V				V	V		V			V	
51	*Micrococcus*	V				V		V		V		V		
52	*Moraxella*							V	V	V				

Table D 1*b* (*cont.*)

		1	2	3	4	5	6	7	8	9	10	11	12	Notes for centre of card
53	*Mycobacterium*	V		V				V		V		V		Does not branch or produce aerial hyphae
56	*Necromonas*						V	V	V	V			V	May produce gas. No growth at 37 °C
57	*Neisseria*					V		V	V	V		V		Carboxyphilic
58a	*Nocardia*	V		V				V		V		V		Feebly acid fast; produce aerial hyphae
58b	*Nocardia*	V						V		V		V		Some spp. (strains) not acid fast
61	*Pasteurella*						V	V	V	V			V	Gas not produced
62	*Pediococcus*	V				V	V	V					V	
63	*Peptococcus*	V				V	V							
64	*Peptostreptococcus*	V				V	V						V	Gas may be produced
65	*Plesiomonas*		V				V	V	V	V			V	Gas not produced; indole +; gelatin −
66	*Propionibacterium*	V					V			V			V	Club shapes; branching
67	*Pseudomonas*		V				V	V	V	V		V		May produce fluorescent or green pigment
71	*Rothia*	V						V		V			V	Filamentous; no mycelium or hyphae. Will grow under microaerophilic conditions
81	*Staphylococcus*	V				V	V	V		V			V	
82	*Streptobacillus*						V	V					V	Needs enrichment (Also *Shigella dysenteriae* 1)
83	*Streptococcus*	V				V	V	V					V	
91a	*Veillonella*					V	V							⎱ Catalase variable
91b	*Veillonella*					V	V			V				⎰
92	*Vibrio*		V				V	V	V	V			V	Gas not produced. Arginine −; lysine +; ornithine +

See Table 5.2 (facing p. 43) for explanations of the symbols used in the right-hand column.

Table D 1*c* *Notching and probing of cards (single row) and disposal after sorting*

Character of unknown strain	Unknown's card	Disposal of cards after probing	
		Cards remaining on probe	Cards that drop out
Positive	Notched	Discard	Keep and retest for other characters
Negative	Not notched	Keep and retest for other characters	Discard

Table D 2*a* *Key to numbered holes, Identicard set no. 2 (card with two rows of holes)*

Hole no.	Character represented
1	Growth in KCN medium
2	Utilization of citrate as C source
3	Gas from glucose
4	VP reaction
5	Gelatin hydrolysis
6	Urease
7	Phenylalanine deaminase (PPA test)
8	Motility
9	H_2S production from TSI
10	Malonate
11	Arginine dihydrolase
12	Lysine decarboxylase
13	Ornithine decarboxylase
14	
15	
16	Adonitol, acid
17	Dulcitol, acid
18	Mannitol, acid
19	Lactose, acid
20	Indole produced

Table D 2b *Notching of master cards for Identicard set no. 2 (card with two rows of holes)*

		1	2	3	4	5	6	7	8	9	10	11	12	13	14	15	16	17	18	19	20
1	*Escherichia coli*			V					o			o	V	o				o	V	V	V
2	A–D group											o	o	o				o	V	o	V
3	*Edwardsiella tarda*			V					V	V			V	V							V
4	*Yersinia pestis*																		V		
5	*Yersinia pseudotuberculosis*						V		V								V		V		
6	*Yersinia enterocolitica*						V		V				V	V					V		o
7	*Shigella dysenteriae* 1																				
8	*Shigella dysenteriae* 2–10																				o
9	*Shigella flexneri* 1–5																		V		o
10	*Shigella flexneri* 6			o								o						o	V		
11	*Shigella boydii*											o							V		o
12	*Shigella sonnei*													V					V	o	
13	*Citrobacter freundii*	V	V	V					V	V		o		o				o	V	o	
14	*Citrobacter koseri*		V	V			V		V		V	o		V			V	o	V	o	o
15	*Levinea* species	V	V	V			V		V		o	V		V			o	o	V	V	o
16	*Salmonella typhi*								V	V		o	V					o	V		
17	*Salmonella pullorum*		o	V								V	V	V					V		
18	*Salmonella gallinarum*		o									o	V					V	V		
19	*Salmonella choleraesuis*		o	V					V	V		o	V	V				o	V		
20	*Salmonella kauffmannii*		V	V					V	V		o	V	V				V	V		
21	*Salmonella salamae*		V	V		o			V	V	V		V	V					V	V	
22	*Salmonella arizonae*		V	V		o			V	V	V		V	V					V	o	
23	*Salmonella houtenae*	V	V	V		o			V	V			V	V					V		
24	*Erwinia herbicola*		V			V		V	V										V	o	
25	*Morganella morganii*	V		V			V	V	V					V						V	
26	*Proteus vulgaris*	V	o	V		V	V	V	V												V
27	*Proteus mirabilis*	V	o	V	o	V	V	V	V					V							
28	*Proteus rettgeri*	V	V	V			V	V	V								V		V		V
29	*Proteus inconstans*	V	V	V				V	V								V				V
30	*Proteus stuartii*	V	V					V	V												V
31	*Hafnia alvei*	V	V	V	V				V		o		V	V					V		
32	*Serratia marcescens*	V	V	o	V	V			V		o		V	V			o		V		
33	*Serratia liquefaciens*	V	V	V	V	V	o		V				o	V					V		
34	*Serratia rubidaea*	V	o	o	V	V	o		V		o		o				V		V	V	
35	*Enterobacter cloacae*	V	V	V	V	o	o		V		o	V		V			o	o	V	o	
36	*Enterobacter aerogenes*	V	V	V	V	o	o		V		V		V	V			V	o	V	V	
37	*Klebsiella aerogenes*	V	V	V	V	o	V				V			V			V	o	V	V	
38	*Klebsiella oxytoca*	V	V	V	V	V	V							V			V	V	V	V	V
39	*Klebsiella pneumoniae* (*s.s.*)		V	V			V				V			V			V	V	V	V	
40	*Klebsiella atlantae*	V	V	V	o		V							V			V		V	o	
41	*Klebsiella edwardsii*	V	o		V		V				o			V			V		V	o	
42	Unnamed klebsiella	o		V	o						V		o				V		V	V	
43	*Klebsiella ozaenae*	V	o	o			o						o				V	o	V	o	
44	*Klebsiella rhinoscleromatis*	V									V						V		V		

V Notched to the inner row (plus line)   o Notched to the outer row (dee line)

Table D 2c *Notching and probing of cards (double row) and disposal after sorting*

Character of unknown strain	Unknown's card	Row tested	Disposal of cards	
			On probe	Drop-out cards
Positive	Notched to inner row	Outer	Discard	Keep for retest
Negative	Not notched	Inner	Keep for retest	Discard

Test organisms

Many of the biochemical tests described in this *Manual* are controlled by test organisms that are known to give either positive or negative reactions under the appropriate conditions. As far as possible we chose species readily available and in Table E1 we give the accession numbers of suitable strains in the National Collection of Type Cultures, Central Public Health Laboratory, Colindale Avenue, London NW9 5HT and, in many cases, in the American Type Culture Collection, 12301 Parklawn Drive, Rockville, Maryland 20852, USA.

Freeze-dried (lyophilized) cultures retain their characters indefinitely, have a long storage life and are much better than ordinary 'stock cultures'. For laboratories that do not have a freeze-drier we recommend the method of drying described by Rhodes (1950) which needs only a vacuum pump and phosphorus pentoxide.

Some workers may prefer to keep a stock culture available for immediate use; in Table E2 we give a list of suitable media and indicate the frequency of subculture to be sure of survival. A more comprehensive list is given by Lapage, Shelton & Mitchell (1970).

Cooked meat is an excellent maintenance medium for many organisms, including anaerobes. Less nutrient media are better than richer media in which cultures die out more quickly.

Shigellas tend to become rough serologically on rich media but salmonellas seem to retain their antigenic structure well on Dorset egg.

Media containing fermentable carbohydrate should be avoided for maintaining cultures, and selective media should never be used for this purpose.

Cultures must not be allowed to dry out, and tightly closed screw-capped containers are preferable to waxed or corked tubes.

Table E1 *Recommended strains of test organisms*

	NCTC	ATCC
Acinetobacter anitratus	7844	15308
Aeromonas hydrophila	7810	9071

	NCTC	ATCC
Alcaligenes bronchisepticus	452[a]	19395
Alcaligenes faecalis	655	—
Bacillus stearothermophilus	10003	—
Bacillus subtilis	3610	6051
Clostridium sporogenes	533	10000
Clostridium tetani (non-toxigenic strain)	6336	
Clostridium welchii	6719	9856
Enterobacter aerogenes	10006	13048
Enterobacter cloacae	10005	13047
Escherichia coli	9001	11775
Klebsiella aerogenes	418	15380
Morganella morganii	10041[b]	—
Mycobacterium avium	8559	19421
Mycobacterium fortuitum	10394	6841
Mycobacterium kansasii	10268	14471
Mycobacterium phlei	8151	—
Mycobacterium smegmatis	8159	—
Nocardia brasiliensis	10300	19295
Nocardia caviae	1934	14629
Proteus vulgaris	4175	13315
Pseudomonas aeruginosa	7244	7700
Salmonella typhi	786	—
Salmonella typhimurium	74	13311
Serratia marcescens	1377	274
Shigella dysenteriae 1	4837	13313
Shigella sonnei	8220	—
Staphylococcus aureus	8532	12600
Staphylococcus epidermidis	4276[c]	—
Streptococcus agalactiae	8181	13813
Streptococcus dysgalactiae	4669	—
Streptococcus faecalis	8213	—
Streptococcus pneumoniae	7465	10015
Streptococcus salivarius	8618[d]	7073
Streptococcus sanguis	7863	10556
Vibrio parahaemolyticus	10903	—

[a] Listed as *Bordetella bronchiseptica* in NCTC Catalogue (1972).
[b] Listed as *Proteus morganii* in NCTC Catalogue (1972).
[c] Listed as *Micrococcus* sp. subgroup I in NCTC Catalogue (1972).
[d] Listed as *Streptococcus hominis* in NCTC Catalogue (1972).

Table E2 *Conditions for maintenance of test organisms*

Genus	Medium	Incubation Temp. (°C)	Time (h)	Storage* (°C)	Interval between subcultures (months)
Acinetobacter	Nutrient agar	37	18	5–25	3
Aeromonas	Nutrient agar	37	18	5–25	3
Alcaligenes	Nutrient agar	37	18	5–25	3
Bacillus	Nutrient agar	30	18	5–25	12
Clostridium	Cooked meat	37	18	5–25	12
Enterobacter	Nutrient agar	37	18	5–25	6
Escherichia	Nutrient agar	37	18	5–25	6
Klebsiella	Nutrient agar	37	18	5–25	3
Mycobacterium	Dorset egg	37	48–72†	15–25	6
Nocardia	Dorset egg	37	48–72	15–25	3
Proteus	Nutrient agar	37	18	5–25	3
Pseudomonas	Peptone water agar	30	18	5–25	3
Salmonella	Dorset egg	37	18	5–25	12
Shigella	Nutrient agar	37	18	5–25	6
Staphylococcus	Nutrient agar	37	18	5–25	3
Streptococcus	Cooked meat or	37	18	5–25	3
	Blood broth	37	18	5	1
Vibrio	Sloppy agar	30	48	22–25	1
Vibrio (marine) (*Beneckea* spp.)	Salt-water agar or 3 % NaCl agar	22	72	15–20	1

* In the dark.
† *M. tuberculosis* and other slow-growing mammalian pathogens should be incubated for 10–20 days or until growth is apparent to the naked eye.

APPENDIX F
Glossary

F1   TAXONOMIC TERMS

We have been unable to avoid the use of some taxonomic jargon in this edition of our *Manual*, and short notes on some of the more commonly used words and terms are given below. Those who would like more help or greater detail will probably find these in *A Dictionary of Microbial Taxonomic Usage* (Cowan, 1968*a*).

Accession number. The number allotted to a culture when it is accessioned (accepted) into a culture collection. Even if the classification (and the name) of the organism changes, the accession number remains the same.

Antibiogram is a record of the sensitivity or resistance of an organism to the different antibiotics listed. It is an essential part of the report made by a bacteriologist to the clinician who sent the specimen. But in cultures from a patient treated with antibiotic(s) the antibiogram cannot play any significant part in the identification of the organism, which is itself a survivor of antibiotic therapy and has almost certainly acquired some resistance to the therapeutic agent. Non-therapeutic substances such as lysozyme or O/129 may assist in the identification of an organism.

Carboxyphilic. Used to describe an organism whose growth is improved, or made possible, by an increase in the CO_2 content of the atmosphere.

Category. In taxonomy indicates RANK in a hierarchical system of classification; genus, species, and so on. Often used with its ordinary meaning of 'kind'.

Description. The characters of a taxon. When a description has been well written and includes all the essential information, it should enable future workers to recognize the taxon, should they meet it in their practice. Descriptions vary greatly in value; older ones, because of the limited development of knowledge at the time they were written, are often inadequate by present standards, and the taxa may not now be recognizable.

Diagnosis in systematics (and taxonomy) is a brief statement of characters that distinguish an organism from its neighbours. It is the equivalent of the term 'differential diagnosis' in clinical medicine.

Diagnostician. In a medical bacteriology laboratory this means one who identifies an organism. It does *not* mean the writer of a DIAGNOSIS or the clinician who sent the specimen to the laboratory.

Effective publication is the term used in the Bacteriological Code for the kind of publication authorized by the Code. Effective publication consists of publication in printed form, distributed for sale or gift to the public and scientific institutions. Reading a paper at a meeting of a learned society does not constitute effective publication for names of bacteria, but publication in the Proceedings (or Transactions) of the Society may well do so.

Genotype, -ic. The hereditary potential of an organism. A theoretical unit from which existing organisms have developed under the influence of their surroundings and possibly changed character to become the PHENOTYPE.

Group. A common term in English and American for a collection of similar objects or biological entities. It is used in taxonomy for a collection of strains not yet allocated to a particular RANK; it may be a collection of strains (eventually they may form a species) or a collection of species (? a potential genus). In serology it may be a collection of serotypes.

Preferably it is written or printed (in English) with a lower case letter g so as not to be confused with Pop or Political Groups.

Halophil(e) describes an organism that can tolerate and grow in a medium with a salt concentration greater than 0.85 %; it is usually applied only to organisms with requirement for a concentration of salt greater than 3 %.

Illegitimate name of an organism is one that has not been formed or published in accordance with the rules of the Bacteriological Code.

Legitimate name is a name applied to an organism; the name has been formed and published in accordance with the rules of the Bacteriological Code.

Neotype. The author of a new name (of a bacterium) should designate a nomenclatural type strain (see TYPE); if he fails to do this a subsequent author may designate a type strain; a neotype is such a designated strain provided it is not one of the strains used by the original author of the name.

There are official recommendations for the choice, proposal, and designation of type strains; the old Recommendation 12e of the 1958 edition of the Bacteriological Code was unintentionally omitted from the 1966 version printed in the *International Journal of Systematic Bacteriology* (IJSB), **16**, 459–90. The point is dealt with fully in the proposed revision of the Code (Lapage *et al.* 1973) in Rule 18e. The most important points for an author who intends to propose a neotype are (i) the proposal must be published in IJSB; (ii) it must be accompanied by a description (or a reference to a published description) of the proposed strain; and (iii) it must include a record of the deposition of the strain in a permanently established culture collection.

Phase should be reserved for phenomena with cyclical or to-and-fro variation, as the phases of the salmonella H antigens.

The three phases in the development of our tables (p. xi) is a misuse of the term that would be allowed to an author only in a non-technical section of a book or paper.

Phenotype, -ic. The characters of an organism that can be determined now; cf. the GENOTYPE which is the theoretical starting point that contains the hereditary potential of the taxon.

Psychrophil(e) describes an organism that grows at temperatures below those used in most medical laboratories; the optimal temperature for psychrophils is usually about 20 °C. Organisms able to grow below 5 °C may be described as psychrotrophic.

Rank. In a hierarchical system of classification organisms are arranged in a series of ranks (or CATEGORIES) each of which includes all members of the ranks immediately below. A taxon with the rank of family includes the lower taxa with the rank of genus, and each genus is made up of taxa with the rank of species; thus a family consists of the genera of that family and the species of those genera. And as in an army, the species are subordinate to taxa of higher rank.

A better analogy is to the shelves of a book-stack;

families near the top, genera in the middle, and species lower down the stack.

Subspecies, a fashionable replacement for VARIETY. A subdivision of a species.

Symbiosis. Often used to mean two organisms living together for mutual benefit. According to R. E. Hungate this usage is incorrect, and we think he has a point. Strictly, symbiosis means physical contact between organisms, each of which is a symbiont. Examples of symbiosis are *Rickettsia prowazekii* and *Pediculus corporis*. See also SYNERGISM.

Synergism. The state in which two or more organisms form an organization for mutual benefit (often called SYMBIOSIS, q.v.). The satellitism shown by colonies of *Haemophilus influenzae* near colonies of *Staphylococcus aureus* growing on blood agar is a one-sided form of synergism.

Synonym. A word with the same meaning as another; synonyms are different words for the same thing. In nomenclature synonyms are different names applied to the same taxon, but this does not mean that the individual units or organisms making up the taxon are identical. Strictly, synonymy applies only to the names; taxa and individual bacteria cannot be synonymous.

Taxon (pl. -a). A taxonomic group of any size greater than a single strain. Two or more similar strains can form a taxon; its RANK may be that of a serotype, species, genus, or even a kingdom, with numerous intermediate ranks between kingdom and genus, none of which has any practical significance.

Type. This common English word meaning 'kind' has a special use in taxonomy, to mean the nomenclatural type of a taxon. The nomenclatural type of a species is a strain (the type strain); of a genus the type is a species (type species), and of a family or higher taxon the type is a genus.

The nomenclatural type is a means of attaching a name to a taxon; actually it merely attaches it to a particular strain, but other strains that are regarded as similar (and that may be a matter of opinion) are entitled to bear the same name. It is a purely nomenclatural device and it is naive of nomenclaturists to think that bacteriologists will not use the word type except in its strict taxonomic sense; it would be impertinent for anyone to say that they must not do so. On the other hand it is reasonable to expect that, in papers on taxonomic subjects, the word will be used only in its taxonomic sense.

GLOSSARY

Valid publication is publication (of a name) in accordance with certain requirements laid down in the Bacteriological Code.

Variant. A strain that shows one or more differences in characters from the parent; largely replaced by the word mutant when the change is believed to be due to a genetic change.

Variety (abbreviated to **var.**) is a term used for a variant that has become stabilized as a regular form. Equivalent to subspecies, but pleasanter English.

F2 ABBREVIATIONS AND ACRONYMS

An expansion of some less well-known abbreviations and acronyms may be useful to readers of this *Manual*. The list is based partly on queries raised by the proofreaders for this edition; it may be parochial and a different selection would be appreciated better by readers in other countries.

ADC albumin + glucose (dextrose) + catalase
ALM *Anaerobe Laboratory Manual*, Virginia Polytechnic Institute
ASS Ammonium salt sugars

B5W *Acinetobacter anitratus*
BSS Buffered single substrate tests
CAMP Test described by Christie, Atkins & Munch-Petersen (1944)
CDC Communicable Disease Center/Center for Disease Control, Atlanta, Georgia, USA
CSU Carbon source utilization tests
FN Fluorescence–denitrification medium of Pickett & Pedersen (1968)
IMViC Indole, methyl red, Voges–Proskauer, citrate utilization tests
KIA Kligler iron agar
LV Lecithovitellin
MHL Modified Hugh & Leifson medium (Park, 1964)
NW Neisser–Wechsberg leucocidin; a manifestation of staphylococcal α-toxin; acts on rabbit but not human leucocytes
PHB Poly-β-hydroxybutyrate
PRAS Pre-reduced anaerobically sterilized
PV Panton–Valentine leucocidin (not part of the α-toxin) of staphylococcus; acts on human leucocytes
29911 group or biotype = *Proteus inconstans*
32011 group or biotype = *Hafnia alvei*

189

APPENDIX G

Proposed revision of the Bacteriological Code

The original Bacteriological Code, approved in 1947, was based on the Botanical Code. It was long and complicated. In attempts to make it more useful in bacteriology, it became longer and more complicated.

A helpful explanation of the Code accompanied the version published in 1958 (Buchanan *et al.* 1958) and reprinted (with corrections) in 1959. The annotations were entirely the work of R. E. Buchanan.

The complexities of the Code remained and a Drafting Committee has attempted to simplify it; the introduction is reprinted below (Lapage *et al.* 1973).

Proposed Revision of the International Code of Nomenclature of Bacteria

S. P. LAPAGE,* W. A. CLARK, E. F. LESSEL, H. P. R. SEELIGER, and P. H. A. SNEATH, Drafting Committee

Introduction

A revision of the *International Code of Nomenclature of Bacteria* (Int. J. Syst. Bacteriol. **16**: 459–490 [1966]) has been undertaken in an attempt to simplify the rules of nomenclature, thus encouraging wider use of the code, and to provide a sound basis for bacterial systematics. When ratified, it will supersede all previous editions of the International Code of Nomenclature of Bacteria.

In order to achieve these aims, certain principles were recently approved by the International Committee on Systematic Bacteriology (ICSB) (Int. J. Syst. Bacteriol. **21**: 100–103 [1971]), and these have been incorporated into the proposed revision. In essence the significant modifications are as follows:

(1) A new starting date (1 January 1980 rather than 1 May 1753) for the nomenclature of bacteria will be instituted so as to put into practice more meaningful requirements for the valid publication of names. Among these are:

(a) New names and combinations must be published in the IJSB or, if published previously else-

* Chairman.

where, an announcement of such publication must be made in the IJSB;

(b) A description or a reference to a previously and effectively published description of the named taxon must also be given in the IJSB.

(c) The type of [a] named taxon must be designated.

Furthermore, it will be recommended that the description of the named taxon contain at least those characters cited for the taxon in the list of minimal standards which will be compiled by the members of the various ICSB taxonomic subcommittees and by other experts. In addition, it will be recommended that, in the case of cultivable organisms, cultures of the type strains of newly named species and subspecies be deposited in culture collections from which they would be available.

(2) For names published prior to 1 January 1980, *Approved Lists of Names of Bacteria* will be compiled by the members of the taxonomic subcommittees and by other experts for approval by the Judicial Commission and the ICSB. Only the names of bacteria which are adequately described and for which there is a type or neotype strain, if the organism is cultivable, will be placed on the approved lists. In determinations of priority after 1 January 1980, then, only those names which appear on the approved lists of names or which are validated by publication in the IJSB after 1 January 1980 need be taken into consideration. Thus it will no longer be necessary to conduct extensive, frequently difficult literature searches merely for the purpose of determining the earliest name which was used for a bacterial taxon. Most important, however, will be the fact that after 1 January 1980 all of the validly published names for the bacteria will have clear and precise applications because the names will be associated with adequate descriptions and type or neotype strains.

The proposed revision of the code has now gone through five drafts, the fourth draft having been circulated to the members of the ICSB for comment. The fifth draft is presented here for consideration and comment by the scientific community prior to submission to the Judicial Commission, the ICSB, and ultimately the Plenary Session of the relevant International Congress for final approval and acceptance.

G1   CONSEQUENCES OF THE REVISION

In general, the proposed revision was accepted at the 1973 International Congress, but the *-ii* ending of specific epithets made from personal names is to be retained (personal communication from S. P. Lapage). It follows that the spellings of epithets made from personal names used in this edition of this *Manual* will be correct until at least 1 January 1980, when the *Approved Lists of Names of Bacteria* will become effective.

Media, chemicals, reagents and laboratory supplies

Table H1 *Media from commercial sources*

Brand	Manufacturer
BBL	BBL Division of Beckton Dickinson & Co. Cockeysville, Maryland 21030, USA
	Beckton Dickinson (UK) Ltd Brindley 74, Astmoor Industrial Estate, Runcorn, Cheshire
Difco	Difco Laboratories Detroit, Michigan 48201, USA
	UK Division of Difco Laboratories Ltd PO Box 14B, Central Avenue, West Molesey, Surrey
Eiken	Eiken Chemical Co. Ltd 8–33 1-chome, Hongo, Bunkyo-ku, Tokyo, Japan
Nissui	Nissui Seiyaku Co. Ltd 2–5–11 Komagome, Toshima-ku, Tokyo, Japan
Oxoid	Oxoid Ltd Southwark Bridge Road, London SE 1
	USA agents: Flow Laboratories Inc., PO Box 2226, 1710 Chapman Avenue, Rockville, Maryland 20852, USA
Wellcome	Wellcome Reagents Ltd Wellcome Research Laboratories, Beckenham, Kent BR3 3BS
	Burroughs Wellcome Company 3030 Cornwallis Road, Research Triangle Park, NC 17709, USA

Table H2 *Chemicals, stains, reagents and other laboratory supplies from commercial sources in the UK*

BDH Limited, Poole, Dorset

T. M. Duche & Sons (UK) Ltd, 50 Mark Lane, London EC3

Flow Laboratories Ltd, Victoria Park, Heatherhouse Road, Irvine, Scotland

Hopkins & Williams Ltd, Freshwater Road, Chadwell Heath, Essex

Koch-Light Laboratories Ltd, Poyle Trading Estate, Colnbrook, Bucks

Kodak Limited, Chemical Division, Kirby, Liverpool L33 7UF. Agents for:
Eastman Kodak Company, Rochester, NY 14650, USA
K & K Laboratories Inc., 121 Express Street, Engineers Hill, Plainview, NY 11803, USA

Miles Laboratories Ltd, Ames Division, Stoke Court, Stoke Poges, Slough, Bucks

G. D. Searle & Co. Ltd, Lane End Road, High Wycombe, Bucks

Sass Scientific Chemicals Ltd, Victoria House, Vernon Place, Holborn, London WC1B 4DR

Sigma London Chemical Co. Ltd, Norbiton Station Yard, Kingston-upon-Thames, Surrey KT2 7BH

Turner–Stayne Laboratories Ltd, Greenfields Road, Tindale Crescent, Bishop Auckland, County Durham

References

Aaronson, S. (1956). A biochemical–taxonomic study of a marine micrococcus, *Gaffkya homari*, and a terrestrial counterpart. *J. gen. Microbiol.* **15**, 478.

Abbot, J. D. & Shannon, R. (1958). A method for typing *Shigella sonnei*, using colicine production as a marker. *J. clin. Path.* **11**, 71.

Abd-el-Malek, Y. & Gibson, T. (1948*a*). Studies in the bacteriology of milk. I. The streptococci of milk. *J. Dairy Res.* **15**, 233.

Abd-el-Malek, Y. & Gibson, T. (1948*b*). Studies in the bacteriology of milk. II. The staphylococci and micrococci of milk. *J. Dairy Res.* **15**, 249.

Abd-el-Malek, Y. & Gibson, T. (1952). Studies in the bacteriology of milk. III. The corynebacteria of milk. *J. Dairy Res.* **19**, 153.

Abrams, E., Zierdt, C. H. & Brown, J. A. (1971). Observations on *Aeromonas hydrophila* septicaemia in a patient with leukaemia. *J. clin. Path.* **24**, 491.

Albert, H. (1921). Modification of stain for diphtheria bacilli. *J. Am. med. Ass.* **76**, 240.

Alder, V. G., Brown, A. M. & Mitchell, R. G. (1966). The tellurite reactions of coagulase negative staphylococci and micrococci. *J. appl. Bact.* **29**, 304.

Alder, V. G., Gillespie, W. A. & Waller, L. J. (1962). The use of tellurite–egg yolk medium for the isolation and identification of staphylococci in hospitals. *J. appl. Bact.* **25**, 436.

Allen, L. A., Pasley, S. M. & Pierce, M. S. F. (1952). Conditions affecting the growth of *Bacterium coli* on bile salts media. Enumeration of this organism in polluted waters. *J. gen. Microbiol.* **7**, 257.

Aluotto, B. B., Wittler, R. G., Williams, C. O. & Faber, J. E. (1970). Standardized bacteriologic techniques for the characterization of *Mycoplasma* species. *Int. J. syst. Bact.* **20**, 35.

Anaerobe Laboratory Manual (1972). Edited by L. V. Holdeman & W. E. C. Moore. Blacksburg, Virginia: VPI Anaerobe Laboratory, Virginia Polytechnic Institute & State University.

Anderson, E. S. (1966). Possible importance of transfer factors in bacterial evolution. *Nature, Lond.* **209**, 637.

Anderson, E. S. & Lewis, M. J. (1965*a*). Drug resistance and its transfer in *Salmonella typhimurium*. *Nature, Lond.* **206**, 579.

Anderson, E. S. & Lewis, M. J. (1965*b*). Characterization of a transfer factor associated with drug resistance in *Salmonella typhimurium*. *Nature, Lond.* **208**, 843.

Anderson, J. D., Gillespie, W. A. & Richmond, M. H. (1973). The effect of antibiotics upon R-factor transfer between strains of *Escherichia coli* in the human gastro-intestinal tract. *J. med. Microbiol.* **6**, P ix.

Anderson, J. S., Cooper, K. E., Happold, F. C. & McLeod, J. W. (1933). Incidence and correlation with clinical severity of gravis, mitis, and intermediate types of diphtheria bacillus in a series of 500 cases at Leeds. *J. Path. Bact.* **36**, 169.

Anderson, J. S., Happold, F. C., McLeod, J. W. & Thomson, J. G. (1931). On the existence of two forms of diphtheria bacillus – *B. diphtheriae gravis* and *B. diphtheriae mitis* – and a new medium for their differentiation and for the bacteriological diagnosis of diphtheria. *J. Path. Bact.* **34**, 667.

Ando, K., Moriya, Y. & Kuwahara, S. (1959). Studies on the effect of Tween 80 on the growth of *Erysipelothrix incidiosa*. *Jap. J. Microbiol.* **3**, 85.

Andrade, E. (1906). Influence of glycerin in differentiating certain bacteria. *J. med. Res.* **14**, 551.

Andrewes, C. H., Burke-Gaffney, H. J. O'D., Cowan, S. T., Fry, R. M., Kelsey, J. C., Oakley, C. L., Standfast, A. F. B. & Sykes, G. (1965). Typography of bacteria. *Nature, Lond.* **208**, 332.

Andrewes, F. W. (1918). Dysentery bacilli: the differentiation of the true dysentery bacilli from allied species. *Lancet*, i, 560.

Andrewes, F. W. & Inman, A. C. (1919). A study of the serological races of the Flexner group of dysentery bacilli. *Spec. Rep. Ser. med. Res. Coun.* no. 42.

Arkwright, J. A. (1909). Varieties of the meningococcus with special reference to a comparison of strains from epidemic and sporadic sources. *J. Hyg., Camb.* **9**, 104.

Arnold, W. M., Jr & Weaver, R. H. (1948). Quick microtechniques for the identification of cultures. I. Indole production. *J. Lab. clin. Med.* **33**, 1334.

Ashley, D. J. B. & Kwantes, W. (1961). Four cases of human infection with *Achromobacter anitratus*. *J. clin. Path.* **14**, 670.

Aubert, E. (1950). 'Cold' stain for acid-fast bacteria. *Can. J. publ. Hlth*, **41**, 31.

Auletta, A. E. & Kennedy, E. R. (1966). Deoxyribonucleic acid base composition of some members of the *Micrococcaceae*. *J. Bact.* **92**, 28.

Austrian, R. & Collins, P. (1966). Importance of carbon dioxide in the isolation of pneumococci. *J. Bact.* **92**, 1281.

Ayers, S. H. & Rupp, P. (1922). Differentiation of hemolytic streptococci from human and bovine sources by the hydrolysis of sodium hippurate. *J. infect. Dis.* **30**, 388.

Bachmann, B. & Weaver, R. H. (1951). Rapid microtechnics for identification of cultures. V. Reduction of nitrates to nitrites. *Am. J. clin. Path.* **21**, 195.

Baer, H. & Washington, L. (1972). Numerical diagnostic key for the identification of *Enterobacteriaceae*. *Appl. Microbiol.* **23**, 108.

Bailey, J. H. (1933). A medium for the isolation of *Bacillus pertussis*. *J. infect. Dis.* **52**, 94.

Bain, N. & Shewan, J. M. (1968). Identification of *Aeromonas*, *Vibrio* and related organisms. In *Identification Methods for Microbiologists*, part B, p. 79. Edited by B. M. Gibbs & D. A. Shapton. London: Academic Press.

Baird-Parker, A. C. (1962). An improved diagnostic and selective medium for isolating coagulase positive staphylococci. *J. appl. Bact.* **25**, 12.

Baird-Parker, A. C. (1963). A classification of micrococci and staphylococci based on physiological and biochemical tests. *J. gen. Microbiol.* **30**, 409.

Baird-Parker, A. C. (1965a). The classification of staphylococci and micrococci from world-wide sources. *J. gen. Microbiol.* **38**, 363.

Baird-Parker, A. C. (1965b). Staphylococci and their classification. *Ann. N.Y. Acad. Sci.* **128**, 4.

Baird-Parker, A. C. (1970). The relationship of cell wall composition to the current classification of staphylococci and micrococci. *Int. J. syst. Bact.* **20**, 483.

Ballard, R. W., Doudoroff, M., Stanier, R. Y. & Mandel, M. (1968). Taxonomy of the aerobic pseudomonads: *Pseudomonas diminuta* and *P. vesiculare*. *J. gen. Microbiol.* **53**, 349.

Barakat, M. Z. & Abd El-Wahab, M. E. (1951). The differentiation of monosaccharides from disaccharides and polysaccharides and identification of fructose. *J. Pharm. Pharmac.* **3**, 511.

Barber, M. (1939). A comparative study of *Listerella* and *Erysipelothrix*. *J. Path. Bact.* **48**, 11.

Barber, M. (1955). Pigment production by staphylococci. *J. gen. Microbiol.* **13**, 338.

Barber, M. & Kuper, S. W. A. (1951). Identification of *Staphylococcus pyogenes* by the phosphatase reaction. *J. Path. Bact.* **63**, 65.

Barksdale, W. L., Li, K., Cummins, C. S. & Harris, H. (1957). The mutation of *Corynebacterium pyogenes* to *Corynebacterium haemolyticum*. *J. gen. Microbiol.* **16**, 749.

Barnes, E. M. (1956). Tetrazolium reduction as a means of differentiating *Streptococcus faecalis* from *Streptococcus faecium*. *J. gen. Microbiol.* **14**, 57.

Barnes, E. M., Impey, C. S. & Goldberg, H. S. (1966). Methods for the characterization of the Bacteroidaceae. In *Identification Methods for Microbiologists*, part A, p. 51. Edited by B. M. Gibbs & F. A. Skinner. London: Academic Press.

Baross, J. & Liston, J. (1970). Occurrence of *Vibrio parahaemolyticus* and related hemolytic vibrios in marine environments of Washington state. *Appl. Microbiol.* **20**, 179.

Barritt, M. M. (1936). The intensification of the Voges–Proskauer reaction by the addition of α-naphthol. *J. Path. Bact.* **42**, 441.

Barrow, G. I. & Miller, D. C. (1969). Marine bacteria in oysters purified for human consumption. *Lancet*, ii, 421.

Barrow, G. I. & Miller, D. C. (1972a). *Vibrio parahaemolyticus*: a potential pathogen from marine sources in Britain. *Lancet*, i, 485.

Barrow, G. I. & Miller, D. C. (1972b). *Vibrio parahaemolyticus* investigations. In *Modern Trends in Microbiology*, Symposium 28 September 1972, sponsored by Beckton Dickinson UK Ltd, Wembley.

Bascomb, S., Lapage, S. P., Willcox, W. R. & Curtis, M. A. (1971). Numerical classification of the tribe Klebsielleae. *J. gen. Microbiol.* **66**, 279.

Bascomb, S., Lapage, S. P., Curtis, M. A. & Willcox, W. R. (1973). Identification of bacteria by computer. Identification of reference strains. *J. gen. Microbiol.* **77**, 291.

Batty, I. (1958). *Actinomyces odontolyticus*, a new species of actinomycete regularly isolated from deep carious dentine. *J. Path. Bact.* **75**, 455.

Batty-Smith, C. G. (1941). The detection of acetyl-methyl-carbinol in bacterial cultures. A comparative study of the methods of O'Meara and of Barritt. *J. Hyg., Camb.* **41**, 521.

Baumann, P., Baumann, L. & Mandel, M. (1971). Taxonomy of marine bacteria: the genus *Beneckea*. *J. Bact.* **107**, 268.

Baumann, P., Doudoroff, M. & Stanier, R. Y. (1968a). Study of the *Moraxella* group. I. Genus *Moraxella* and the *Neisseria catarrhalis* group. *J. Bact.* **95**, 58.

Baumann, P., Doudoroff, M. & Stanier, R. Y. (1968b). A study of the *Moraxella* group. II. Oxidative [sic]-negative species (genus *Acinetobacter*). *J. Bact.* **95**, 1520.

Becker, B., Lechevalier, M. P., Gordon, R. E. & Lechevalier, H. A. (1964). Rapid differentiation between *Nocardia* and *Streptomyces* by paper chromatography of whole-cell hydrolysates. *Appl. Microbiol.* **12**, 421.

Beerens, H. & Tahon-Castel, M. (1965). *Infections Humaines à Bactéries Anaérobies non toxigènes.* Brussels: Presses Academiques Européennes.

Beijerinck, M. W. (1900). Schwefelwasserstoffbildung in den Stadtgräben und Aufstellung der Gattung Aërobacter. *Zentbl. Bakt. ParasitKde II Abt.* **6**, 193.

Berger, U. (1960a). *Neisseria haemolysans* (Thjötta und Böe, 1938): Untersuchungen zur Stellung im System. *Z. Hyg. InfektKrankh.* **146**, 253.

Berger, U. (1960b). *Neisseria animalis* nov. spec. *Z. Hyg. InfektKrankh.* **147**, 158.

Berger, U. (1961). A proposed new genus of Gram-negative cocci: *Gemella*. *Int. Bull. bact. Nomencl. Taxon.* **11**, 17.

Berger, U. (1962). Über das Vorkommen von Neisserien bei einigen Tieren. *Z. Hyg. InfektKrankh.* **148**, 445.

Bergey's Manual of Determinative Bacteriology (1923–74). Eight edns: **1**, 1923; **2**, 1925; **3**, 1930; **4**, 1934; **5**, 1939; **6**, 1948; **7**, 1957; **8**, 1974. Baltimore: The Williams & Wilkins Co.

Beveridge, W. I. B. (1934). A study of twelve strains of *Bacillus necrophorus*, with observations on the oxygen intolerance of the organism. *J. Path. Bact.* **38**, 467.

Biberstein, E. L. & Gills, M. G. (1962). The relation of the antigenic types to the A and T types of *Pasteurella haemolytica*. *J. comp. Path. Ther.* **72**, 316.

Biberstein, E. L., Gills, M. & Knight, H. (1960). Serological types of *Pasteurella haemolytica*. *Cornell Vet.* **50**, 283.

Biberstein, E. L. & White, D. C. (1969). A proposal for the establishment of two new *Haemophilus* species. *J. med. Microbiol.* **2**, 75.

Billing, E. (1955). Studies on a soap tolerant organism: a new variety of *Bacterium anitratum*. *J. gen. Microbiol.* **13**, 252.

Billing, E. & Luckhurst, E. R. (1957). A simplified method for the preparation of egg yolk media. *J. appl. Bact.* **20**, 90.

Black, W. A., Hodgson, R. & McKechnie, A. (1971). Evaluation of three methods using deoxyribonuclease production as a screening test for *Serratia marcescens*. *J. clin. Path.* **24**, 313.

Blair, J. E. & Carr, M. (1953). The bacteriophage typing of staphylococci. *J. infect. Dis.* **93**, 1.

Board, R. G. & Holding, A. J. (1960). The utilization of glucose by aerobic Gram-negative bacteria. *J. appl. Bact.* **23**, xi.

Bojalil, L. F., Cerbón, J. & Trujillo, A. (1962). Adansonian classification of mycobacteria. *J. gen. Microbiol.* **28**, 333.

Bordet, J. & Gengou, O. (1906). Le microbe de la coqueluche. *Annls Inst. Pasteur, Paris*, **20**, 731.

Borman, E. K., Stuart, C. A. & Wheeler, K. M. (1944). Taxonomy of the family Enterobacteriaceae. *J. Bact.* **48**, 351.

Boswell, P. A., Batstone, G. F. & Mitchell, R. G. (1972). The oxidase reaction in the classification of the Micrococcaceae. *J. med. Microbiol.* **5**, 267.

Bouley, G. (1965). Épreuve de C.A.M.P. et distinction rapide entre *Pasteurella multocida* et *Pasteurella haemolytica*. *Annls Inst. Pasteur, Paris*, **108**, 129.

Bøvre, K., Fiandt, M. & Szybalski, W. (1969). DNA base composition of *Neisseria*, *Moraxella*, and *Acinetobacter*, as determined by measurement of buoyant density in CsCl gradients. *Can. J. Microbiol.* **15**, 335.

Bøvre, K. & Henriksen, S. D. (1967a). A new *Moraxella* species, *Moraxella osloensis*, and a revised description of *Moraxella nonliquefaciens*. *Int. J. syst. Bact.* **17**, 127.

Bøvre, K. & Henriksen, S. D. (1967b). A revised description of *Moraxella polymorpha* Flamm 1957, with a proposal of a new name, *Moraxella phenylpyrouvica* for the species. *Int. J. syst. Bact.* **17**, 343.

Bøvre, K. & Holten, E. (1970). *Neisseria elongata* sp. nov., a rod-shaped member of the genus *Neisseria*. Re-evaluation of cell shape as a criterion in classification. *J. gen. Microbiol.* **60**, 67.

Bøvre, K. & Tønjum, A. M. (1963). Non-pigmented *Serratia marcescens* var. *kielensis* [sic] as a probable cause of bronchopneumonia. *Acta path. microbiol. scand.* **58**, 251.

Bowen, M. K., Thiele, L. C., Stearman, B. D. & Schaub, I. G. (1957). The optochin sensitivity test: a reliable method for identification of pneumococci. *J. Lab. clin. Med.* **49**, 641.

Bowers, E. F. & Jeffries, L. R. (1955). Optochin in the identification of *Str. pneumoniae*. *J. clin. Path.* **8**, 58.

Boyce, J. M. H., Frazer, J. & Zinnemann, K. (1969). The growth requirements of *Haemophilus aphrophilus*. *J. med. Microbiol.* **2**, 55.

Boyd, J. S. K. (1938). The antigenic structure of the mannitol-fermenting dysentery bacilli. *J. Hyg., Camb.* **38**, 477.

Branham, S. E. (1930). A new meningococcus-like organism (*Neisseria flavescens*, n. sp.) from epidemic meningitis. *Publ. Hlth Rep., Wash.* **45**, 845.

Bray, J. (1945). A method of suppressing Proteus and coliform bacteria on routine blood agar plates. *J. Path. Bact.* **57**, 395.

Breed, R. S. (1952). The type species of the genus *Micrococcus. Int. Bull. bact. Nomencl. Taxon.* **2**, 85.

Brenner, D. J. (1973). Deoxyribonucleic acid reassociation in the taxonomy of enteric bacteria. *Int. J. syst. Bact.* **23**, 298.

Brenner, D. J., Fanning, G. R., Miklos, G. V. & Steigerwalt, A. G. (1973). Polynucleotide sequence relatedness among *Shigella* species. *Int. J. syst. Bact.* **23**, 1.

Brenner, D. J., Steigerwalt, A. G. & Fanning, G. R. (1972). Differentiation of *Enterobacter aerogenes* from klebsiellae by deoxyribonucleic acid reassociation. *Int. J. syst. Bact.* **22**, 193.

Brewer, J. H. (1940). Clear liquid mediums for the 'aerobic' cultivation of anaerobes. *J. Am. med. Ass.* **115**, 598.

Bridson, E. Y. & Brecker, A. (1970). Design and formulation of microbial culture media. In *Methods in Microbiology*, vol. 3A, p. 229. Edited by J. R. Norris & D. W. Ribbons. London: Academic Press.

Briggs, M. (1953a). An improved medium for lactobacilli. *J. Dairy Res.* **20**, 36.

Briggs, M. (1953b). The classification of lactobacilli by means of physiological tests. *J. gen. Microbiol.* **9**, 234.

Brindle, C. S. & Cowan, S. T. (1951). Flagellation and taxonomy of Whitmore's bacillus. *J. Path. Bact.* **63**, 571.

Brisou, J. (1953). Essai sur la systématique du genre *Achromobacter. Annls Inst. Pasteur, Paris*, **84**, 812.

Brisou, J. & Morichau-Beauchant, R. (1952). Identité biochimique entre certaines souches de *B. anitratum* et *Moraxella lwoffi. Annls Inst. Pasteur, Paris*, **82**, 640.

Brisou, J. & Prévot, A. R. (1954). Étude de systématique bactérienne. X. Révision des espèces réunies dans le genre *Achromobacter. Annls Inst. Pasteur, Paris*, **86**, 722.

Brisou, J., Tysset, C., Rautlin de la Roy, Y. de & Jarriault, J. (1962). Intérêt taxinomique des oxydases et cytochromeoxydases microbiennes. *C. r. Séanc. Soc. Biol., Paris*, **156**, 1904.

British Pharmacopoeia (1963). London: The Pharmaceutical Press.

British Standard (1934). B.S. 541:1934. Determining the Rideal–Walker coefficients of disinfectants. London: British Standards Institution.

British Standard (1952). B.S. 611:1952. Petri dishes. London: British Standards Institution.

British Standard (1959). B.S. 757:1959. Methods of sampling and testing gelatines. London: British Standards Institution.

Brock, T. D. (1961). *Milestones in Microbiology.* London: Prentice-Hall International Inc.

Brooks, M. E. & Epps, H. B. G. (1959). Taxonomic studies of the genus *Clostridium: Clostridium bifermentans* and *C. sordellii. J. gen. Microbiol.* **21**, 144.

Brooks, M. E., Sterne, M. & Warrack, G. H. (1957). A re-assessment of the criteria used for type differentiation of *Clostridium perfringens. J. Path. Bact.* **74**, 185.

Brough, F. K. (1950). A rapid microtechnique for the determination of nitrate reduction by micro-organisms. *J. Bact.* **60**, 365.

Brown, A. E. (1961). A simple and efficient method of filtering agar. *J. med. Lab. Technol.* **18**, 109.

Brown, A. E. & Harris, H. R. (1963). The effect of carbohydrates on the production of staphylococcal pigment. *J. clin. Path.* **16**, 261.

Brown, J. A. (1959). Preparing egg base media for tubercle bacilli in the autoclave. *Am. J. med. Technol.* **25**, 53.

Brown, J. H. (1919). The use of blood agar for the study of streptococci. *Monogr. Rockefeller Inst. med. Res.* no. 9.

Brown, R. L. & Evans, J. B. (1963). Comparative physiology of antibiotic-resistant strains of *Staphylococcus aureus. J. Bact.* **85**, 1409.

Brown, W. R. L. & Ridout, C. W. (1960). An investigation of some sterilization indicators. *Pharm. J.* **184**, 5.

Bryce, D. M. (1956). The design and interpretation of sterility tests. *J. Pharm. Pharmac.* **8**, 561.

Brzin, B. (1964). Studies on the *Corynebacterium acnes. Acta path. microbiol. scand.* **60**, 599.

Brzin, B. (1965). Spheroplasty effect of the temperature of incubation on the cells of *Bacterium antitratum. Acta path. microbiol. scand.* **63**, 404.

Buchanan, B. B. & Pine, L. (1962). Characterization of a propionic acid producing actinomycete, *Actinomyces propionicus*, sp. nov. *J. gen. Microbiol.* **28**, 305.

Buchanan, R. E. (1918). Studies in the nomenclature and classification of the bacteria. V. Subgroups and genera of the Bacteriaceae. *J. Bact.* **3**, 27.

Buchanan, R. E., Cowan, S. T., Wikén, T. & Clark, W. A. (1958). *International Code of Nomenclature of Bacteria and Viruses.* Ames, Iowa: State College Press. Reprinted with corrections 1959: Iowa State University Press.

Buchanan, R. E., Holt, J. G. & Lessel, E. F., Jr (1966). *Index Bergeyana. An Annotated Alphabetic Listing of Names of the Taxa of the Bacteria*. Baltimore: The Williams & Wilkins Co.

Buchanan, R. E., St John-Brooks, R. & Breed, R. S. (1948). International bacteriological code of nomenclature. *J. Bact.* **55**, 287. Reprinted 1949, *J. gen. Microbiol.* 3, 444.

Buissière, J. & Nardon, P. (1968). Microméthode d'identification des bactéries. I. Intérêt de la quantification des caractères biochimiques. *Annls Inst. Pasteur, Paris*, **115**, 218.

Bulloch, W. (1938). *The History of Bacteriology*. London: Oxford University Press.

Bulmash, J. M., Fulton, M. & Jiron, J. (1965). Lactose and sulfide reactions of an aberrant *Salmonella* strain. *J. Bact.* **89**, 259.

Burdon, K. L. & Wende, R. D. (1960). On the differentiation of anthrax bacilli from *Bacillus cereus*. *J. infect. Dis.* **107**, 224.

Burman, N. P. (1955). The standardisation and selection of bile salt and peptone for culture media used in the bacteriological examination of water. *Proc. Soc. Wat. Treat. Exam.* **4**, 10.

Burrows, T. W., Farrell, J. M. F. & Gillett, W. A. (1964). The catalase activities of *Pasteurella pestis* and other bacteria. *Br. J. exp. Path.* **45**, 579.

Buttiaux, R., Osteux, R., Fresnoy, R. & Moriamez, J. (1954). Les propriétés biochimiques caractéristiques du genre *Proteus*. Inclusion souhaitable des *Providencia* dans celui-ci. *Annls Inst. Pasteur, Paris*, **87**, 375.

Cabrera, H. A. & Davis, G. H. (1961). Epidemic meningitis of the newborn caused by flavobacteria. I. Epidemiology and bacteriology. *Am. J. Dis. Child.* **101**, 289.

Cadness-Graves, B., Williams, R., Harper, G. J. & Miles, A. A. (1943). Slide-test for coagulase-positive staphylococci. *Lancet*, i, 736.

Carpenter, K. P. (1961). The relationship of the enterobacterium A 12 (Sachs) to *Shigella boydii* 14. *J. gen. Microbiol.* **26**, 535.

Carpenter, K. P., Cowan, S. T., Lapage, S. P., Lautrop, H., Le Minor, L., Ørskov, F., Ørskov, I., Rohde, R., Sakazaki, R., Sedlák, J., Taylor, J., Thal, E., Floyd, T. M., Mollaret, H. H., Makela, P. H., Seeliger, H., Lachowicz, K., Rauss, K. & van Oye, E. (1970). Request to the Judicial Commission that *Aerobacter* Beijerinck 1900 and *Aerobacter* Hormaeche and Edwards 1958 be declared rejected generic names. *Int. J. syst. Bact.* **20**, 221.

Carpenter, K. P., Hart, J. M., Hatfield, J. & Wicks, G. (1968). Identification of human vibrios and allied organisms. In *Identification Methods for Microbiologists*, part B, p. 9. Edited by B. M. Gibbs & D. A. Shapton. London: Academic Press.

Carpenter, K. P. & Lachowicz, K. (1959). The catalase activity of *Shigella flexneri*. *J. Path. Bact.* **77**, 645.

Carpenter, K. P., Lapage, S. P. & Steel, K. J. (1966). Biochemical identification of Enterobacteriaceae. In *Identification Methods for Microbiologists*, part A, p. 21. Edited by B. M. Gibbs & F. A. Skinner. London: Academic Press.

Carson, F., Kingsley, W. B., Haberman, S. & Race, G. J. (1964). Unclassified mycobacteria contaminating acid-fast stains of tissue sections. *Am. J. clin. Path.* **41**, 561.

Castellani, A. & Chalmers, A. J. (1919). *Manual of Tropical Medicine*, edn 3. London: Baillière, Tindall & Cox.

Catlin, B. W. (1970). Transfer of the organism named *Neisseria catarrhalis* to *Branhamella* gen. nov. *Int. J. syst. Bact.* **20**, 155.

Catsaras, M. & Buttiaux, R. (1963). Au sujet de quelques réactions biochimiques pour l'identification des Enterobacteriaceae. *Annls Inst. Pasteur, Lille*, **14**, 111.

Chapman, G. H. (1946). A single culture medium for selective isolation of plasma-coagulating staphylococci and for improved testing of chromogenesis, plasma coagulation, mannite fermentation, and the Stone reaction. *J. Bact.* **51**, 409.

Chapman, G. H. (1952). A simple method for making multiple tests of a microorganism. *J. Bact.* **63**, 147.

Cheeseman, G. C. & Fuller, R. (1966). A study by high voltage electrophoresis of the amino acid decarboxylases and arginine dihydrolase of bacteria isolated from the alimentary tract of pigs. *J. appl. Bact.* **29**, 596.

Cherry, W. B. & Moody, M. D. (1965). Fluorescent-antibody techniques in diagnostic bacteriology. *Bact. Rev.* **29**, 222.

Chester, F. D. (1901). *A Manual of Determinative Bacteriology*. New York: The Macmillan Co.

Childs, E. & Allen, L. A. (1953). Improved methods for determining the most probable number of *Bacterium coli* and of *Streptococcus faecalis*. *J. Hyg., Camb.* **51**, 468.

Chilton, M. L. & Fulton, M. (1946). A presumptive medium for differentiating paracolon from Salmonella organisms. *J. Lab. clin. Med.* **31**, 824.

Christensen, W. B. (1946). Urea decomposition as a means of differentiating Proteus and paracolon cultures from each other and from Salmonella and Shigella. *J. Bact.* **52**, 461.

Christensen, W. B. (1949). Hydrogen sulfide production

and citrate utilization in the differentiation of the enteric pathogens and the coliform bacteria. *Res. Bull., Weld County Hlth Dept.* **1**, 3.

Christie, R., Atkins, N. E. & Munch-Petersen, E. (1944). A note on a lytic phenomenon shown by group B streptococci. *Aust. J. exp. Biol. med. Sci.* **22**, 197.

Christie, R. & Keogh, E. V. (1940). Physiological and serological characteristics of staphylococci. *J. Path. Bact.* **51**, 189.

Clark, F. E. (1952). The generic classification of the soil corynebacteria. *Int. Bull. bact. Nomencl. Taxon.* **2**, 45.

Clark, W. M. & Lubs, H. A. (1915). The differentiation of bacteria of the colon-aerogenes family by the use of indicators. *J. infect. Dis.* **17**, 160.

Clarke, P. H. (1953*a*). Hydrogen sulphide production by bacteria. *J. gen. Microbiol.* **8**, 397.

Clarke, P. H. (1953*b*). Growth of streptococci in a glucose phenolphthalein broth. *J. gen. Microbiol.* **9**, 350.

Clarke, P. H. & Cowan, S. T. (1952). Biochemical methods for bacteriology. *J. gen. Microbiol.* **6**, 187.

Clarke, P. H. & Steel, K. J. (1966). Rapid and simple biochemical tests for bacterial identification. In *Identification Methods for Microbiologists*, part A, p. 111. Edited by B. M. Gibbs & F. A. Skinner. London: Academic Press.

Clausen, O. G. (1964). The discovery, isolation, and classification of various α-haemolytic micrococci which resemble aerococci. *J. gen. Microbiol.* **35**, 1.

Cobb, R. W. (1963). Cultural characteristics of some corynebacteria of animal origin, with special reference to *C. bovis* and *C. pyogenes*. *J. med. Lab. Technol.* **20**, 199.

Cobb, R. W. (1966). *Corynebacterium bovis*: fermentation of sugars in the presence of serum or Tween 80. *Vet. Rec.* **78**, 33.

Cohen, R. L., Wittler, R. G. & Faber, J. E. (1968). Modified biochemical tests for characterization of L-phase variants of bacteria. *Appl. Microbiol.* **16**, 1655.

Cohn, F. (1872). Untersuchungen über Bacterien. *Beitr. Biol. Pfl.* **1**, Heft 2, 127.

Colbeck, J. C. & Proom, H. (1944). Use of dried rabbit plasma for the staphylococcus coagulase test. *Br. med. J.* ii, 471.

Cole, S. W. & Onslow, H. (1916). On a substitute for peptone and a standard nutrient medium for bacteriological purposes. *Lancet*, ii, 9.

Collee, J. G. & Watt, B. (1972). Perspectives in clinical anaerobic bacteriology – Where do we go from here?

In *Modern Trends in Microbiology*, Symposium 28 September 1972, sponsored by Beckton Dickinson UK Ltd, Wembley.

Collins, C. H. & Massey, M. L. (1963). The laboratory diagnosis of mycobacterial infections. In *Progress in Medical Laboratory Technique*, vol. 2. Edited by F. J. Baker. London: Butterworth & Co.

Colman, G. (1968). The application of computers to the classification of streptococci. *J. gen. Microbiol.* **50**, 149.

Colman, G. (1969). Transformation of viridans-like streptococci. *J. gen. Microbiol.* **57**, 247.

Colman, G. & Williams, R. E. O. (1965). The cell walls of streptococci. *J. gen. Microbiol.* **41**, 375.

Colman, G. [incorrectly spelt Coleman] & Williams, R. E. O. (1967). Classification of nonhaemolytic streptococci. *Int. J. syst. Bact.* **17**, 306.

Colman, G. & Williams, R. E. O. (1972). Taxonomy of some human viridans streptococci. In *Streptococci and Streptococcal Diseases: Recognition, Understanding and Management*, p. 281. Edited by L. W. Wannamaker & J. M. Matsen. New York: Academic Press.

Colwell, R. R. (1970). Polyphasic taxonomy of the genus *Vibrio*: numerical taxonomy of *Vibrio cholerae*, *Vibrio parahaemolyticus*, and related *Vibrio* species. *J. Bact.* **104**, 410.

Conn, H. J. (1930). The identity of *Bacillus subtilis*. *J. infect. Dis.* **46**, 341.

Conn, H. J. (1936). On the detection of nitrate reduction. *J. Bact.* **31**, 225.

Conn, H. J. (1942). Validity of the genus *Alcaligenes*. *J. Bact.* **44**, 353.

Conn, H. J. (1947). A protest against the misuse of the generic name *Corynebacterium*. *J. Bact.* **54**, 10.

Conn, H. J. & Conn, J. E. (1941). Value of pigmentation in classifying actinomycetes: a preliminary note. *J. Bact.* **42**, 791.

Conn, H. J., Darrow, M. A. & Emmel, V. M. (1960). *Staining Procedures used by the Biological Stain Commission*, edn 2. Baltimore: The Williams & Wilkins Co.

Conn, H. J. & Dimmick, I. (1947). Soil bacteria similar in morphology to *Mycobacterium* and *Corynebacterium*. *J. Bact.* **54**, 291.

Conn, H. J., Wolfe, G. E. & Ford, M. (1940). Taxonomic relationships of *Alcaligenes* spp. to certain soil saprophytes and plant parasites. *J. Bact.* **39**, 207.

Conn, H. W. (1900). Classification of dairy bacteria. *Twelfth Ann. Rep. Storrs Agric. Exp. Sta., Storrs, Conn. 1899*, 13.

Conn, H. W., Esten, W. M. & Stocking, W. A. (1907).

A classification of dairy bacteria. *Ann. Rep. Storrs Agric. Exp. Sta., Storrs, Conn. 1906*, 91.

Cook, A. M. & Steel, K. J. (1959*a*). The stability of thioglycollate solutions. Part I. Effects of method of preparation of solutions, pH and temperature upon the oxidation of thioglycollate. *J. Pharm. Pharmac.* **11**, 216.

Cook, A. M. & Steel, K. J. (1959*b*). The stability of thioglycollate solutions. Part II. Miscellaneous factors associated with the oxidation and stability. *J. Pharm. Pharmac.* **11**, 434.

Cook, G. T. (1948). Urease and other biochemical reactions of the Proteus group. *J. Path. Bact.* **60**, 171.

Cook, G. T. (1950). A plate test for nitrate reduction. *J. clin. Path.* **3**, 359.

Cook, G. T. & Jebb, W. H. H. (1952). Starch-fermenting, gelatin-liquefying corynebacteria and their differentiation from *C. diphtheriae gravis*. *J. clin. Path.* **5**, 161.

Corlett, D. A., Jr, Lee, J. S. & Sinnhuber, R. O. (1965). Application of replica plating and computer analysis for rapid identification of bacteria in some foods. Identification scheme. *Appl. Microbiol.* **13**, 808.

Corper, H. J. (1928). The certified diagnosis of tuberculosis. Practical evaluation of a new method for cultivating tubercle bacilli for diagnostic purposes. *J. Am. med. Ass.* **91**, 371.

Coster, E. & White, H. R. (1964). Further studies of the genus *Pediococcus*. *J. gen. Microbiol.* **37**, 15.

Costin, I. D. (1965). Biochemical differentiation of *Salmonella gallinarum* and *Salmonella pullorum* cultures. *Path. Microbiol.* **28**, 303.

Cowan, S. T. (1938*a*). Unusual infections following cerebral operations. With a description of *Diplococcus mucosus* (von Lingelsheim). *Lancet*, ii, 1052.

Cowan, S. T. (1938*b*). The classification of staphylococci by precipitation and biological reactions. *J. Path. Bact.* **46**, 31.

Cowan, S. T. (1939). Classification of staphylococci by slide agglutination. *J. Path. Bact.* **48**, 169.

Cowan, S. T. (1956*a*). 'Ordnung in das Chaos' Migula. *Can. J. Microbiol.* **2**, 212.

Cowan, S. T. (1956*b*). Taxonomic rank of Enterobacteriaceae 'groups'. *J. gen. Microbiol.* **15**, 345.

Cowan, S. T. (1962*a*). The microbial species – a macromyth? *Symp. Soc. gen. Microbiol.* **12**, 433.

Cowan, S. T. (1962*b*). An introduction to chaos, or the classification of micrococci and staphylococci. *J. appl. Bact.* **25**, 324.

Cowan, S. T. (1965*a*). Principles and practice of bacterial taxonomy – a forward look. *J. gen. Microbiol.* **39**, 143.

Cowan, S. T. (1965*b*). Development of coding schemes for microbial taxonomy. *Adv. appl. Microbiol.* **7**, 139.

Cowan, S. T. (1968*a*). *A Dictionary of Microbial Taxonomic Usage*. Edinburgh: Oliver & Boyd.

Cowan, S. T. (1968*b*). An assessment of the value of biochemical and serological techniques in microbial taxonomy. In *Chemotaxonomy and Serotaxonomy*, p. 269. Edited by J. G. Hawkes. London: Academic Press.

Cowan, S. T. (1970*a*). Heretical taxonomy for bacteriologists. *J. gen. Microbiol.* **61**, 145.

Cowan, S. T. (1970*b*). Are some characters more equal than others? *Int. J. syst. Bact.* **20**, 541.

Cowan, S. T. (1971). Sense and nonsense in bacterial taxonomy. *J. gen. Microbiol.* **67**, 1.

Cowan, S. T. & Steel, K. J. (1960). A device for the identification of microorganisms. *Lancet*, i, 1172.

Cowan, S. T. & Steel, K. J. (1961). Diagnostic tables for the common medical bacteria. *J. Hyg., Camb.* **59**, 357.

Cowan, S. T. & Steel, K. J. (1964). Comparison of differentiating criteria for staphylococci and micrococci. *J. Bact.* **88**, 804.

Cowan, S. T., Steel, K. J., Shaw, C. & Duguid, J. P. (1960). A classification of the Klebsiella group. *J. gen. Microbiol.* **23**, 601.

Craigie, J. (1931). Studies on the serological reactions of the flagella of *B. typhosus*. *J. immun.* **21**, 417.

Cross, T. (1970). The diversity of bacterial spores. *J. appl. Bact.* **33**, 95.

Cruickshank, J. C. (1935). A study of the so-called *Bacterium typhi flavum*. *J. Hyg., Camb.* **35**, 354.

Cruickshank, R. (1937). Staphylocoagulase. *J. Path. Bact.* **45**, 295.

Cummins, C. S. (1962). Chemical composition and antigenic structure of cell walls of *Corynebacterium*, *Mycobacterium*, *Nocardia*, *Actinomyces* and *Arthrobacter*. *J. gen. Microbiol.* **28**, 35.

Cummins, C. S. (1970). Cell wall composition in the classification of Gram positive anaerobes. *Int. J. syst. Bact.* **20**, 413.

Cummins, C. S. (1971). Catalase activity in *Corynebacterium pyogenes*. *Can. J. Microbiol.* **17**, 1001.

Cummins, C. S. & Harris, H. (1956). The chemical composition of the cell wall in some Gram-positive bacteria and its possible value as a taxonomic character. *J. gen. Microbiol.* **14**, 583.

Cummins, C. S. & Harris, H. (1958). Studies on the cell-wall composition and taxonomy of Actinomycetales and related groups. *J. gen. Microbiol.* **18**, 173.

Cummins, C. S. & Johnson, J. L. (1974). *Corynebacterium parvum*: a synonym for *Propionibacterium acnes*? *J. gen. Microbiol.* **80**, 433.

Cunliffe, A. C., Gillam, G. G. & Williams, R. (1943). Bacterial endocarditis associated with a coagulase-negative *Staphylococcus albus*. *Lancet*, ii, 355.

Cure, G. L. & Keddie, R. M. (1973). Methods for the morphological examination of aerobic coryneform bacteria. In *Sampling – Microbiological Monitoring of Environments*, p. 123. Edited by R. G. Board & D. W. Lovelock. London: Academic Press.

Dacre, J. C. & Sharpe, M. E. (1956). Catalase production by lactobacilli. *Nature, Lond.* **178**, 700.

Darmady, E. M., Hughes, K. E. A. & Jones, J. D. (1958). Thermal death-time of spores in dry heat in relation to sterilisation of instruments and syringes. *Lancet*, ii, 766.

Daubner, I. (1962). Die Reduktion der Nitrate durch Bakterien der Familie Enterobacteriaceae. *Arch. Hyg. Bakt.* **146**, 147.

Davis, D. H., Doudoroff, M., Stanier, R. Y. & Mandel, M. (1969). Proposal to reject the genus *Hydrogenomonas*: taxonomic implications. *Int. J. syst. Bact.* **19**, 375.

Davis, G. H. G. (1955). The classification of lactobacilli from the human mouth. *J. gen. Microbiol.* **13**, 481.

Davis, G. H. G. (1960). Lactobacilli of the human mouth. *J. appl. Bact.* **22**, 350.

Davis, G. H. G., Fomin, L., Wilson, E. & Newton, K. G. (1969). Numerical taxonomy of *Listeria*, streptococci and possibly related bacteria. *J. gen. Microbiol.* **57**, 333.

Davis, G. H. G. & Hoyling, B. (1973). Use of a rapid acetoin test in the identification of staphylococci and micrococci. *Int. J. syst. Bact.* **23**, 281.

Davis, G. H. G. & Newton, K. G. (1969). Numerical taxonomy of some named coryneform bacteria. *J. gen. Microbiol.* **56**, 195.

Davis, G. H. G. & Park, R. W. A. (1962). A taxonomic study of certain bacteria currently classified as *Vibrio* species. *J. gen. Microbiol.* **27**, 101.

Davis, J. G. (1939). A rapid, simple and reproducible method for the determination of bacterial sugar fermentations. *Zentbl. Bakt. ParasitKde Abt. II*, **101**, 97.

Davis, J. G. (1960). The lactobacilli – I. *Prog. industr. Microbiol.* **2**, 1.

Davis, J. G. & Rogers, H. J. (1939). The effect of sterilization upon sugars. *Zentbl. Bakt. ParasitKde Abt II*, **101**, 102.

Dawson, B., Farnworth, E. H., McLeod, J. W. & Nicholson, D. E. (1951). Observations on the value

of Bordet–Gengou medium for the cultivation of *Haemophilus pertussis*. *J. gen. Microbiol.* **5**, 408.

De, S. N., Bhattacharyya, K. & Roychandhury, P. K. (1954). The haemolytic activities of *Vibrio cholerae* and related vibrios. *J. Path. Bact.* **67**, 117.

De Bord, G. G. (1939). Organisms invalidating the diagnosis of gonorrhoea by the smear method. *J. Bact.* **38**, 119.

De Bord, G. G. (1942). Descriptions of Mimeae Trib. nov. with three genera and three species and two new species of Neisseria from conjunctivitis and vaginitis. *Iowa St. Coll. J. Sci.* **16**, 471.

De Bord, G. G. (1943). Species of the tribes Mimeae, Neisseriae, and Streptococceae which confuse the diagnosis of gonorrhoea by smears. *J. Lab. clin. Med.* **28**, 710.

De Bord, G. G. (1948). *Mima polymorpha* meningitis. *J. Bact.* **55**, 764.

Deibel, R. H., Lake, D. E. & Niven, C. F., Jr (1963). Physiology of the enterococci as related to their taxonomy. *J. Bact.* **86**, 1275.

Deibel, R. H. & Niven, C. F., Jr (1960). Comparative study of *Gaffkya homari*, *Aerococcus viridans*, tetrad-forming cocci from meat curing brines, and the genus *Pediococcus*. *J. Bact.* **79**, 175.

Deibel, R. H., Yao, J., Jacobs, N. J. & Niven, C. F., Jr (1964). Group E streptococci. I. Physiological characterization of strains isolated from swine cervical abscesses. *J. infect. Dis.* **114**, 327.

De Ley, J. (1968). DNA base composition and taxonomy of some *Acinetobacter* strains. *Antonie van Leeuwenhoek*, **34**, 109.

De Waart, J., Mossel, D. A. A., ten Broeke, R. & van de Moosdijk, A. (1968). Enumeration of *Staphylococcus aureus* in foods with special reference to egg-yolk reaction and mannitol negative mutants. *J. appl. Bact.* **31**, 276.

Difco Manual of Dehydrated Culture Media and Reagents for Microbiological and Clinical Laboratory Procedures (1953). Anonymous, edn 9. Detroit: Difco Laboratories Inc.

Dighero, M. W., Bradstreet, C. M. P. & Andrews, B. E. (1970). Dried paper discs for serological identification of human mycoplasmas. *J. appl. Bact.* **33**, 750.

Doetsch, R. N. & Pelczar, M. J., Jr (1948). The microbacteria. I. Morphological and physiological characteristics. *J. Bact.* **56**, 37.

Douglas, H. C. & Gunter, S. E. (1946). The taxonomic position of *Corynebacterium acnes*. *J. Bact.* **52**, 15.

Douglas, S. R. (1922). A new medium for the isolation of *B. diphtheriae*. *Br. J. exp. Path.* **3**, 263.

Downie, A. W. (1937). A comparison of the value of

heat-killed vaccines and toxoid as immunising agents against experimental staphylococcal infection in the rabbit. *J. Path. Bact.* **44**, 573.

Downie, A. W., Stent, L. & White, S. M. (1931). The bile solubility of pneumococcus, with special reference to the chemical structure of various bile salts. *Br. J. exp. Path.* **12**, 1.

Downie, A. W., Wade, E. & Young, J. A. (1933). An organism resembling the Newcastle type of dysentery bacillus associated with cases of dysentery. *J. Hyg., Camb.* **33**, 196.

Drea, W. F. (1942). Growth of small numbers of tubercle bacilli, H 37, in Long's liquid synthetic medium and some interfering factors. *J. Bact.* **44**, 149.

Drucker, D. B. & Melville, T. H. (1969). Computer classification of streptococci, mostly of oral origin. *Nature, Lond.* **221**, 664.

Duguid, J. P. (1951). The demonstration of bacterial capsules and slime. *J. Path. Bact.* **63**, 673.

Dunkelberg, W. E., Jr & McVeigh, I. (1969). Growth requirements of *Haemophilus vaginalis*. *Antonie van Leeuwenhoek*, **35**, 129.

Durham, H. E. (1898). A simple method for demonstrating the production of gas by bacteria. *Br. med. J.* i, 1387.

Durlakowa, I., Lachowicz, Z. & Ślopek, S. (1967). Biochemical properties of *Klebsiella* bacilli. *Arch. Immun. Ther. exp.* **15**, 490.

Dybowski, W. & Franklin, D. A. (1968). Conditional probability and the identification of bacteria: a pilot study. *J. gen. Microbiol.* **54**, 215.

Eddy, B. P. (1960). Cephalotrichous, fermentative Gram-negative bacteria: the genus *Aeromonas*. *J. appl. Bact.* **23**, 216.

Eddy, B. P. (1961). The Voges–Proskauer reaction and its significance: a review. *J. appl. Bact.* **24**, 27.

Eddy, B. P. (1962). Further studies on *Aeromonas*. I. Additional strains and supplementary biochemical tests. *J. appl. Bact.* **25**, 137.

Eddy, B. P. & Carpenter, K. P. (1964). Further studies on Aeromonas. II. Taxonomy of Aeromonas and C 27 strains. *J. appl. Bact.* **27**, 96.

Edward, D. G. ff. & Freundt, E. A. (1967). Proposal for Mollicutes as name of the class established for the order Mycoplasmatales. *Int. J. syst. Bact.* **17**, 267.

Edward, D. G. ff. & Freundt, E. A. (1970). Amended nomenclature for strains related to *Mycoplasma laidlawii*. *J. gen. Microbiol.* **62**, 1.

Edwards, P. R. & Bruner, D. W. (1942). Serological identification of salmonella cultures. *Circ. Ky agric. Exp. Sta.* no. 54.

Edwards, P. R. & Ewing, W. H. (1962, 1972). *Identifica-tion of Enterobacteriaceae*, edn 2, 1962; edn 3, 1972. Minneapolis: Burgess Publishing Co.

Edwards, P. R. & Kauffmann, F. (1952). A simplification of the Kauffmann–White schema. *Am. J. clin. Path.* **22**, 692.

Eiken, M. (1958). Studies on an anaerobic, rod-shaped, Gram-negative microorganism: *Bacteroides corrodens* n. sp. *Acta path. microbiol. scand.* **43**, 404.

Eisenberg, R. C. & Evans, J. B. (1963). Energy and nitrogen requirements of *Micrococcus roseus*. *Can. J. Microbiol.* **9**, 633.

Elek, S. D. (1948). Rapid identification of Proteus. *J. Path. Bact.* **60**, 183.

Elek, S. D. & Levy, E. (1954). The nature of discrepancies between haemolysins in culture filtrates and plate haemolysin patterns of staphylococci. *J. Path. Bact.* **68**, 31.

Elliott, S. D. (1945). A proteolytic enzyme produced by group A streptococci with special reference to its effect on the type-specific M antigen. *J. exp. Med.* **81**, 573.

Ellis, G. (1971). *Units, Symbols and Abbreviations. A Guide for Biological and Medical Editors and Authors.* London: Royal Society of Medicine.

Elrod, R. P. (1942). The erwinia–coliform relationship. *J. Bact.* **44**, 433.

Elston, H. R. (1961). *Kurthia bessonii* isolated from clinical material. *J. Path. Bact.* **81**, 245.

Elston, H. R. & Fitch, D. M. (1964). Determination of potential pathogenicity of staphylococci. *Am. J. clin. Path.* **42**, 346.

Eltinge, E. T. (1956). Nitrate reduction in the genus *Chromobacterium*. *Antonie van Leeuwenhoek*, **22**, 139.

Eltinge, E. T. (1957). Status of the genus *Chromobacterium*. *Int. Bull. bact. Nomencl. Taxon.* **7**, 37.

Engbaek, H. C., Runyon, E. H. & Karlson, A. G. (1971). *Mycobacterium avium* Chester. Designation of the neotype strain. *Int. J. syst. Bact.* **21**, 192.

Evans, J. B., Bradford, W. L., Jr & Niven, C. F., Jr (1955). Comments concerning the taxonomy of the genera *Micrococcus* and *Staphylococcus*. *Int. Bull. bact. Nomencl. Taxon.* **5**, 61.

Evans, J. B., Buettner, L. G. & Niven, C. F., Jr (1952). Occurrence of streptococci that give a false-positive coagulase test. *J. Bact.* **64**, 433.

Evans, J. B. & Kloos, W. E. (1972). Use of shake cultures in a semisolid thioglycolate medium for differentiating staphylococci from micrococci. *Appl. Microbiol.* **23**, 326.

Evans, J. B. & Schultes, L. M. (1969). DNA base composition and physiological characteristics of the genus *Aerococcus*. *Int. J. syst. Bact.* **19**, 159.

Eveland, W. C. & Faber, J. E., Jr (1953). Antigenic studies of a group of paracolon bacteria (32011 group). *J. infect. Dis.* **93**, 226.

Ewing, W. H. (1949*a*). The relationship of *Bacterium anitratum* and members of the tribe Mimeae (de Bord). *J. Bact.* **57**, 659.

Ewing, W. H. (1949*b*). The relationship of *Shigella dispar* to certain coliform bacteria. *J. Bact.* **58**, 497.

Ewing, W. H. (1953). Serological relationships between shigella and coliform cultures. *J. Bact.* **66**, 333.

Ewing, W. H. (1962). The tribe Proteeae: its nomenclature and taxonomy. *Int. Bull. bact. Nomencl. Taxon.* **12**, 93.

Ewing, W. H. (1963). An outline of nomenclature for the family Enterobacteriaceae. *Int. Bull. bact. Nomencl. Taxon.* **13**, 95.

Ewing, W. H. & Ball, M. M. (1966). *The Biochemical Reactions of Members of the Genus Salmonella.* Atlanta, Georgia: National Communicable Disease Center.

Ewing, W. H. & Davis, B. R. (1971). *Biochemical Characterization of Citrobacter freundii and Citrobacter diversus.* Atlanta, Georgia: Center for Disease Control, Laboratory Division.

Ewing, W. H. & Davis, B. R. (1972*a*). Biochemical characterization of *Citrobacter diversus* (Burkey) Werkman and Gillen and designation of the neotype strain. *Int. J. syst. Bact.* **22**, 12.

Ewing, W. H. & Davis, B. R. (1972*b*). Biochemical characterization of *Serratia marcescens.* *Publ. Hlth Lab.* **30**, 211.

Ewing, W. H., Davis, B. R. & Fife, M. A. (1972). *Biochemical Characterization of Serratia liquefaciens and Serratia rubidaea.* Atlanta, Georgia: Center for Disease Control, Laboratory Division.

Ewing, W. H., Davis, B. R. & Martin, W. J. (1972). *Biochemical Characterization of Escherichia coli.* Atlanta, Georgia: Center for Disease Control, Laboratory Division.

Ewing, W. H., Davis, B. R. & Reavis, R. W. (1957). Phenylalanine and malonate media and their use in enteric bacteriology. *Publ. Hlth Lab.* **15**, 153.

Ewing, W. H. & Fife, M. A. (1972). *Enterobacter agglomerans* (Beijerinck) comb. nov. (the herbicola–lathyri bacteria). *Int. J. syst. Bact.* **22**, 4.

Ewing, W. H., Hugh, R. & Johnson, J. G. (1961). *Studies on the Aeromonas group.* Atlanta, Georgia: Communicable Disease Center.

Ewing, W. H., Jaugstetter, J. E., Martin, W. J., Sikes, J. V. & Wathen, H. G. (1971). *Biochemical Reactions of Shigella.* Atlanta, Georgia: Center for Disease Control, Laboratory Division.

Ewing, W. H. & Johnson, J. G. (1960). The differentiation of *Aeromonas* and C 27 cultures from Enterobacteriaceae. *Int. Bull. bact. Nomencl. Taxon.* **10**, 223.

Ewing, W. H., McWhorter, A. C., Escobar, M. R. & Lubin, A. H. (1965). *Edwardsiella*, a new genus of Enterobacteriaceae based on a new species, *E. tarda*. *Int. Bull. bact. Nomencl. Taxon.* **15**, 33.

Extra Pharmacopoeia (Martindale) (1955). Vol. II, edn 23. London: The Pharmaceutical Press.

Falkow, S. (1958). Activity of lysine decarboxylase as an aid in the identification of salmonellae and shigellae. *Am. J. clin. Path.* **29**, 598.

Fallon, R. J. (1973). The relationship between the biotype of Klebsiella species and their pathogenicity. *J. clin. Path.* **26**, 523.

Farmer, J. J., III & Herman, L. G. (1969). Epidemiological fingerprinting of *Pseudomonas aeruginosa* by the production of and sensitivity to pyocin and bacteriophage. *Appl. Microbiol.* **18**, 760.

Feeley, J. C. (1965). Classification of *Vibrio cholerae* (*Vibrio comma*), including el Tor vibrios, by infrasubspecific characteristics. *J. Bact.* **89**, 665.

Feeley, J. C. & Pittman, M. (1963). Studies on the haemolytic activity of El Tor vibrios. *Bull. Wld Hlth Org.* **28**, 347.

Felton, E. A., Evans, J. B. & Niven, C. F., Jr (1953). Production of catalase by pediococci. *J. Bact.* **65**, 481.

Ferguson, W. W. & Henderson, N. D. (1947). Description of strain C 27: a motile organism with the major antigen of *Shigella sonnei* phase I. *J. Bact.* **54**, 179.

Ferguson, W. W. & Hook, A. E. (1943). Urease activity of Proteus and Salmonella organisms. *J. Lab. clin. Med.* **28**, 1715.

Fey, H. (1959). Differenzierungsschema für gram-negative aerobe Stäbchen. *Schweiz. Z. allg. Path. Bakt.* **22**, 641.

Fife, M. A., Ewing, W. H & Davis, B. R. (1965). *The Biochemical Reactions of the Tribe Klebsielleae.* Atlanta, Georgia: National Communicable Disease Center, Laboratory Branch.

Fildes, P. (1920). A new medium for the growth of *B. influenzae*. *Br. J. exp. Path.* **1**, 129.

Fishbein, M., Mehlman, I. J. & Pitcher, J. (1970). Isolation of *Vibrio parahaemolyticus* from the processed meat of Chesapeake Bay blue crab. *Appl. Microbiol.* **20**, 176.

Fisk, R. T. (1942). Studies on staphylococci: II. Identification of *Staphylococcus aureus* strains by means of bacteriophage. *J. infect. Dis.* **71**, 161.

Fleming, A. (1922). On a remarkable bacteriolytic element found in tissues and secretions. *Proc. R. Soc.* B. **93**, 306.

Floch, H. (1953). Etude comparative des genres *Moraxella, Achromobacter* et *Alcaligenes. Annls Inst. Pasteur, Paris*, **85**, 675.

Floodgate, G. D. [printed C. D.] (1962). Some comments on the Adansonian taxonomic method. *Int. Bull. bact. Nomencl. Taxon.* **12**, 171.

Focht, D. D. & Lockhart, W. R. (1965). Numerical survey of some bacterial taxa. *J. Bact.* **90**, 1314.

Ford, W. W. (1916). Studies on aerobic spore-bearing non-pathogenic bacteria. Part II. Classification. *J. Bact.* **1**, 527.

Forsdike, J. L. (1950). A comparative study of agars from various geographical sources. *J. Pharm. Pharmac.* **2**, 796.

Foster, A. R. & Cohn, C. (1945). A method for the rapid preparation of Loffler's and Petroff's media. *J. Bact.* **50**, 561.

Foster, W. D. & Bragg, J. (1962). Biochemical classification of Klebsiella correlated with the severity of the associated disease. *J. clin. Path.* **15**, 478.

Fraser, G. (1961). Haemolytic activity of *Corynebacterium ovis. Nature, Lond.* **189**, 246.

Frazer, J., Zinnemann, K. & Boyce, J. M. H. (1969). The effect of different environmental conditions on some characters of *Haemophilus paraphrophilus. J. med. Microbiol.* **2**, 563.

Frazier, W. C. (1926). A method for the detection of changes in gelatin due to bacteria. *J. infect. Dis.* **39**, 302.

Frederiksen, W. (1964). A study of some Yersinia pseudotuberculosis-like bacteria ('Bacterium enterocoliticum' and 'Pasteurella X'). *Proc. XIV Scand. Congr. Path. Microbiol.* 1964, 103.

Frederiksen, W. (1970). *Citrobacter koseri* (n. sp.) a new species within the genus *Citrobacter*, with a comment on the taxonomic position of *Citrobacter intermedium* (Werkman and Gillen). *Publ. Fac. Sci. J. E. Purkyne, Brno*, **47**, 89.

Frederiksen, W. (1971). A taxonomic study of *Pasteurella* and *Actinobacillus* strains. *J. gen. Microbiol.* **69**, viii.

Frost, A. J. (1967). Phage typing of *Staphylococcus aureus* from dairy cattle in Australia. *J. Hyg., Camb.* **65**, 311.

Fuller, A. T. (1938). The formamide method for the extraction of polysaccharides from haemolytic streptococci. *Br. J. exp. Path.* **19**, 130.

Fuller, A. T. & Maxted, W. R. (1939). The production of haemolysins and peroxide by haemolytic streptococci in relation to the non-haemolytic variants of group A. *J. Path. Bact.* **49**, 83.

Fulton, M. (1943). The identity of *Bacterium columbensis* Castellani. *J. Bact.* **46**, 79.

Fulton, M., Halkias, D. & Yarashus, D. A. (1960). Voges–Proskauer test using ɪ-naphthol purified by steam distillation. *Appl. Microbiol.* **8**, 361.

Gaby, W. L. & Hadley, C. (1957). Practical laboratory test for the identification of *Pseudomonas aeruginosa. J. Bact.* **74**, 356.

Gagnon, M., Hunting, W. M. & Esselen, W. B. (1959). New method for catalase determination. *Analyt. Chem.* **31**, 144.

Gardner, A. D. & Venkatraman, K. V. (1935). The antigens of the cholera group of vibrios. *J. Hyg., Camb.* **35**, 262.

Garvie, E. I. (1960). The genus *Leuconostoc* and its nomenclature. *J. Dairy Res.* **27**, 283.

Gasser, F. (1970). Electrophoretic characterization of lactic dehydrogenases in the genus *Lactobacillus. J. gen. Microbiol.* **62**, 223.

Gasser, F., Mandel, M. & Rogosa, M. (1970). *Lactobacillus jensenii* sp. nov., a new representative of the subgenus *Thermobacterium. J. gen. Microbiol.* **62**, 219.

Gaughran, E. R. L. (1969). From superstition to science: the history of a bacterium. *Trans. N.Y. Acad. Sci.* **31**, 3.

Gekker, V. D., Ravitch-Birger, E. D. & Belaya, J. A. (1965). The position of Newcastle bacteria in the classification of the shigellae. *Int. Bull. bact. Nomencl. Taxon.* **15**, 133.

Gemmel, M. & Hodgkiss, W. (1964). The physiological characters and flagellar arrangement of motile homofermentative lactobacilli. *J. gen. Microbiol.* **35**, 519.

Georg, L. K. & Brown, J. M. (1967). *Rothia*, gen. nov. an aerobic genus of the family *Actinomycetaceae. Int. J. syst. Bact.* **17**, 79.

Georg, L. K., Robertstad, G. W., Brinkman, S. A. & Hicklin, M. D. (1965). A new pathogenic anaerobic *Actinomyces* species. *J. infect. Dis.* **115**, 88.

Georgala, D. L. & Boothroyd, M. (1965). A system for detecting salmonellae in meat and meat products. *J. appl. Bact.* **28**, 206.

Georgala, D. L. & Boothroyd, M. (1968). Immunofluorescence – a useful technique for microbial identification. In *Identification Methods for Microbiologists*, part B, p. 187. Edited by B. M. Gibbs & D. A. Shapton. London: Academic Press.

Gerencser, M. A. & Slack, J. M. (1967). Isolation and characterization of *Actinomyces propionicus. J. Bact.* **94**, 109.

Gershman, M. (1961). Use of a tetrazolium salt for an easily discernible KCN reaction. *Can. J. Microbiol.* **7**, 286.

Gibbons, N. E. (1972). *Listeria* Pirie – whom does it honor? *Int. J. syst. Bact.* **22**, 1.

Gibson, T. (1944). A study of *Bacillus subtilis* and related organisms. *J. Dairy Res.* **13**, 248.

Gibson, T. & Abd-el-Malek, Y. (1945). The formation of carbon dioxide by lactic acid bacteria and *Bacillus licheniformis* and a cultural method of detecting the process. *J. Dairy Res.* **14**, 35.

Gilardi, G. L. (1969). Characterization of the oxidase-negative, Gram-negative coccobacilli (the *Achromobacter–Acinetobacter* group). *Antonie van Leeuwenhoek* **35**, 421.

Gilardi, G. L. (1970). Characterization of EO-1 strains (*Pseudomonas kingii*) isolated from clinical specimens and the hospital environment. *Appl. Microbiol.* **20**, 521.

Gilardi, G. L. (1971*a*). Characterization of non-fermentative nonfastidious Gram negative bacteria encountered in medical bacteriology. *J. appl. Bact.* **34**, 623.

Gilardi, G. L. (1971*b*). Characterization of *Pseudomonas* species isolated from clinical specimens. *Appl. Microbiol.* **21**, 414.

Gilardi, G. L. (1971*c*). Antimicrobial susceptibility as a diagnostic aid in the identification of nonfermenting Gram-negative bacteria. *Appl. Microbiol.* **22**, 821.

Gilardi, G. L. (1972*a*). Practical schema for the identification of nonfermentative Gram negative bacteria encountered in medical bacteriology. *Am. J. med. Technol.* **38**, 65.

Gilardi, G. L. (1972*b*). Infrequently encountered *Pseudomonas* species causing infection in humans. *Ann. intern. Med.* **77**, 211.

Gilardi, G. L., Bottone, E. & Birnbaum, M. (1970*a*). Unusual fermentative, Gram-negative bacilli isolated from clinical specimens. I. Characterization of *Erwinia* strains of the 'lathyri–herbicola group'. *Appl. Microbiol.* **20**, 151.

Gilardi, G. L., Bottone, E. & Birnbaum, M. (1970*b*). Unusual fermentative, Gram-negative bacilli isolated from clinical specimens. II. Characterization of *Aeromonas* species. *Appl. Microbiol.* **20**, 156.

Gilardi, G. L. & Hirschl, S. (1969). Morphological and biochemical characterization of *Alcaligenes odorans* var. *viridans*. *Int. J. syst. Bact.* **19**, 167.

Gilbert, R. & Stewart, F. C. (1926–7). *Corynebacterium ulcerans*: a pathogenic microorganism resembling *C. diphtheriae*. *J. Lab. clin. Med.* **12**, 756.

Gillespie, E. H. (1943). The routine use of the coagulase test for staphylococci. *Mon. Bull. Emerg. publ. Hlth Lab. Serv.* **2**, 19.

Gillespie, E. H. (1948). Chloral hydrate plates for the inhibition of swarming of proteus. *J. clin. Path.* **1**, 99.

Gillies, R. R. (1956). An evaluation of two composite media for preliminary identification of Shigella and Salmonella. *J. clin. Path.* **9**, 368.

Gnezda, J. (1899). Sur des réactions nouvelles des bases indoliques et des corps albuminoides. *C. r. hebd. Séanc. Acad. Sci., Paris*, **128**, 1584.

Goldin, M. & Glenn, A. (1962). A simple phenylalanine paper strip method for identification of *Proteus* strains. *J. Bact.* **84**, 870.

Goldsworthy, N. E. & Still, J. L. (1936). The effect of meat extract and other substances upon pigment production. *J. Path. Bact.* **43**, 555.

Goldsworthy, N. E. & Still, J. L. (1938). The effect of various meat extracts on pigment production by *B. prodigiosus*. *J. Path. Bact.* **46**, 634.

Goldsworthy, N. E., Still, J. L. & Dumaresq, J. A. (1938). Some sources of error in the interpretation of fermentation reactions, with special reference to the effects of serum enzymes. *J. Path. Bact.* **46**, 253.

Gooder, H. (1970). Cell wall composition in the classification of streptococci. *Int. J. syst. Bact.* **20**, 475.

Goodfellow, M. (1971). Numerical taxonomy of some nocardioform bacteria. *J. gen. Microbiol.* **69**, 33.

Goodfellow, M., Fleming, A. & Sakin, M. J. (1972). Numerical classification of '*Mycobacterium*' rhodochrous and Runyon's group IV mycobacteria. *Int. J. syst. Bact.* **22**, 81.

Gordon, J. & McLeod, J. W. (1928). The practical application of the direct oxidase reaction in bacteriology. *J. Path. Bact.* **31**, 185.

Gordon, R. E. (1966*a*). Some strains in search of a genus – *Corynebacterium, Mycobacterium, Nocardia* or what? *J. gen. Microbiol.* **43**, 329.

Gordon, R. E. (1966*b*). Some criteria for the recognition of *Nocardia madurae* (Vincent) Blanchard. *J. gen. Microbiol.* **45**, 355.

Gordon, R. E. (1967). The taxonomy of soil bacteria. In *The Ecology of Soil Bacteria*, p. 293. Edited by T. R. G. Gray & D. Parkinson. Liverpool: Liverpool University Press.

Gordon, R. E., Haynes, W. C. & Pang, C. H.-N. (1973). The genus *Bacillus*. Agriculture Handbook no. 427. US Dept Agric.

Gordon, R. E. & Mihm, J. M. (1957). A comparative study of some strains received as nocardiae. *J. Bact.* **73**, 15.

Gordon, R. E. & Mihm, J. M. (1959). A comparison of four species of mycobacteria. *J. gen. Microbiol.* **21**, 736.

Gordon, R. E. & Mihm, J. M. (1961). The specific identity of *Jensenia canicruria*. *Can. J. Microbiol.* **7**, 108.

Gordon, R. E. & Mihm, J. M. (1962*a*). The type species of the genus *Nocardia*. *J. gen. Microbiol.* **27**, 1.

Gordon, R. E. & Mihm, J. M. (1962b). Identification of *Nocardia caviae* (Erikson) *nov. comb. Ann. N.Y. Acad. Sci.* **98**, 628.

Gordon, R. E. & Rynearson, T. K. (1963). Variation in pigmentation by a strain of *Mycobacterium smegmatis. Can. J. Microbiol.* **9**, 737.

Gordon, R. E. & Smith, M. M. (1953). Rapidly growing, acid fast bacteria. I. Species' descriptions of *Mycobacterium phlei* Lehmann and Neumann and *Mycobacterium smegmatis* (Trevisan) Lehmann and Neumann. *J. Bact.* **66**, 41.

Gordon, R. E. & Smith, M. M. (1955). Rapidly growing, acid fast bacteria. II. Species' description of *Mycobacterium fortuitum* Cruz. *J. Bact.* **69**, 502.

Graham, D. C. & Hodgkiss, W. (1967). Identity of Gram negative, yellow pigmented, fermentative bacteria isolated from plants and animals. *J. appl. Bact.* **30**, 175.

Gratia, A. (1920). Nature et genèse de l'agent coagulant du Staphylocoque ou 'Staphylocoagulase'. *C. r. Séanc. Soc. Biol.* **83**, 584.

Greene, R. A. & Larks, G. G. (1955). A quick method for the detection of gelatin liquefying bacteria. *J. Bact.* **69**, 224.

Grimont, P. A. D. & Dulong de Rosnay, H. L. C. (1972). Numerical study of 60 strains of *Serratia. J. gen. Microbiol.* **72**, 259.

Grossgebauer, K., Schmidt, B. & Langmaack, H. (1968). Lysozyme production as an aid for identification of potentially pathogenic strains of staphylococci. *Appl. Microbiol.* **16**, 1745.

Günther, H. L. & White, H. R. (1961). The cultural and physiological characters of the pediococci. *J. gen. Microbiol.* **26**, 185.

Gurr, E. (1956). *A Practical Manual of Medical and Biological Staining Techniques*, edn 2. London: Leonard Hill Ltd.

Gurr, G. T. (1963). *Biological Staining Methods*, edn 7. London: George T. Gurr Ltd.

Gutekunst, R. R., Delwiche, E. A. & Seeley, H. W. (1957). Catalase activity in *Pediococcus cerevisiae* as related to hydrogen ion activity. *J. Bact.* **74**, 693.

Gutiérrez-Vázquez, J. M. (1960). Further studies on the spot test for the differentiation of tubercle bacilli of human origin from other mycobacteria. *Am. Rev. resp. Dis.* **81**, 412.

Habeeb, A. F. S. A. (1960a). A study of bacteriological media. The examination of Proteose–Peptone. *J. Pharm. Pharmac.* **12**, 119.

Habeeb, A. F. S. A. (1960b). A study of bacteriological media: the examination of peptides in Casamin E. *Can. J. Microbiol.* **6**, 237.

Habs, H. & Schubert, R. H. W. (1962). Über die biochemischen Merkmale und die taxonomische Steelung von *Pseudomonas shigelloides* (Bader). *Zentbl. Bakt. ParasitKde Abt. II*, **186**, 316.

Hájek, V. & Maršálek, E. (1971). The differentiation of pathogenic staphylococci and a suggestion for their taxonomic classification. *Zentbl. Bakt. ParasitKde Abt I*, A **217**, 176.

Hájek, V., Maršálek, E. & Černá, I. (1968). Plazmakoagulázová aktivita stafylokoků různého původu. *Cslka epid. Mikrobiol. Immunol.* **17**, 39 [Summary in English].

Hajna, A. A. (1950). A semi-solid medium suitable for both motility and hydrogen sulfide tests. *Publ. Hlth Lab.* **8**, 36.

Hajna, A. A. & Damon, S. R. (1934). Differentiation of *Aerobacter aerogenes* and *A. cloacae* on the basis of the hydrolysis of sodium hippurate. *Am. J. Hyg.* **19**, 545.

Halvorsen, J. F. (1963). Gliding motility in the organisms *Bacterium anitratum* (B5W), *Moraxella lwoffi* and *Alkaligenes haemolysans*, as compared to *Moraxella nonliquefaciens. Acta path. microbiol. scand.* **59**, 200.

Hansen, P. A. (1968). *Type Strains of Lactobacillus species.* Rockville, Maryland: American Type Culture Collection.

Harden, A. & Norris, D. (1912). The bacterial production of acetylmethylcarbinol and 2,3-butylene glycol from various substances. *Proc. R. Soc. B.* **84**, 492.

Harding, H. A. (1910). The constancy of certain physiological characters in the classification of bacteria. *N.Y. Agric. exp. Sta. Tech. Bull.* no. 13.

Hare, R. & Colebrook, L. (1934). The biochemical reactions of haemolytic streptococci from the vagina of febrile and afebrile parturient women. *J. Path. Bact.* **39**, 429.

Hare, R., Wildy, P., Billett, F. S. & Twort, D. N. (1952). The anaerobic cocci: gas formation, fermentation reactions, sensitivity to antibiotics and sulphonamides. Classification. *J. Hyg., Camb.* **50**, 295.

Harper, E. M. & Conway, N. S. (1948). Clotting of human citrated plasma by Gram-negative organisms. *J. Path. Bact.* **60**, 247.

Harrington, B. J. (1966). A numerical taxonomical study of some corynebacteria and related organisms. *J. gen. Microbiol.* **45**, 31.

Harrison, A. P., Jr & Hansen, P. A. (1950). A motile lactobacillus from cecal feces of turkeys. *J. Bact.* **59**, 444.

Hartley, P (1922). The value of Douglas's medium for the production of diphtheria toxin. *J. Path. Bact.* **25**, 479.

Hartman, P. A., Reinbold, G. W. & Saraswat, D. S. (1966). Indicator organisms – a review. I. Taxonomy of the fecal streptococci. *Int. J. syst. Bact.* **16**, 197.

Harvey, R. W. S. & Thomson, S. (1953). Optimum temperature of incubation for isolation of salmonellae. *Mon. Bull. Minist. Hlth*, **12**, 149.

Hastings, E. G. (1903). Milchagar als Medium zur Demonstration der Erzeugung proteolytischer Enzyme. *Zentbl. Bakt. ParasitKde Abt. II*, **10**, 384.

Hastings, E. G. (1904). The action of various classes of bacteria on casein as shown by milk-agar plates. *Zentbl. Bakt. ParasitKde Abt. II*, **12**, 590.

Hatt, H. D. & Zvirbulis, E. (1967). Status of names of bacterial taxa not evaluated in *Index Bergeyana* (1966). I. Names published *circa* 1950–1967 exclusive of the genus *Salmonella*. *Int. J. syst. Bact.* **17**, 171.

Hauduroy, P., Hovanessian, A. & Roussianos, D. (1965). Instabilité de la chromogénéité des souches de *Mycobacterium kansasii*. *Annls Inst. Pasteur, Paris*, **109**, 142.

Hawn, C. V. Z. & Beebe, E. (1965). Rapid method for demonstrating bile solubility of *Diplococcus pneumoniae*. *J. Bact.* **90**, 549.

Haynes, W. C. (1951). *Pseudomonas aeruginosa* – its characterization and identification. *J. gen. Microbiol.* **5**, 939.

Hayward, N. J. & Miles, A. A. (1943). Inhibition of Proteus in cultures from wounds. *Lancet*, ii, 116.

Heiberg, B. (1936). The biochemical reactions of vibrios. *J. Hyg., Camb.* **36**, 114.

Henderson, A. (1967a). The urease activity of *Acinetobacter lwoffii* and *A. anitratus*. *J. gen. Microbiol.* **46**, 399.

Henderson, A. (1967b). The saccharolytic activity of *Acinetobacter lwoffii* and *A. anitratus*. *J. gen. Microbiol.* **49**, 487.

Hendrie, M. S., Mitchell, T. G. & Shewan, J. M. (1968). The identification of yellow-pigmented rods. In *Identification Methods for Microbiologists*, part B, p. 67. Edited by B. M. Gibbs & D. A. Shapton. London: Academic Press.

Hendrie, M. S., Shewan, J. M. & Véron, M. (1971). *Aeromonas shigelloides* (Bader) Ewing *et al.*: a proposal that it be transferred to the genus *Vibrio*. *Int. J. syst. Bact.* **21**, 25.

Hendry, C. B. (1938). The effect of serum maltase on fermentation reactions with gonococci. *J. Path. Bact.* **46**, 383.

Henriksen, S. D. (1950). A comparison of the phenylpyruvic acid reaction and the urease test in the differentiation of Proteus from other enteric organisms. *J. Bact.* **60**, 225.

Henriksen, S. D. (1952). *Moraxella*: classification and taxonomy. *J. gen. Microbiol.* **6**, 318.

Henriksen, S. D. (1960). *Moraxella*. Some problems of taxonomy and nomenclature. *Int. Bull. bact. Nomencl. Taxon.* **10**, 23.

Henriksen, S. D. (1962). Some Pasteurella strains from the human respiratory tract. A correction and supplement. *Acta path. microbiol. scand.* **55**, 355.

Henriksen, S. D. (1963). Mimae. The standing in nomenclature of the names of this tribus and of its genera and species. *Int. Bull. bact. Nomencl. Taxon.* **13**, 51.

Henriksen, S. D. & Bøvre, K. (1968a). *Moraxella kingii* sp. nov., a haemolytic, saccharolytic species of the genus *Moraxella*. *J. gen. Microbiol.* **51**, 377.

Henriksen, S. D. & Bøvre, K. (1968b). The taxonomy of the genera *Moraxella* and *Neisseria*. *J. gen. Microbiol.* **51**, 387.

Henriksen, S. D. & Closs, K. (1938). The production of phenylpyruvic acid by bacteria. *Acta path. microbiol. scand.* **15**, 101.

Henriksen, S. D. & Grelland, R. (1952). Toxigenicity, serological reactions and relationships of the diphtheria-like corynebacteria. *J. Path. Bact.* **64**, 503.

Henriksen, S. D. & Jyssum, K. (1960). A new variety of *Pasteurella haemolytica* from the human respiratory tract. *Acta path. microbiol scand.* **50**, 443.

Heyl, J. G. (1963). A study of Pasteurella strains from animal sources. *Antonie van Leeuwenhoek*, **29**, 79.

Hill, L. R. (1959). The Adansonian classification of the staphylococci. *J. gen. Microbiol.* **20**, 277.

Hill, L. R. (1966). An index to deoxyribonucleic acid base compositions of bacterial species. *J. gen. Microbiol.* **44**, 419.

Hill, L. R., Snell, J. J. S. & Lapage, S. P. (1970). Identification and characterisation of *Bacteroides corrodens*. *J. med. Microbiol.* **3**, 483.

Hill, L. R., Turri, M., Gilardi, E. & Silvestri, L. G. (1961). Quantitative methods in the systematics of Actinomycetales. II. *G. Microbiol.* **9**, 56.

Hitchens, A. P. & Leikind, M. C. (1939). The introduction of agar-agar into bacteriology. *J. Bact.* **37**, 485.

Hitchner, E. R. & Snieszko, S. F. (1947). A study of a microorganism causing a bacterial disease of lobsters. *J. Bact.* **54**, 48.

Hobbs, B. C. (1948). A study of the serological type differentiation of *Staphylococcus pyogenes*. *J. Hyg., Camb.* **46**, 222.

Hobbs, B. C. & Allison, V. D. (1945). Studies on the isolation of *Bact. typhosum* and *Bact. paratyphosum* B. *Mon. Bull. Minist. Hlth* **4**, 63.

Hodgkiss, W. (1960). The interpretation of flagella stains. *J. appl. Bact.* **23**, 398.

Hodgkiss, W. & Ordal, Z. J. (1966). Morphology of the spore of some strains of *Clostridium botulinum* type E. *J. Bact.* **91**, 2031.

Hok, T. T. (1962). A simple and rapid cold-staining method for acid-fast bacteria. *Am. Rev. resp. Dis.* **85**, 753.

Holdeman, L. V. & Moore, W. E. C. (1972). Eds, *Anaerobe Laboratory Manual.* Blacksburg, Virginia: Anaerobe Laboratory, Virginia Polytechnic Institute & State University.

Holding, A. J. & Collee, J. G. (1971). Routine biochemical tests. In *Methods in Microbiology*, vol. 6A, p. 1. Edited by J. R. Norris & D. W. Ribbons. London: Academic Press.

Hollis, D. G., Wiggins, G. L. & Weaver, R. E. (1969). *Neisseria lactamicus* sp. n., a lactose-fermenting species resembling *Neisseria meningitidis. Appl. Microbiol.* **17**, 71.

Holman, W. L. & Gonzales, F. L. (1923). A test for indol based on the oxalic reaction of Gnezda. *J. Bact.* **8**, 577.

Holmberg, K. & Hallander, H. O. (1973). Numerical taxonomy and laboratory identification of *Bacterionema matruchotii, Rothia dentocariosa, Actinomyces naeslundii, Actinomyces viscosus*, and some related bacteria. *J. gen. Microbiol.* **76**, 43.

Holt, R. (1969). The classification of staphylococci from colonized ventriculoatrial shunts. *J. clin. Path.* **22**, 475.

Hormaeche, E. & Edwards, P. R. (1958). Observations on the genus *Aerobacter* with a description of two species. *Int. Bull. bact. Nomencl. Taxon.* **8**, 111.

Hormaeche, E. & Edwards, P. R. (1960). A proposed genus *Enterobacter. Int. Bull. bact. Nomencl. Taxon.* **10**, 71.

Hormaeche, E. & Munilla, M. (1957). Biochemical tests for the differentiation of *Klebsiella* and *Cloaca. Int. Bull. bact. Nomencl. Taxon.* **7**, 1.

Howell, A., Jr & Jordan, H. V. (1963). A filamentous microorganism isolated from periodontal plaque in hamsters. II. Physiological and biochemical characteristics. *Sabouraudia*, **3**, 93.

Howell, A., Murphy, W. C., Paul, F. & Stephan, R. M. (1959). Oral strains of *Actinomyces. J. Bact.* **78**, 82.

Hoyle, L. (1941). A tellurite blood-agar medium for the rapid diagnosis of diphtheria. *Lancet*, i, 175.

Hoyt, R. E. (1951). Tableted substrates in the detection of indol and urease production by bacteria. *Am. J. clin. Path.* **21**, 892.

Hoyt, R. E. & Pickett, M. J. (1957). Use of 'rapid substrate' tablets in the recognition of enteric bacteria. *Am. J. clin. Path.* **27**, 343.

Hsu, S. T., Liu, C. H. & Liao, C. L. (1964). A new differential medium for enteropathogenic vibrios and other Gram-negative intestinal organisms. *Bull. Wld Hlth Org.* **31**, 136.

Hubálek, Z. (1969). Numerical taxonomy of genera *Micrococcus* Cohn and *Sarcina* Goodsir. *J. gen. Microbiol.* **57**, 349.

Hucker, G. J. (1924a). Studies on the Coccaceae. II. A study of the general characters of the micrococci. *Tech. Bull. N.Y. St. agric. Exp. Sta.* no. 100.

Hucker, G. J. (1924b). Studies on the Coccaceae. IV. The classification of the genus *Micrococcus* Cohn. *Tech. Bull. N.Y. St. agric. Exp. Sta.* no. 102.

Hucker, G. J. & Conn, H. J. (1923). Methods of Gram staining. *Tech. Bull. N.Y. St. agric. Exp. Sta.* no. 93.

Hugh, R. (1959). Oxytoca group organisms isolated from the oropharyngeal region. *Canad. J. Microbiol.* **5**, 251.

Hugh, R. & Ellis, M. A. (1968). The neotype strain for *Staphylococcus epidermidis* (Winslow and Winslow 1908) Evans 1916. *Int. J. syst. Bact.* **18**, 231.

Hugh, R. & Feeley, J. C. (1972a). Report (1966–1970) of the Subcommittee on Taxonomy of Vibrios to the International Committee on [the] Nomenclature of Bacteria. *Int. J. syst. Bact.* **22**, 123.

Hugh, R. & Feeley, J. C. (1972b). International Committee on Systematic Bacteriology Subcommittee on Taxonomy of Vibrios; Minutes of the Meeting, 22 July 1971. *Int. J. syst. Bact.* **22**, 189.

Hugh, R. & Leifson, E. (1953). The taxonomic significance of fermentative versus oxidative metabolism of carbohydrates by various Gram negative bacteria. *J. Bact.* **66**, 24.

Hugh, R. & Leifson, E. (1963). A description of the type strain of *Pseudomonas maltophilia. Int. Bull. bact. Nomencl. Taxon.* **13**, 133.

Hugh, R. & Reese, R. (1968). A comparison of 120 strains of *Bacterium anitratum* Schaub and Hauber with the type strain of this species. *Int. J. syst. Bact.* **18**, 207.

Hugh, R. & Ryschenkow, E. (1961). *Pseudomonas maltophilia*, an Alcaligenes-like species. *J. gen. Microbiol.* **26**, 123.

Hugh, R. & Sakazaki, R. (1972). Minimal number of characters for the identification of *Vibrio* species, *Vibrio cholerae*, and *Vibrio parahaemolyticus. Publ. Hlth Lab.* **30**, 133.

Hutner, S. H. (1942). Some growth requirements of Erysipelothrix and Listerella. *J. Bact.* **43**, 629.

Ikari, P. & Hugh, R. (1963). *Pseudomonas alcaligenes* Monias (1928), a polar monotrichous dextrose non-oxidizer. *Bact. Proc.* 41.

Index Bergeyana (1966). Edited by R. E. Buchanan, J. G. Holt & E. F. Lessel, Jr. Baltimore: The Williams & Wilkins Co.

International Code of Nomenclature of Bacteria (1966). *Int. J. syst. Bact.* **16**, 459. [Earlier editions known as *International Bacteriological Code of Nomenclature* (1948); *International Code of Nomenclature of Bacteria and Viruses*, approved 1953, published 1958 (Buchanan, Cowan, Wikén & Clark). Short title of all versions is *Bacteriological Code*. 1966 version is imperfect as some paragraphs were unintentionally omitted from the code as printed. See Lapage, Clark, Lessel, Seeliger & Sneath (1973) for proposed revision.]

Jackson, F. L. & Goodman, Y. E. (1972). Transfer of the facultatively anaerobic organism *Bacteroides corrodens* Eiken to a new genus, *Eikenella. Int. J. syst. Bact.* **22**, 73.

Jameson, J. E. (1965). A modified Elek test for toxigenic *Corynebacterium diphtheriae. Mon. Bull. Minist. Hlth*, **24**, 55.

Jameson, J. E. & Emberley, N. W. (1956). A substitute for bile salts in culture media. *J. gen. Microbiol.* **15**, 198.

Jawetz, E. (1950). A pneumotropic pasteurella of laboratory animals. I. Bacteriological and serological characteristics of the organism. *J. infect. Dis.* **86**, 172.

Jayne-Williams, D. J. & Cheeseman, G. C. (1960). The differentiation of bacterial species by paper chromatography. IX. The genus *Bacillus*: a preliminary investigation. *J. appl. Bact.* **23**, 250.

Jayne-Williams, D. J. & Skerman, T. M. (1966). Comparative studies on coryneform bacteria from milk and dairy sources. *J. appl. Bact.* **29**, 72.

Jeffries, C. D., Holtman, D. F. & Guse, D. G. (1957). Rapid method for determining the activity of microorganisms on nucleic acids. *J. Bact.* **73**, 590.

Jennens, M. G. (1954). The methyl red test in peptone media. *J. gen. Microbiol.* **10**, 121.

Jensen, H. L. (1952). The coryneform bacteria. *A. Rev. Microbiol.* **6**, 77.

Jensen, K. A. (1932). Reinzüchtung und Typenbestimmung von Tuberkelbazillenstämmen. Eine Vereinfachung der Methoden für die Praxis. *Zentbl. Bakt. ParasitKde Abt. I*, **125**, 222.

Jensen, W. I., Owen, C. R. & Jellison, W. L. (1969). *Yersinia philomiragia* sp. n., a new member of the Pasteurella group of bacteria, naturally pathogenic for the muskrat (*Ondatra zibethica*). *J. Bact.* **100**, 1237.

Johnson, J. L. & Cummins, C. S. (1972). Cell wall composition and deoxyribonucleic acid similarities among the anaerobic coryneforms, classical propionibacteria, and strains of *Arachnia propionica. J. Bact.* **109**, 1047.

Johnson, R. & Sneath, P. H. A. (1973). Taxonomy of *Bordetella* and related organisms of the families *Achromobacteraceae*, *Brucellaceae*, and *Neisseriaceae. Int. J. syst. Bact.* **23**, 381.

Johnston, M. A. & Delwiche, E. A. (1962). Catalase of the Lactobacillaceae. *J. Bact.* **83**, 936.

Johnston, W. (1895). On grouping water bacteria. *Publ. Hlth Pap. Rep., N.Y.* **20**, 445.

Jones, D., Deibel, R. H. & Niven, C. F., Jr (1963a). Identity of *Staphylococcus epidermidis. J. Bact.* **85**, 62.

Jones, D., Deibel, R. H. & Niven, C. F., Jr (1963b). Apparent pigment production by *Streptococcus faecalis* in the presence of metallic ions. *J. Bact.* **86**, 171.

Jones, D., Deibel, R. H. & Niven, C. F., Jr (1964). Catalase activity of two *Streptococcus faecalis* strains and its enhancement by aerobiosis and added cations. *J. Bact.* **88**, 602.

Jones, D. M. (1962). A pasteurella-like organism from the human respiratory tract. *J. Path. Bact.* **83**, 143.

Jones, L. M. (1964). Use of safranin O for characterization of *Brucella* species. *J. Bact.* **88**, 1527.

Jones, L. M. & Morgan, W. J. B. (1958). A preliminary report on a selective medium for the culture of Brucella, including fastidious types. *Bull. Wld Hlth Org.* **19**, 200.

Jones, L. M. & Wundt, W. (1971). International Committee on Nomenclature of Bacteria. Subcommittee on the taxonomy of *Brucella. Int. J. syst. Bact.* **21**, 126.

Jones, N. R. (1956). A tentative method for the determination of the grade strength of agars. *Analyst*, **81**, 243.

Jonsson, V. (1970). Proposal of a new species *Pseudomonas kingii. Int. J. syst. Bact.* **20**, 255.

Jordan, E. O. (1890). A report on certain species of bacteria observed in sewage. *Rep. Mass. St. Bd Hlth*, part II, 821.

Jordan, E. O., Crawford, R. R. & McBroom, J. (1935). The Morgan bacillus. *J. Bact.* **29**, 131.

Julianelle, L. A. (1941). Biological and immunological studies of Listerella. *J. Bact.* **42**, 367.

Kampelmacher, E. H. (1959). On antigenic O-relationships between the groups Salmonella, Arizona, Escherichia and Shigella. *Antonie van Leeuwenhoek*, **25**, 289.

Kampelmacher, E. H., Mossel, D. A. A., van Noorle Jansen, L. M. & Vincentie, H. A. (1970). A survey on the occurrence of *Vibrio parahaemolyticus* on fish and shellfish, marketed in The Netherlands. *J. Hyg., Camb.* **68**, 189.

Kandler, O. (1970). Amino acid sequence of the murein and taxonomy of the genera *Lactobacillus, Bifidobacterium, Leuconostoc* and *Pediococcus. Int. J. syst. Bact.* **20**, 491.

Kanetsuna, F. & Bartoli, A. (1972). A simple chemical method to differentiate *Mycobacterium* from *Nocardia. J. gen. Microbiol.* **70**, 209.

Karlson, A. G. & Lessel, E. F. (1970). *Mycobacterium bovis* nom. nov. *Int. J. syst. Bact.* **20**, 273.

Kauffmann, F. (1953). On the classification and nomenclature of Enterobacteriaceae. *Riv. Ist. sieroter. ital.* **28**, 485.

Kauffmann, F. (1954). *Enterobacteriaceae*, edn 2. Copenhagen: Ejnar Munksgaard.

Kauffmann, F. (1959*a*). On the principles of classification and nomenclature of Enterobacteriaceae. *Int. Bull. bact. Nomencl. Taxon.* **9**, 1.

Kauffmann, F. (1959*b*). Definition of genera and species of Enterobacteriaceae. Request for an Opinion. *Int. Bull. bact. Nomencl. Taxon.* **9**, 7.

Kauffmann, F. (1963*a*). Zur Differentialdiagnose der Salmonella-Sub-genera I, II und III. *Acta path. microbiol. scand.* **58**, 109.

Kauffmann, F. (1963*b*). On the species-definition. *Int. Bull. bact. Nomencl. Taxon.* **13**, 181.

Kauffmann, F. & Edwards, P. R. (1952). Classification and nomenclature of Enterobacteriaceae. *Int. Bull. bact. Nomencl. Taxon.* **2**, 2.

Kauffmann, F., Edwards, P. R. & Ewing, W. H. (1956). The principles of group differentiation within the Enterobacteriaceae by biochemical methods. *Int. Bull. bact. Nomencl. Taxon.* **6**, 29.

Keddie, R. M., Leask, B. G. S. & Grainger, J. M. (1966). A comparison of coryneform bacteria from soil and herbage: cell wall composition and nutrition. *J. appl. Bact.* **29**, 17.

Keilty, R. A. (1917). The problem of acid-fast organisms in distilled water. *J. med. Res.* **37**, 183.

Keleti, J., Lüderitz, O., Mlynarčík, D. & Sedlák, J. (1971). Immunochemical studies on *Citrobacter* O antigens (lipopolysaccharides). *Eur. J. Biochem.* **20**, 237.

Kellerman, K. F. & McBeth, I. G. (1912). The fermentation of cellulose. *Zentbl. Bakt. ParasitKde Abt. II*, **34**, 485.

Kelly, A. T. & Fulton, M. (1953). Use of triphenyl tetrazolium in motility test medium. *Am. J. clin. Path.* **23**, 512.

Kelsey, J. C. (1958). The testing of sterilizers. *Lancet*, i, 306.

Kelsey, J. C. (1961). The testing of sterilizers. 2. Thermophilic spore papers. *J. clin. Path.* **14**, 313.

Kendal, A. I. & Ryan, M. (1919). A double sugar medium for the cultural diagnosis of intestinal and other bacteria. *J. infect. Dis.* **24**, 400.

Khairat, O. (1940). Endocarditis due to a new species of *Haemophilus. J. Path. Bact.* **50**, 497.

Kharasch, M. S., Conway, E. A. & Bloom, W. (1936). Some chemical factors influencing growth and pigmentation of certain microörganisms. *J. Bact.* **32**, 533.

King, B. M. & Adler, D. L. (1964). A previously undescribed group of Enterobacteriaceae. *Am. J. clin. Path.* **41**, 230.

King, B. M., Ranck, B. A., Daugherty, F. D. & Rau, C. A. (1963). *Clostridium tertium* septicemia. *New Engl. J. Med.* **269**, 467.

King, E. O. (1959). Studies on a group of previously unclassified bacteria associated with meningitis in infants. *Am. J. clin. Path.* **31**, 241.

King, E. O. (1962). The laboratory recognition of *Vibrio fetus* and a closely related *Vibrio* isolated from cases of human vibriosis. *Ann. N.Y. Acad. Sci.* **98**, 700.

King, E. O. (1964, 1972). *The Identification of Unusual Pathogenic Gram negative Bacteria.* Revised (1972) by Weaver, R. E., Tatum, H. W. & Hollis, D. G. Atlanta, Georgia: Center for Disease Control, US Dept. of Health, Education, and Welfare, Public Health Service.

King, E. O. & Tatum, H. W. (1962). *Actinobacillus actinomycetemcomitans* and *Hemophilus aphrophilus. J. infect. Dis.* **111**, 85.

King, E. O., Ward, M. K. & Raney, D. E. (1954). Two simple media for the demonstration of pyocyanin and fluorescin. *J. Lab. clin. Med.* **44**, 301.

Kingsbury, D. T. (1967). Deoxyribonucleic acid homologies among species of the genus *Neisseria. J. Bact.* **94**, 870.

Kingsbury, D. T., Fanning, G. R., Johnson, K. E. & Brenner, D. J. (1969). Thermal stability of interspecies Neisseria DNA duplexes. *J. gen. Microbiol.* **55**, 201.

Kligler, I. J. (1917). A simple medium for the differentiation of members of the typhoid–paratyphoid group. *Am. J. publ. Hlth*, **7**, 1042.

Kligler, I. J. (1918). Modifications of culture media used in the isolation and differentiation of typhoid, dysentery, and allied bacilli. *J. exp. Med.* **28**, 319.

Kligler, I. J. & Defandorf, J. (1918). The Endo medium for the isolation of *B. dysenteriae* and a double sugar medium for the differentiation of *B. dysenteriae*, Shiga and Flexner. *J. Bact.* **3**, 437.

Knapp, W. (1965). Neuere experimentelle Untersuchungen mit *Pasteurella pseudotuberculosis* (*Yersinia pseudotuberculosis*). *Arch. Hyg. Bakt.* **149**, 715.

Knapp, W. & Thal, E. (1973). Die biochemische Charakterisierung von Yersinia enterocolitica (syn. 'Pasteurella X') als Grundlage eines vereinfachten O-Antigenschemas. *Zentbl. Bakt. ParasitKde Abt. I*, **A223**, 88.

Knight, B. C. J. G. & Proom, H. (1950). A comparative survey of the nutrition and physiology of mesophilic species in the genus *Bacillus. J. gen. Microbiol.* **4**, 508.

Knox, R. (1949). A screening plate for the rapid identification of faecal organisms. *J. Path. Bact.* **61**, 343.

Kocur, M., Bergan, T. & Mortensen, N. (1971). DNA base composition of Gram-positive cocci. *J. gen. Microbiol.* **69**, 167.

Kocur, M. & Martinec, T. (1962). A contribution to the taxonomy of the genus Staphylococcus. *Publs Fac. Sci. Univ. J. E. Purkyne, Brno*, **28**, 492.

Kocur, M. & Martinec, T. (1972). Taxonomic status of *Micrococcus varians* Migula 1900 and designation of the neotype strain. *Int. J. syst. Bact.* **22**, 228.

Kocur, M. & Páčová, Z. (1970). The taxonomic status of *Micrococcus roseus* Flügge, 1886. *Int. J. syst. Bact.* **20**, 233.

Kocur, M., Páčová, Z. & Martinec, T. (1972). Taxonomic status of *Micrococcus luteus* (Schroeter 1872) Cohn 1872, and designation of the neotype strain. *Int. J. syst. Bact.* **22**, 218.

Kohn, J. (1953). A preliminary report of a new gelatin liquefaction method. *J. clin. Path.* **6**, 249.

Kohn, J. (1954). A two-tube technique for the identification of organisms of the Enterobacteriaceae group. *J. Path. Bact.* **67**, 286.

Koontz, F. B. & Faber, J. E. (1963). A taxonomic study of some Gram-negative, non-fermenting bacteria. *Can. J. Microbiol.* **9**, 499.

Kopper, P. H. (1962). Effect of sodium chloride concentration on the swarming tendency of *Proteus. J. Bact.* **84**, 1119.

Koser, S. A. (1923). Utilization of the salts of organic acids by the colon-aerogenes group. *J. Bact.* **8**, 493.

Kovács, N. (1928). Eine vereinfachte Methode zum Nachweis der Indolbildung durch Bakterien. *Z. ImmunForsch. exp. Ther.* **55**, 311.

Kovács, N. (1956). Identification of *Pseudomonas pyocyanea* by the oxidase reaction. *Nature, Lond.* **178**, 703.

Kriebel, R. M. (1934). A comparative bacteriological study of a group of non-lactose-fermenting bacteria isolated from stools of healthy food-handlers. *J. Bact.* **27**, 357.

Kubica, G. P. (1973). Differential identification of mycobacteria. VII. Key features for identification of clinically significant mycobacteria. *Am. Rev. resp. Dis.* **107**, 9.

Kubica, G. P., Baess, I., Gordon, R. E., Jenkins, P. A., Kwapinski, J. B. G., McDurmont, C., Pattyn, S. R., Saito, H., Silcox, V., Stanford, J. L., Takeya, K. & Tsukamura, M. (1972). A co-operative numerical analysis of rapidly growing mycobacteria. *J. gen. Microbiol.* **73**, 55.

Kubica, G. P. & Dye, W. E. (1967). Laboratory methods for clinical and public health mycobacteriology. *Publ. Hlth Ser. Publ.* no. 1547. Washington, DC: US Government Printing Office.

Kubica, G. P. & Pool, G. L. (1960). Studies on the catalase activity of acid-fast bacilli. I. An attempt to subgroup these organisms on the basis of their catalase activities at different temperatures and pH. *Am. Rev. resp. Dis.* **81**, 387.

Kubica, G. P. & Silcox, V. A. (1973). Numerical taxonomic analysis of some slowly growing mycobacteria using hypothetical median strain patterns. *J. gen. Microbiol.* **74**, 149.

Kulp, W. L. & White, V. (1932). A modified medium for plating *L. acidophilus. Science, N.Y.* **76**, 17.

Küster, E. (1972). Simple working key for the classification and identification of named taxa included in the International *Streptomyces* Project. *Int. J. syst. Bact.* **22**, 139.

Lacey, B. W. (1951). Selective media for *Haemophilus pertussis* and *parapertussis. J. gen. Microbiol.* **5**, vi.

Lakso, J. U. & Starr, M. P. (1970). Comparative injuriousness to plants of *Erwinia* spp. and other enterobacteria from plants and animals. *J. appl. Bact.* **33**, 692.

Lambert, M. A., Hollis, D. G., Moss, C. W., Weaver, R. E. & Thomas, M. L. (1971). Cellular fatty acids of nonpathogenic *Neisseria. Can. J. Microbiol.* **17**, 1491.

Lancefield, R. C. (1928). The antigenic complex of *Streptococcus haemolyticus*: I. Demonstration of a type-specific substance in extracts of *Streptococcus haemolyticus. J. exp. Med.* **47**, 91.

Lancefield, R. C. (1933). A serological differentiation of human and other groups of hemolytic streptococci. *J. exp. Med.* **57**, 571.

Lancefield, R. C. (1940). The significance of M and T antigens in the cross reactions between certain types of group A hemolytic streptococci. *J. exp. Med.* **71**, 539.

Langston, C. W., Gutierrez, J. & Bouma, C. (1960*a*). Catalase-producing strains of streptococci. *J. Bact.* **80**, 693.

Langston, C. W., Gutierrez, J. & Bouma, C. (1960*b*). Motile enterococci (*Streptococcus faecium* var. *mobilis* var. n.) isolated from grass silage. *J. Bact.* **80**, 714.

Langston, C. W. & Williams, P. P. (1962). Reduction of nitrate by streptococci. *J. Bact.* **84**, 603.

Lányi, B. & Ádám, M. M. (1960). Agar diffusion test and micromethods for the rapid biochemical differentiation of enteric bacteria. *Acta microbiol. Acad. Sci. hung.* **7**, 313.

Lapage, S. P. (1961). *Haemophilus vaginalis* and its role in vaginitis. *Acta path. microbiol. scand.* **52**, 34.

Lapage, S. P. & Bascomb, S. (1968). Use of selenite reduction in bacterial classification. *J. appl. Bact.* **31**, 568.

Lapage, S. P., Bascomb, S., Willcox, W. R. & Curtis, M. A. (1970). Computer identification of bacteria. In *Automation, Mechanization and Data Handling in Microbiology*, p. 1. Edited by A. Baillie & R. J. Gilbert. London: Academic Press.

Lapage, S. P., Bascomb, S., Willcox, W. R. & Curtis, M. A. (1973). Identification of bacteria by computer. General aspects and perspectives. *J. gen. Microbiol.* **77**, 273.

Lapage, S. P., Clark, W. A., Lessel, E. F., Seeliger, H. P. R. & Sneath, P. H. A. (1973). Proposed revision of the International Code of Nomenclature of Bacteria. *Int. J. syst. Bact.* **23**, 83.

Lapage, S. P., Efstratiou, A. & Hill, L. R. (1973). The ortho-nitrophenol (ONPG) test and acid from lactose in Gram-negative genera. *J. clin. Path.* **26**, 821.

Lapage, S. P., Hill, L. R. & Reeve, J. D. (1968). *Pseudomonas stutzeri* in pathological material. *J. med. Microbiol.* **1**, 195.

Lapage, S. P., Shelton, J. E. & Mitchell, T. G. (1970). Media for the maintenence and preservation of bacteria. In *Methods in Microbiology*, vol. 3A, p. 1. Edited by J. R. Norris & D. W. Ribbons. London: Academic Press.

Lapage, S. P. & Zinnemann, K. (1971). Internationa Committee on Nomenclature of Bacteria subcommittee on the Taxonomy of Haemophilus. Minutes of meeting, 11 August, 1970. *Int. J. syst. Bact.* **21**, 132.

Larkin, J. M. & Stokes, J. L. (1967). Taxonomy of psychrophilic strains of *Bacillus. J. Bact.* **94**, 889.

Lautrop, H. (1956*a*). A modified Kohn's test for the demonstration of bacterial gelatin liquefaction. *Acta path. microbiol. scand.* **39**, 357.

Lautrop, H. (1956*b*). Gelatin-liquefying Klebsiella strains (*Bacterium oxytocum* (Flügge)). *Acta path. microbiol. scand.* **39**, 375.

Lautrop, H. (1960). Laboratory diagnosis of whooping cough or *Bordetella* infections. *Bull. Wld Hlth Org.* **23**, 15.

Lautrop, H. (1961). *Bacterium anitratum* transferred to the genus *Cytophaga. Int. Bull. bact. Nomencl. Taxon.* **11**, 107.

Lautrop, H. (1965). Gliding motility in bacteria as a taxonomic criterion. *Publs Fac. Sci. Univ. J. E. Purkyne, Brno,* **K35**, 322.

Lautrop, H., Bøvre, K. & Frederiksen, W. (1970). A *Moraxella*-like microorganism isolated from the genito-urinary tract of man. *Acta path. microbiol. scand.* **78 B**, 255.

Laybourn, R. L. (1924). A modification of Albert's stain for the diphtheria bacilli. *J. Am. med. Ass.* **83**, 121.

Lazar, I. (1968). Serological relationships of corynebacteria. *J. gen. Microbiol.* **52**, 77.

Leach, P. A., Bullen, J. J. & Grant, I. D. (1971). Anaerobic CO_2 cabinet for the cultivation of strict anaerobes. *Appl. Microbiol.* **22**, 824.

Leclerc, H. & Beerens, H. (1962). Une technique simple de mise en évidence de l'oxydase chez les bactéries. *Annls Inst. Pasteur, Lille,* **13**, 187.

Lederberg, J. (1950). The beta-D-galactosidase of *Escherichia coli,* strain K-12. *J. Bact.* **60**, 381.

Lederberg, J. & Lederberg, E. M. (1952). Replica plating and indirect selection of bacterial mutants. *J. Bact.* **63**, 399.

Lee, W. H. & Riemann, H. (1970). The genetic relatedness of proteolytic *Clostridium botulinum* strains. *J. gen. Microbiol.* **64**, 85.

Leffmann, H. & La Wall, C. H. (1911). Sulphur dioxide in commercial gelatins. *Analyst,* **36**, 271.

Legroux, R. & Genevray, J. (1933). Étude comparative entre le bacille de Whitmore et le bacille pyocyanique. *Annls Inst. Pasteur, Paris,* **51**, 249.

Leifson, E. (1933). The fermentation of sodium malonate as a means of differentiating *Aerobacter* and *Escherichia. J. Bact.* **26**, 329.

Leifson, E. (1935). New culture media based on sodium desoxycholate for the isolation of intestinal pathogens and for the enumeration of colon bacilli in milk and water. *J. Path. Bact.* **40**, 581.

Leifson, E. (1951). Staining, shape, and arrangement of bacterial flagella. *J. Bact.* **62**, 377.

Leifson, E. (1956). Morphological and physiological characteristics of the genus *Chromobacterium. J. Bact.* **71**, 393.

Leifson, E. (1960). *Atlas of Bacterial Flagellation.* New York: Academic Press.

Leifson, E. (1961). The effect of formaldehyde on the shape of bacterial flagella. *J. gen. Microbiol.* **25**, 131.

Leifson, E. (1963). Determination of carbohydrate metabolism of marine bacteria. *J. Bact.* **85**, 1183.

Leise, J. M., Carter, C. H., Friedlander, H. & Freed, S. W. (1959). Criteria for the identification of *Bacillus anthracis. J. Bact.* **77**, 655.

Lemcke, R. M. & Leach, R. H. (1968). Methods for the identification of mycoplasmas. In *Identification Methods for Microbiologists*, part B, p. 125. Edited by B. M. Gibbs & D. A. Shapton. London: Academic Press.

Le Minor, L. & Ben Hamida, F. (1962). Avantages de la recherche de la *β*-galactosidase sur celle de la fermentation du lactose en milieu complexe dans le diagnostic bactériologique, en particulier des Enterobacteriaceae. *Annls Inst. Pasteur, Paris*, **102**, 267.

Le Minor, L. & Piéchaud, M. (1963). Note technique. Une méthode rapide de recherche de la protéolyse de la gélatine. *Annls Inst Pasteur, Paris*, **105**, 792.

Le Minor, L., Rohde, R. & Taylor, J. (1970). Nomenclature des *Salmonella. Annls Inst. Pasteur, Paris*, **119**, 206.

Lepper, E. & Martin, C. J. (1929). The chemical mechanisms exploited in the use of meat media for the cultivation of anaerobes. *Br. J. exp. Path.* **10**, 327.

Levin, M. (1943). Two agar-less media for the rapid isolation of *Corynebacterium* and *Neisseria. J. Bact.* **46**, 233.

Levine, M. (1918). A statistical classification of the colon–cloacae group. *J. Bact.* **3**, 253.

Levine, M., Epstein, S. S. & Vaughn, R. H. (1934). Differential reactions in the colon group of bacteria. *Am. J. publ. Hlth*, **24**, 505.

Lewis, B. (1961). Phosphatase production by staphylococci – a comparison of two methods. *J. med. Lab. Technol.* **18**, 112.

Lewis, P. A. & Shope, R. E. (1931). Swine influenza. II. A hemophilic bacillus from the respiratory tract of infected swine. *J. exp. Med.* **54**, 361.

Lillie, R. D. (1928). The Gram stain. I. A quick method for staining Gram-positive organisms in the tissues. *Arch. Path.* **5**, 828.

Lindqvist, K. (1960). A Neisseria species associated with infectious kerato-conjunctivitis of sheep – *Neisseria ovis* nov. spec. *J. infect. Dis.* **106**, 162.

Lingappa, Y. & Lockwood, J. L. (1961). A chitin medium for isolation, growth and maintenance of actinomycetes. *Nature, Lond.* **189**, 158.

Lingelsheim, W. von (1906). Die bakteriologischen Arbeiten der Kgl. Hygienischen Station zu Beuthen O.-Schl. während der Genickstarreepidemie in Oberschlesien im Winter 1904/5. *Klin. Jahrb.* **15**, 373.

Lingelsheim, W. von (1908). Beiträge zur Ätiologie der epidemischen Genickstarre nach den Ergebnessen der letzten Jahre. *Z. Hyg. InfectKrankh.* **59**, 457.

Linton, C. S. (1925). A note on the Voges–Proskauer reaction. *J. Am. Wat. Wks Ass.* **13**, 547.

Liston, J., Wiebe, W. & Colwell, R. R. (1963). Quantitative approach to the study of bacterial species. *J. Bact.* **85**, 1061.

Live, I. (1972). Differentiation of *Staphylococcus aureus* of human and canine origins: coagulation of human and canine plasma, fibrinolysin activity, and serologic reaction. *Am. J. vet. Res.* **33**, 385.

Lockhart, W. R. (1967). Factors affecting reproducibility of numerical classifications. *J. Bact.* **94**, 826.

Lockhart, W. R. & Hartman, P. A. (1963). Formation of monothetic groups in quantitative bacterial taxonomy. *J. Bact.* **85**, 68.

Loeb, L. (1903). The influence of certain bacteria on the coagulation of the blood. *J. med. Res.* **10**, 407.

Loesche, W. J., Gibbons, R. J. & Socransky, S. S. (1965). Biochemical characteristics of *Vibrio sputorum* and relationship to *Vibrio bubulus* and *Vibrio fetus. J. Bact.* **89**, 1109.

Love, R. M. (1953). A qualitative test for monosaccharides. *Analyst*, **78**, 732.

Lovell, R. (1946). Studies on *Corynebacterium renale*. I. A systematic study of a number of strains. *J. comp. Path.* **56**, 196.

Lowe, G. H. (1962). The rapid detection of lactose fermentation in paracolon organisms by the demonstration of *β*-D-galactosidase. *J. med. Lab. Technol.* **19**, 21.

Lowe, G. H. & Evans, J. H. (1957). A simple medium for the rapid detection of salmonella-like paracolon organisms. *J. clin. Path.* **10**, 318.

Lund, B. M. (1967). A study of some motile group D streptococci. *J. gen. Microbiol.* **49**, 67.

Luria, S. E. & Burrous, J. W. (1957). Hybridization between *Escherichia coli* and Shigella. *J. Bact.* **74**, 461.

Lwoff, A. (1939). Revision et démembrement des Hemophilae, le genre *Moraxella nov. gen. Annls Inst. Pasteur, Paris*, **62**, 168.

Lwoff, A. (1958). L'espèce bactérienne. *Annls Inst. Pasteur, Paris*, **94**, 137.

Lysenko, O. (1961). *Pseudomonas* – An attempt at a general classification. *J. gen. Microbiol.* **25**, 379.

MacConkey, A. T. (1908). Bile salt media and their advantages in some bacteriological examinations. *J. Hyg., Camb.* **8**, 322.

Macfarlane, R. G., Oakley, C. L. & Anderson, C. G.

(1941). Haemolysis and the production of opalescence in serum and lecitho-vitellin by the α toxin of *Clostridium welchii. J. Path. Bact.* **52**, 99.

McGaughey, C. A. & Chu, H. P. (1948). The egg-yolk reaction of aerobic sporing bacilli. *J. gen. Microbiol.* **2**, 334.

McIntosh, J. (1920). A litmus solution suitable for bacteriological purposes. *Br. J. exp. Path.* **1**, 70.

McIntosh, J., James, W. W. & Lazarus-Barlow, P. (1922). An investigation into the aetiology of dental caries. I: The nature of the destructive agent and the production of artificial caries. *Br. J. exp. Path.* **3**, 138.

Maclean, P. D., Liebow, A. A. & Rosenberg, A. A. (1946). A hemolytic corynebacterium resembling *Corynebacterium ovis* and *Corynebacterium pyogenes* in man. *J. infect. Dis.* **79**, 69.

McLeod, J. W. (1947). Smear and culture diagnosis in gonorrhoea. *Br. J. vener. Dis.* **23**, 53.

McLeod, J. W., Coates, J. C., Happold, F. C., Priestly, D. P. & Wheatley, B. (1934). Cultivation of the gonococcus as a method in the diagnosis of gonorrhoea with special reference to the oxydase reaction and to the value of air reinforced in its carbon dioxide content. *J. Path. Bact.* **39**, 221.

Madison, R. R. (1935). Fibrinolytic staphylococci. *Proc. Soc. exp. Biol. Med.* **33**, 209.

Madison, R. R. & Dart, E. E. (1936). Veterinary staphylo-fibrinolysin. *Proc. Soc. exp. Biol. Med.* **34**, 299.

Mahl, M. C., Wilson, P. W., Fife, M. A. & Ewing, W. H. (1965). Nitrogen fixation by members of the tribe Klebsielleae. *J. Bact.* **89**, 1482.

Mair, W. (1917). The preparation of desoxycholic acid. *Biochem. J.* **11**, 11.

Málek, I., Radochová, M. & Lysenko, O. (1963). Taxonomy of the species *Pseudomonas odorans. J. gen. Microbiol.* **33**, 349.

Man, J. C. de, Rogosa, M. & Sharpe, M. E. (1960). A medium for the cultivation of lactobacilli. *J. appl. Bact.* **23**, 130.

Manclark, C. R. & Pickett, M. J. (1961). Diagnostic bacteriological screening procedures. *Lab. Wld*, **12**, 446.

Marandon, J.-L. & Oeding, P. (1966). Investigations on animal *Staphylococcus aureus* strains. 1. Biochemical characteristics and phage typing. *Acta path. microbiol. scand.* **67**, 149.

Marcus, S. & Greaves, C. (1950). Danger of false results using screw-capped tubes in diagnostic bacteriology. *J. Lab. clin. Med.* **36**, 134.

Marks, J. & Richards, M. (1962). Classification of the anonymous mycobacteria as a guide to their significance. *Mon. Bull. Minist. Hlth* **21**, 200.

Marks, J. & Trollope, D. R. (1960). A study of the 'anonymous' mycobacteria. I. Introduction; colonial characteristics and morphology; growth rates; biochemical tests. *Tubercle, Lond.* **41**, 51.

Marmur, J., Falkow, S. & Mandel, M. (1963). New approaches to bacterial taxonomy. *A. Rev. Microbiol.* **17**, 329.

Marshall, J. H. & Kelsey, J. C. (1960). A standard culture medium for general bacteriology. *J. Hyg., Camb.* **58**, 367.

Martin, W. J., Bartes, S. F. & Ball, M. M. (1971). Evaluation of reagent-impregnated strips for identification of Enterobacteriaceae. *Am. J. med. Technol.* **37**, 99.

Martin, W. J., Mock, W. E. & Ewing, W. H. (1968). Antigenic analysis of *Shigella sonnei* by gel diffusion technics. *Can. J. Microbiol.* **14**, 737.

Matsen, J. M. (1970). Ten-minute test for differentiating between *Klebsiella* and *Enterobacter* isolates. *Appl. Microbiol.* **19**, 438.

Matsen, J. M., Blazevic, D. J., Ryan, J. A. & Ewing, W. H. (1972). Characterization of indole-positive *Proteus mirabilis. Appl. Microbiol.* **23**, 592.

Matthews, P. R. J. & Pattison, I. H. (1961). The identification of a Haemophilus-like organism associated with pneumonia and pleurisy in the pig. *J. comp. Path. Ther.* **71**, 44.

Maxted, W. R. (1948). Preparation of streptococcal extracts for Lancefield grouping. *Lancet*, ii, 255.

Maxted, W. R. (1953). The use of bacitracin for identifying group A haemolytic streptococci. *J. clin. Path.* **6**, 224.

Mayr, E. (1968). The role of systematics in biology. *Science, N.Y.* **159**, 595.

Medrek, T. F. & Barnes, E. M. (1962). The influence of the growth medium on the demonstration of a group D antigen in faecal streptococci. *J. gen. Microbiol.* **28**, 701.

Melville, T. H. (1965). A study of the overall similarity of certain actinomycetes mainly of oral origin. *J. gen. Microbiol.* **40**, 309.

Merkel, J. R., Traganza, E. D., Mukherjee, B. B., Griffin, T. B. & Prescott, J. M. (1964). Proteolytic activity and general characteristics of a marine bacterium, *Aeromonas proteolytica* sp. n. *J. Bact.* **87**, 1227.

Merlino, C. P. (1924). Bartolomeo Bizio's letter to the most eminent priest, Angelo Bellani, concerning the phenomenon of the red-colored polenta. *J. Bact.* **9**, 527.

Messer, A. I. (1947). Formalin in filter paper. *Mon. Bull. Minist. Hlth* **6**, 94.

Meyer, M. E. & Cameron, H. S. (1961*a*). Metabolic characterization of the genus *Brucella*. I. Statistical evaluation of the oxidative rates by which type I of each species can be identified. *J. Bact.* **82**, 387.

Meyer, M. E. & Cameron, H. S. (1961*b*). Metabolic characterization of the genus *Brucella*. II. Oxidative metabolic patterns of the described species. *J. Bact.* **82**, 396.

Meyer, W. (1967*a*). *Staphylococcus aureus* strains of phage-group IV. *J. Hyg., Camb.* **65**, 439.

Meyer, W. (1967*b*). A proposal for subdividing the species *Staphylococcus aureus*. *Int. J. syst. Bact.* **17**, 387.

Meynell, G. G. & Meynell, E. (1965). *Theory and Practice in Experimental Bacteriology*, **1** edn, 1965; **2** edn, 1970. London: Cambridge University Press.

Middlebrook, G., Dubos, R. J. & Pierce, C. (1947). Virulence and morphological characteristics of mammalian tubercle bacilli. *J. exp. Med.* **86**, 175.

Middleton, G. & Stuckey, R. E. (1951). The standardisation of the digestion process in the Kjeldahl determination of nitrogen. *J. Pharm. Pharmac.* **3**, 829.

Midgley, J. (1966). The sensitivity to basic dyes of *Pasteurella* and some other Gram-negative genera. *Publs Fac. Sci. Univ. J. E. Purkyne, Brno*, **K 38**, 282.

Midgley, J., Lapage, S. P., Jenkins, B. A. G., Barrow, G. I., Roberts, M. E. & Buck, A. G. (1970). *Cardiobacterium hominis* endocarditis. *J. med. Microbiol.* **3**, 91.

Miles, A. A. (1965). Introductory essay on microbiological media: Good Food Guide. *Lab. Pract.* **14**, 688.

Miles, A. A. & Misra, S. S. (1938). The estimation of the bactericidal power of the blood. *J. Hyg., Camb.* **38**, 732.

Mirick, G. S., Thomas, L., Curnen, E. C. & Horsfall, F. L., Jr (1944). Studies of a non-hemolytic streptococcus isolated from the respiratory tract of human beings. I. Biological characteristics of Streptococcus MG. *J. exp. Med.* **80**, 391.

Mitchell, M. S., Rhoden, D. L. & King, E. O. (1965). Lactose-fermenting organisms resembling *Neisseria meningitidis*. *J. Bact.* **90**, 560.

Mitchell, R. G. & Clarke, S. K. R. (1965). An Alcaligenes species with distinctive properties isolated from human sources. *J. gen. Microbiol.* **40**, 343.

Moeller, H. (1891). Ueber eine neue Methode der Sporenfärbung. *Zentbl. Bakt. ParasitKde Abt. I,* **10**, 273.

Mollaret, H. H. & Chevalier, A. (1964). Contribution a l'étude d'un nouveau groupe de germes proches du bacille du Malassez et Vignal. I. Caractères culturaux et biochimiques. *Annls Inst. Pasteur, Paris,* **107**, 121.

Mollaret, H. H. & Lucas, A. (1965). Sur les particularités biochimiques des souches de *Yersinia enterocolitica* isolées chez les lièvres. *Annls Inst. Pasteur, Paris,* **108**, 121.

Møller, V. (1954*a*). Activity determination of amino acid decarboxylases in Enterobacteriaceae. *Acta path. microbiol. scand.* **34**, 102.

Møller, V. (1954*b*). Diagnostic use of the Braun KCN test within the Enterobacteriaceae. *Acta path. microbiol. scand.* **34**, 115.

Møller, V. (1954*c*). Distribution of amino acid decarboxylases in Enterobacteriaceae. *Acta path. microbiol. scand.* **35**, 259.

Møller, V. (1955). Simplified tests for some amino acid decarboxylases and for the arginine dihydrolase system. *Acta path. microbiol. scand.* **36**, 158.

de Moor, C. E. (1949). Paracholera (El Tor): enteritis choleriformis El Tor van Loghem. *Bull. World Hlth Org.* **2**, 5.

Moore, H. B. & Pickett, M. J. (1960). Organisms resembling *Alcaligenes faecalis*. *Can. J. Microbiol.* **6**, 43.

Moore, H. F. (1915). The action of ethylhydrocuprein (optochin) on type strains of pneumococci in vitro and in vivo, and on some other microorganisms in vitro. *J. exp. Med.* **22**, 269.

Moore, W. E. C. & Cato, E. P. (1963). Validity of *Propionibacterium acnes* (Gilchrist) Douglas and Gunter comb. nov. *J. Bact.* **85**, 870.

Moore, W. E. C., Cato, E. P. & Holdeman, L. V. (1966). Fermentation patterns of some *Clostridium* species. *Int. J. syst. Bact.* **16**, 383.

Moore, W. E. C., Holdeman, L. V. & Cummins, C. S. (1968). Objection: *Corynebacterium acnes* is not the sole legitimate anaerobic species of *Corynebacterium*. *Int. J. syst. Bact.* **18**, 273.

Mordarska, H., Mordarski, M. & Goodfellow, M. (1972). Chemotaxonomic characters and classification of some nocardioform bacteria. *J. gen. Microbiol.* **71**, 77.

Moreira-Jacob, M. (1963). Safranine O: reliable selective dye for characterization of *Brucella suis*. *J. Bact.* **86**, 599.

Morgan, H. de R. (1906). Upon the bacteriology of the summer diarrhoea of infants. *Br. med. J.* i, 908.

Morgan, W. J. B. & Gower, S. G. M. (1966). Techniques in the identification and classification of *Brucella*. In *Identification Methods for Microbiologists*, part A, p. 35. Edited by B. M. Gibbs & F. A. Skinner. London: Academic Press.

Morse, M. L. & Weaver, R. H. (1950). Rapid micro-technics for identification of cultures. III. Hydrogen sulfide production. *Am. J. clin. Path.* **20**, 481.

Moussa, R. S. (1959). Antigenic formulae for *Clostridium septicum* and *Clostridium chauvoei*. *J. Path. Bact.* **77**, 341.

Much, H. (1908). Über eine Vorstufe des Fibrinfermentes in Kulturen von Staphylokokkus aureus. *Biochem. Z.* **14**, 143.

Mudge, C. S. (1917). The effect of sterilization upon sugars in culture media. *J. Bact.* **2**, 403.

Mukerjee, S. (1963). The bacteriophage-susceptibility test in differentiating *Vibrio cholerae* and *Vibrio el tor*. *Bull. Wld Hlth Org.* **28**, 333.

Mulczyk, M. & Szewczuk, A. (1970). Pyrrolidonyl peptidase in bacteria: a new col[o]rimetric test for differentiation of Enterobacteriaceae. *J. gen. Microbiol.* **61**, 9.

Muraschi, T. F., Friend, M. & Bolles, D. (1965). *Erwinia*-like microorganisms isolated from animal and human hosts. *Appl. Microbiol.* **13**, 128.

Murray, E. G. D. (1918). An attempt at classification of *Bacillus dysenteriae*, based upon an examination of the agglutinating properties of fifty-three strains. *J.R. Army med. Cps*, **31**, 257, 353.

Murray, E. G. D., Webb, R. A. & Swann, M. B. R. (1926). A disease of rabbits characterized by a large mononuclear leucocytosis, caused by a hitherto undescribed bacillus *Bacterium monocytogenes* (n. sp.). *J. Path. Bact.* **29**, 407.

Nagler, F. P. O. (1939). Observations on a reaction between the lethal toxin of *Cl. welchii* (type A) and human serum. *Br. J. exp. Path.* **20**, 473.

Nakagawa, A. & Kitahara, K. (1959). Taxonomic studies on the genus *Pediococcus*. *J. gen. appl. Microbiol., Tokyo*, **5**, 95.

Nakhla, L. S. (1973). A serological method for distinguishing coagulase-negative staphylococci from micrococci. *J. clin. Path.* **26**, 511.

Narayan, K. G., Guinée, P. A. M. & Mossel, D. A. A. (1967). Use of reagent-impregnated ('Patho-Tec') test papers in the identification of Enterobacteriaceae and similar bacteria. *Antonie van Leeuwenhoek*, **33**, 184.

National Collection of Type Cultures (1972). *Catalogue*. London: Her Majesty's Stationery Office.

Newsom, I. E. & Cross, F. (1932). Some bipolar organisms found in pneumonia in sheep. *J. Am. vet. med. Ass.* **80**, 715.

Nielsen, B. B. (1971). Et nyt engangs-forgæringssystem til identifikation af salmonellabakterier (Enterobacteriaceae). *Særtryk af Medlemsblad for Den danske Dyrlægeforening*, **54**, 951.

Niléhn, B. (1967). Studies on *Yersinia enterocolitica*. Characterization of 28 strains from human and animal sources. *Acta path. microbiol. scand.* **69**, 83.

Niven, C. F., Jr, Kiziuta, Z. & White, J. C. (1946). Synthesis of a polysaccharide from sucrose by Streptococcus s.b.e. *J. Bact.* **51**, 711.

Niven, C. F., Jr, Smiley, K. L. & Sherman, J. M. (1941). The production of large amounts of a polysaccharid by *Streptococcus salivarius*. *J. Bact.* **41**, 479.

Niven, C. F., Jr, Smiley, K. L. & Sherman, J. M. (1942). The hydrolysis of arginine by streptococci. *J. Bact.* **43**, 651.

Nowlan, S. S. & Deibel, R. H. (1967). Group Q streptococci. I. Ecology, serology, physiology, and relationships to established enterococci. *J. Bact.* **93**, 291.

Nyberg, C. (1934–5). *Bacillus faecalis alcaligenes* Petruschky. *Zentbl. Bakt. ParasitKde Abt. I*, **133**, 443.

Oakley, C. L. & Warrack, G. H. (1959). The soluble antigens of *Clostridium oedematiens* type D (*Cl. haemolyticum*). *J. Path. Bact.* **78**, 543.

Oakley, C. L., Warrack, G. H. & Clarke, P. H. (1947). The toxins of *Clostridium oedematiens* (*Cl. novyi*). *J. gen. Microbiol.* **1**, 91.

Oberhofer, T. R. & Maddox, L. (1970). Combined medium to determine deoxyribonuclease activity and phenylalanine deamination. *Appl. Microbiol.* **19**, 385.

Obituary: Robert E. Buchanan, 1883–1973. (1973). *J. gen. Microbiol.* **77**, 1.

O'Connor, J. J., Willis, A. T. & Smith, J. A. (1966). Pigmentation of *Staphylococcus aureus*. *J. Path. Bact.* **92**, 585.

Oeding, P. (1952). Serological typing of staphylococci. *Acta path. microbiol. scand.* Suppl. **93**, 356.

Oeding, P. (1960). Antigenic properties of *Staphylococcus aureus*. *Bact. Rev.* **24**, 374.

Okell, C. C. & Parish, H. J. (1926). The virulence testing of the diphtheria bacillus and its practical application. *J. Hyg., Camb.* **25**, 355.

Oldroyd, H. (1966). The future of taxonomic entomology. *Syst. Zool.* **15**, 253.

Olds, R. J. (1966). An information sorter for identifying bacteria. In *Identification Methods for Microbiologists*, part A, p. 131. Edited by B. M. Gibbs & F. A. Skinner. London: Academic Press.

Olds, R. J. (1970). Identification of bacteria with the aid of an improved information sorter. In *Automation, Mechanization and Data Handling in Microbiology*, p. 85. Edited by A. Baillie & R. J. Gilbert. London: Academic Press.

O'Meara, R. A. Q. (1931). A simple delicate and rapid method of detecting the formation of acetylmethylcarbinol by bacteria fermenting carbohydrate. *J. Path. Bact.* **34**, 401.

O'Meara, R. A. Q. & MacSween, J. C. (1936). The failure of staphylococcus to grow from small inocula in routine laboratory media. *J. Path. Bact.* **43**, 373.

O'Meara, R. A. Q. & MacSween, J. C. (1937). The influence of copper in peptones on the growth of certain pathogens in peptone broth. *J. Path. Bact.* **44**, 225.

Opinion A (1958). Conservation of the generic name *Bacillus* Cohn 1872, designation of the type species, and of the type strain of the species. In *International Code of Nomenclature of Bacteria and Viruses.* Ames: Iowa State College Press.

Opinion 4 (revised) (1954). Rejection of the generic name *Bacterium*. *Int. Bull. bact. Nomencl. Taxon.* **4**, 141.

Opinion 16 (1958). Conservation of the generic name *Chromobacterium* Bergonzini 1880 and designation of the type species and the neotype culture of the type species. *Int. Bull. bact. Nomencl. Taxon.* **8**, 151.

Opinion 32 (1970). Conservation of the specific epithet *rhusiopathiae* in the scientific name of the organism known as *Erysipelothrix rhusiopathiae* (Migula 1900) Buchanan 1918. *Int. J. syst. Bact.* **20**, 9.

Opinion 46 (1971). Rejection of the generic name *Aerobacter* Beijerinck. *Int. J. syst. Bact.* **21**, 110.

Orcutt, M. L. & Howe, P. E. (1922). Hemolytic action of a staphylococcus due to a fat-splitting enzyme. *J. exp. Med.* **35**, 409.

Orfila, J. & Courden, B. (1961). Contribution au diagnostic différentiel d'*Hemophilus influenzae* et d'*Hemophilus aegyptius*. *Annls Inst. Pasteur, Paris*, **100**, 252.

Orla-Jensen, S. (1919). *The lactic acid bacteria.* Copenhagen: Andr. Fred. Høst & Søn.

Orr Ewing, J. & Taylor, J. (1945). Variations in the fermentative reactions of antigenically identical strains of *Bact. newcastle*. *Mon. Bull. Emerg. publ. Hlth Lab. Serv.* **4**, 130.

Ørskov, I. (1955). The biochemical properties of Klebsiella (Klebsiella–aerogenes) strains. *Acta path. microbiol. scand.* **37**, 353.

Ørskov, I. (1957). Biochemical types in the Klebsiella group. *Acta path. microbiol. scand.* **40**, 155.

Ortali, V. & Samarani, E. (1955). Micrometodi in microbiologia – I. Determinazione della ureasi. *Rc. Ist. sup. Sanità*, **18**, 1301.

Ottens, H. & Winkler, K. C. (1962). Indifferent and haemolytic streptococci possessing group-antigen F. *J. gen. Microbiol.* **28**, 181.

Owens, J. D. & Keddie, R. M. (1969). The nitrogen nutrition of soil and herbage coryneform bacteria. *J. appl. Bact.* **32**, 338.

Page, M. I. & King, E. O. (1966). Infection due to *Actinobacillus actinomycetemcomitans* and *Haemophilus aphrophilus*. *New Engl. J. Med.* **275**, 181.

Paine, F. S. (1927). The destruction of acetyl-methyl-carbinol by members of the colon-aerogenes group. *J. Bact.* **13**, 269.

Panton, P. N. & Valentine, F. C. O. (1932). Staphylococcal toxin. *Lancet*, i, 506.

Park, R. W. A. (1967). A comparison of two methods for detecting attack on glucose by pseudomonads and achromobacters. *J. gen. Microbiol.* **46**, 355.

Park, R. W. A. & Billing, E. (1965). Media for *Pseudomonas* and related organisms. *Lab. Pract.* **14**, 702.

Park, R. W. A., Munro, I. B., Melrose, D. R. & Stewart, D. L. (1962). Observations on the ability of two biochemical types of *Vibrio fetus* to proliferate in the genital tract of cattle and their importance with respect to infertility. *Br. vet. J.* **118**, 411.

Parnas, J. (1961). Differentiation of brucellae by the aid of phages. *J. Bact.* **82**, 319.

Parr, L. W. (1936). Sanitary significance of the succession of coli–aerogenes organisms in fresh and stored feces. *Am. J. publ. Hlth*, **26**, 39.

Pattyn, S. R. (1965). Comportement de diverses espèces de mycobactéries après injection dans la patte de la souris. *Annls Inst. Pasteur, Paris*, **109**, 309.

Payne, L. C. (1963). Towards medical automation. *Wld med. Electron.* **2**, 6.

Pedersen, M. M., Marso, E. & Pickett, M. J. (1970). Nonfermentative bacilli associated with man: III. Pathogenicity and antibiotic susceptibility. *Am. J. clin. Path.* **54**, 178.

Pederson, C. S. (1949). The genus *Pediococcus*. *Bact. Rev.* **13**, 225.

Pederson, C. S. & Breed, R. S. (1928). The fermentation of glucose by organisms of the genus *Serratia*. *J. Bact.* **16**, 163.

Peffers, A. S. R., Bailey, J., Barrow, G. I. & Hobbs, B. C. (1973). *Vibrio parahaemolyticus* gastroenteritis and international air travel. *Lancet*, i, 143.

Pelczar, M. J., Jr (1953). *Neisseria caviae* nov. spec. *J. Bact.* **65**, 744.

Phillips, J. E. (1960). The characterisation of *Actinobacillus lignieresi*. *J. Path. Bact.* **79**, 331.

Phillips, J. E. (1961). The commensal role of *Actinobacillus lignieresi*. *J. Path. Bact.* **82**, 205.

Pickett, M. J. (1955). Fermentation tests for identification of Brucellae. *Am. J. med. Technol.* **21**, 166.

Pickett, M. J. (1970). Buffered substrates in determinative bacteriology. In *Rapid Diagnostic Methods in Medical Microbiology*. Edited by C. D. Graber. Baltimore: The Williams & Wilkins Co.

Pickett, M. J. & Goodman, R. E. (1966). β-galacto-sidase for distinguishing between *Citrobacter* and *Salmonella*. *Appl. Microbiol.* **14**, 178.

Pickett, M. J. & Manclark, C. R. (1965). Tribe Mimeae. An illegitimate epithet. *Am. J. clin. Path.* **43**, 161.

Pickett, M. J. & Manclark, C. R. (1970). Nonfermenta-tive bacilli associated with man: I. Nomenclature. *Am. J. clin. Path.* **54**, 155.

Pickett, M. J. & Nelson, E. L. (1955). Speciation within the genus *Brucella*. IV. Fermentation of carbohy-drates. *J. Bact.* **69**, 333.

Pickett, M. J. & Pedersen, M. M. (1968). Screening procedure for partial identification of nonfermentative bacilli associated with man. *Appl. Microbiol.* **16**, 1631.

Pickett, M. J. & Pedersen, M. M. (1970a). Nonfer-mentative bacilli associated with man: II. Detection and identification. *Am. J. clin. Path.* **54**, 164.

Pickett, M. J. & Pedersen, M. M. (1970b). Character-ization of saccharolytic nonfermentative bacteria associated with man. *Can. J. Microbiol.* **16**, 351.

Pickett, M. J. & Pedersen, M. M. (1970c). Salient features of nonsaccharolytic and weakly saccharolytic nonfermentative rods. *Can. J. Microbiol.* **16**, 401.

Pickett, M. J. & Scott, M. L. (1955). A medium for rapid VP tests. *Bact. Proc.* p. 110.

Pickett, M. J., Scott, M. L. & Hoyt, R. E. (1955). Tableted mediums for biochemical tests in diagnostic bacteriology. *Am. J. med. Technol.* **21**, 170.

Pickford, G. E. & Dorris, F. (1934). Micro-methods for the detection of proteases and amylases. *Science, N.Y.* **80**, 317.

Piéchaud, M. (1963). Mobilité chez les *Moraxella*. *Annls Inst. Pasteur, Paris*, **104**, 291.

Piéchaud, D. & Szturm-Rubinsten, S. (1963). Étude de quelques enterobactéries n'utilisant pas l'acide citrique. *Annls Inst. Pasteur, Paris*, **105**, 460.

Piéchaud, M. & Szturm-Rubinsten, S. (1965). De quelques caractères différentiels entre *Bordetella bronchiseptica* et *Bordetella parapertussis*. *Annls Inst. Pasteur, Paris*, **108**, 391.

Pine, L. (1970). Classification and phylogenetic rela-tionship of microaerophilic actinomycetes. *Int. J. syst. Bact.* **20**, 445.

Pine, L. & Georg, L. K. (1969). Reclassification of *Actinomyces propionicus*. *Int. J. syst. Bact.* **19**, 267.

Pine, L., Howell, A., Jr & Watson, S. J. (1960). Studies of the morphological, physiological, and biochemical characters of *Actinomyces bovis*. *J. gen. Microbiol.* **23**, 403.

Pitt, T. L. & Dey, D. (1970). A method for the detection of gelatinase production by bacteria. *J. appl. Bact.* **33**, 687.

Pittman, M. (1953). A classification of the hemolytic bacteria of the genus *Haemophilus*: *Haemophilus haemolyticus* Bergey *et al.* and *Haemophilus para-haemolyticus* nov. spec. *J. Bact.* **65**, 750.

Pittman, M. & Davis, D. J. (1950). Identification of the Koch–Weeks bacillus (*Hemophilus aegyptius*). *J. Bact.* **59**, 413.

Plimmer, H. G. & Paine, S. G. (1921). A new method for the staining of bacterial flagella. *J. Path. Bact.* **24**, 286.

Pollock, M. R. (1948). Unsaturated fatty acids in cotton wool plugs. *Nature, Lond.* **161**, 853.

Pope, C. G. & Smith, M. L. (1932). The routine preparation of diphtheria toxin of high value. *J. Path. Bact.* **35**, 573.

Pope, C. G. & Stevens, M. F. (1939). The determination of amino-nitrogen using a copper method. *Biochem. J.* **33**, 1070.

Pope, H. & Smith, D. T. (1946). Synthesis of B-complex vitamins by tubercle bacilli when grown on synthetic media. *Am. Rev. Tuberc.* **54**, 559.

Porterfield, J. S. (1950). Classification of the strepto-cocci of subacute bacterial endocarditis. *J. gen. Microbiol.* **4**, 92.

Pownall, M. (1935). A motile streptococcus. *Br. J. exp. Path.* **16**, 155.

Prefontaine, G. & Jackson, F. L. (1972). Cellular fatty acid profiles as an aid to the classification of 'corrod-ing bacilli' and certain other bacteria. *Int. J. syst. Bact.* **22**, 210.

Prentice, A. W. (1957). *Neisseria flavescens* as a cause of meningitis. *Lancet*, i, 613.

Preston, N. W. & Maitland, H. B. (1952). The influence of temperature on the motility of *Pasteurella pseudo-tuberculosis*. *J. gen. Microbiol.* **7**, 117.

Preston, N. W. & Morrell, A. (1962). Reproducible results with the Gram stain. *J. Path. Bact.* **84**, 241.

Prevorsek, M., Kronish, D. P. & Schwartz, B. S. (1968). Rapid presumptive identification of enterics with reagent impregnated paper strips. *Am. J. med. Technol.* **34**, 271.

Prévot, A.-R. (1961). *Traité de Systématique Bactérienne*. Paris: Dunod.

Priest, F. G., Somerville, H. J., Cole, J. A. & Hough, J. S. (1973). The taxonomic position of *Obesum-bacterium proteus*, a common brewery contaminant. *J. gen. Microbiol.* **75**, 295.

Proom, H. & Knight, B. C. J. G. (1955). The minimal nutritional requirements of some species in the genus *Bacillus*. *J. gen. Microbiol.* **13**, 474.

Proom, H. & Woiwod, A. J. (1951). Amine production in the genus *Proteus*. *J. gen. Microbiol.* **5**, 930.

Pugh, G. W., Jr, Hughes, D. E. & McDonald, T. J. (1966). The isolation and characterization of *Moraxella bovis*. *Am. J. vet. Res.* **27**, 957.

Puhvel, S. M. (1968). Characterization of *Corynebacterium acnes*. *J. gen. Microbiol.* **50**, 313.

Pulverer, G. & Ko, H. L. (1970). *Actinobacillus actinomycetem-comitans*: fermentative capabilities of 140 strains. *Appl. Microbiol.* **20**, 693.

Rahn, O. (1929). Contributions to the classification of bacteria. IV. Intermediate forms. *Zentbl. Bakt. ParasitKde Abt. II*, **78**, 8.

Rahn, O. (1937). New principles for the classification of bacteria. *Zentbl. Bakt. ParasitKde Abt. II*, **96**, 273.

Ralston, E., Palleroni, N. J. & Doudoroff, M. (1973). *Pseudomonas pickettii*, a new species of clinical origin related to *Pseudomonas solanacearum*. *Int. J. syst. Bact.* **23**, 15.

Rammell, C. G. (1962). Inhibition by citrate of the growth of coagulase-positive staphylococci. *J. Bact.* **84**, 1123.

Rauss, K. (1962). A proposal for the nomenclature and classification of the Proteus and Providencia groups. *Int. Bull. bact. Nomencl. Taxon.* **12**, 53.

Rauss, K. & Vörös, S. (1959). The biochemical and serological properties of *Proteus morganii*. *Acta microbiol. Acad. Sci. hung.* **6**, 233.

Rauss, K. F. (1936). The systematic position of Morgan's bacillus. *J. Path. Bact.* **42**, 183.

Reddish, G. F. & Rettger, L. F. (1924). A morphological, cultural and biochemical study of representative spore-forming anaerobic bacteria. *J. Bact.* **9**, 13.

Redfearn, M. S., Palleroni, N. J. & Stanier, R. Y. (1966). A comparative study of *Pseudononas pseudomallei* and *Bacillus mallei*. *J. gen. Microbiol.* **43**, 293.

Redmond, D. L. & Kotcher, E. (1963). Cultural and serological studies on *Haemophilus vaginalis*. *J. gen. Microbiol.* **33**, 77.

Reed, G. B. & Orr, J. H. (1941). Rapid identification of gas gangrene anaerobes. *War. Med., Chicago*, **1**, 493.

Reed, R. W. (1942). Nitrate, nitrite and indole reactions of gas gangrene anaerobes. *J. Bact.* **44**, 425.

Report (1953). Diphtheria and pertussis vaccination. Report of a conference of heads of laboratories producing diphtheria and pertussis vaccines. *Tech. Rep. Wld Hlth Org.* no. 61.

Report (1954a). Reports of the Enterobacteriaceae Sub-Committee on the groups Salmonella, Shigella, Arizona, Bethesda, Ballerup, Escherichia, Alkalescens–Dispar, Klebsiella, and Proteus in Rio de Janeiro, August, 1950. *Int. Bull. bact. Nomencl. Taxon.* **4**, 1.

Report (1954b). Reports on the groups: Salmonella, Shigella, Arizona, Bethesda, Escherichia, Klebsiella (Aerogenes, Aerobacter), Providence (29911 of Stuart *et al.*). *Int. Bull. bact. Nomencl. Taxon.* **4**, 47.

Report (1956a). *Constituents of Bacteriological Culture Media*. Special report Society for General Microbiology. London: Cambridge University Press.

Report (1956b). The nomenclature of coli–aerogenes bacteria. Report of the Coli–aerogenes (1956) Sub-Committee of the Society for Applied Bacteriology. *J. appl. Bact.* **19**, 108.

Report (1956c). The bacteriological examination of water supplies. *Rep. publ. Hlth med. Subj., Lond.* no. 71. (Revised 1969.)

Report (1958). Report of the Enterobacteriaceae Sub-committee of the Nomenclature Committee of the International Association of Microbiological Societies. *Int. Bull. bact. Nomencl. Taxon.* **8**, 25.

Reuter, G. (1971). Designation of type strains for *Bifidobacterium* species. *Int. J. syst. Bact.* **21**, 273.

Reyn, A. (1970). Taxonomic position of *Neisseria haemolysans* (Thjøtta & Bøe, 1938). *Int. J. syst. Bact.* **20**, 19.

Rhodes, M. (1950). Viability of dried bacterial cultures. *J. gen. Microbiol.* **4**, 450.

Rhodes, M. E. (1958). The cytology of *Pseudomonas* spp. as revealed by a silver-plating staining method. *J. gen. Microbiol.* **18**, 639.

Richard, C. (1965). Mesure de l'activité ureasique des *Proteus* au moyen de la réaction phénol-hypochlorite de Berthelot. Intérêt taxinomique. *Annls Inst. Pasteur, Paris*, **109**, 516.

Richard, C. (1966). Caractères biochimiques des biotypes de *Providencia*; leurs rapports avec le genre *Rettgerella*. *Annls Inst. Pasteur, Paris*, **110**, 105.

Richard, C. (1968). Techniques rapides de recherche des lysine-décarboxylase, ornithine-décarboxylase et arginine-dihydrolase dans les genres *Pseudomonas*, *Alcaligenes* et *Moraxella*. *Annls Inst. Pasteur, Paris*, **114**, 425.

Riddle, J. W., Kabler, P. W., Kenner, B. A., Bordner, R. H., Rockwood, S. W. & Stevenson, H. J. R. (1956). Bacterial identification by infrared spectrophotometry. *J. Bact.* **72**, 593.

Rifkind, D. & Cole, R. M. (1962). Non-beta-hemolytic group M-reacting streptococci of human origin. *J. Bact.* **84**, 163.

Riley, P. S., Tatum, H. W. & Weaver, R. E. (1973). Identity of HB-1 of King and *Eikenella corrodens* (Eiken) Jackson and Goodman. *Int. J. syst. Bact.* **23**, 75.

Roberts, G. A. & Charles, H. P. (1970). Mutants of *Neurospora crassa*, *Escherichia coli* and *Salmonella typhimurium* specifically inhibited by carbon dioxide. *J. gen. Microbiol.* **63**, 21.

Roberts, R. J. (1968). Biochemical reactions of *Corynebacterium pyogenes. J. Path. Bact.* **95**, 127.

Robertson, M. (1916). Notes upon certain anaerobes isolated from wounds. *J. Path. Bact.* **20**, 327.

Robinson, D. T. & Peeney, A. L. P. (1936). The serological types amongst *gravis* strains of *C. diphtheriae* and their distribution. *J. Path. Bact.* **43**, 403.

Robinson, W. & Woolley, P. B. (1957). Pseudohaemoptysis due to *Chromobacterium prodigiosum. Lancet*, i, 819.

Roche, A. & Marquet, F. (1935). Recherches sur le vieillissement du sérum. *C. r. Séanc. Soc. Biol.* **119**, 1147.

Rogers, K. B. & Taylor, J. (1961). Laboratory diagnosis of gastro-enteritis due to *Escherichia coli. Bull. Wld Hlth Org.* **24**, 59.

Rogosa, M. (1970). Characters used in the classification of lactobacilli. *Int. J. syst. Bact.* **20**, 519.

Rogosa, M., Franklin, J. G. & Perry, K. D. (1961). Correlation of the vitamin requirements with cultural and biochemical characters of *Lactobacillus* spp. *J. gen. Microbiol.* **25**, 473.

Rogosa, M. & Hansen, P. A. (1971). Nomenclatural considerations of certain species of *Lactobacillus* Beijerinck. Request for an Opinion. *Int. J. syst. Bact.* **21**, 177.

Rogosa, M. & Sharpe, M. E. (1959). An approach to the classification of the lactobacilli. *J. appl. Bact.* **22**, 329.

Rogosa, M. & Sharpe, M. E. (1960). Species differentiation of human vaginal lactobacilli. *J. gen. Microbiol.* **23**, 197.

Rolfe, R. & Meselson, M. (1959). The relative homogeneity of microbial DNA. *Proc. natn. Acad. Sci. U.S.A.* **45**, 1039.

Ross, H. E. (1965). *Clostridium putrefaciens*: a neglected anaerobe. *J. appl. Bact.* **28**, 49.

Ross, R. F., Hall, J. E., Orning, A. P. & Dale, S. E. (1972). Characterization of an *Actinobacillus* isolated from the sow vagina. *Int. J. syst. Bact.* **22**, 39.

Rowatt, E. (1957). The growth of *Bordetella pertussis*: a review. *J. gen. Microbiol.* **17**, 297.

Ruchhoft, C. C., Kallas, J. G., Chinn, B. & Coulter, E. W. (1931). Coli-aerogenes differentiation in water analysis. II. The biochemical differential tests and their interpretation. *J. Bact.* **22**, 125.

Russell, F. F. (1911). The isolation of typhoid bacilli from urine and feces with the description of a new double sugar tube medium. *J. med. Res.* **25**, 217.

Rustigian, R. & Stuart, C. A. (1945). The biochemical and serological relationships of the organisms of the genus *Proteus. J. Bact.* **49**, 419.

Ryan, W. J. (1964). Moraxella commonly present on the conjunctiva of guinea pigs. *J. gen. Microbiol.* **35**, 361.

Ryan, W. J. (1968). An X-factor requiring Haemophilus species. *J. gen. Microbiol.* **52**, 275.

Sakaguchi, K. & Mori, H. (1969). Comparative study on *Pediococcus halophilus, P. soyae, P. homari, P. urinae-equi* and related species. *J. gen. appl. Microbiol., Tokyo*, **15**, 159.

Sakazaki, R. (1961). Studies on the Hafnia group of Enterobacteriaceae. *Jap. J. med. Sci. Biol.* **14**, 223.

Sakazaki, R. (1965a). *Vibrio parahaemolyticus*, a non-choleragenic enteropathogenic vibrio. *Proc. Cholera Res. Symposium*, 24–9 January 1965, Honolulu. Washington, DC: US Government Printing Office.

Sakazaki, R. (1965b). *Vibrio parahaemolyticus. Isolation and Identification.* Toyko: Nihon Eiyo Kagaku.

Sakazaki, R. (1967). Studies on the Asakusa group of Enterobacteriaceae (*Edwardsiella tarda*). *Jap. J. med. Sci. Biol.* **20**, 205.

Sakazaki, R. (1968). Proposal of *Vibrio alginolyticus* for the biotype 2 of *Vibrio parahaemolyticus. Jap. J. med. Sci. Biol.* **21**, 359.

Sakazaki, R. (1969). Halophilic vibrio infections. In *Food-borne Infections and Intoxications*, p. 115. Edited by H. Riemann. New York: Academic Press.

Sakazaki, R., Gomez, C. Z. & Sebald, M. (1967). Taxonomical studies of the so-called NAG vibrios. *Jap. J. med. Sci. Biol.* **20**, 265.

Sakazaki, R., Iwanami, S. & Fukumi, H. (1963). Studies on the enteropathogenic, facultatively halophilic bacteria, *Vibrio parahaemolyticus*. I. Morphological, cultural and biochemical properties and its taxonomical position. *Jap. J. med. Sci. Biol.* **16**, 161.

Sakazaki, R., Iwanami, S. & Tamura, K. (1968). Studies on the enteropathogenic, facultatively halophilic bacteria, *Vibrio parahaemolyticus*. II. Serological characteristics. *Jap. J. med. Sci. Biol.* **21**, 313.

Sakazaki, R. & Tamura, K. (1971). Somatic antigen variation in *Vibrio cholerae. Jap. J. med. Sci. Biol.* **24**, 93.

Sakazaki, R., Tamura, K., Gomez, C. Z. & Sen, R. (1970). Serological studies on the cholera group of vibrios. *Jap. J. med. Sci. Biol.* **23**, 13.

Sakazaki, R., Tamura, K., Kato, T., Obara, Y., Yamai, S. & Hobo, K. (1968). Studies on the enteropathogenic, facultatively halophilic bacteria, *Vibrio parahaemolyticus*. III. Enteropathogenicity. *Jap. J. med. Sci. Biol.* **21**, 325.

Salmonella Subcommittee of the Nomenclature Committee of the International Society for Microbiology (1934). The genus *Salmonella* Lignières, 1900. *J. Hyg., Camb.* **34**, 333.

Samuels, S. B., Pittman, B., Tatum, H. W. & Cherry, W. B. (1972). Report on a study set of moraxellae and allied bacteria. *Int. J. syst. Bact.* **22**, 19.

Sanyal, S. C., Sakazaki, R., Prescott, L. M. & Sinha, R. (1973). Isolation of rapidly lactose-fermenting *Vibrio cholerae* strains. *J. med. Microbiol.* **6**, 119.

Sanyal, S. C., Sil, J. & Sakazaki, R. (1973). Laboratory infection by *Vibrio parahaemolyticus. J. med. Microbiol.* **6**, 121.

Scardovi, V., Trovatelli, L. D., Zani, G., Crociani, F. & Matteuzzi, D. (1971). Deoxyribonucleic acid homology relationships among species of the genus *Bifidobacterium. Int. J. syst. Bact.* **21**, 276.

Schaeffer, A. B. & Fulton, M. (1933). A simplified method of staining endospores. *Science, N.Y.* **77**, 194.

Scharmann, W. & Blobel, H. (1968). Serologische Unterschiede von Staphylokokken-Nucleasen. *Z. Naturf.* **23b**, 1230.

Schaub, I. G. & Hauber, F. D. (1948). A biochemical and serological study of a group of identical unidentifiable Gram-negative bacilli from human sources. *J. Bact.* **56**, 379.

Schindler, C. A. & Schuhardt, V. T. (1964). Lysostaphin: a new bacteriolytic agent for the staphylococcus. *Proc. natn. Acad. Sci. U.S.A.* **51**, 414.

Schneierson, S. S. & Amsterdam, D. (1964). A punch card system for identification of bacteria. *Am. J. clin. Path.* **42**, 328.

Schubert, R. H. W. (1967a). The taxonomy and nomenclature of the genus *Aeromonas* Kluyver and van Niel 1936. Part I. Suggestions on the taxonomy and nomenclature of the aerogenic *Aeromonas* species. *Int. J. syst. Bact.* **17**, 23.

Schubert, R. H. W. (1967b). The taxonomy and nomenclature of the genus *Aeromonas* Kluyver and van Niel 1936. Part II. Suggestions on the taxonomy and nomenclature of the anaerogenic aeromonads. *Int. J. syst. Bact.* **17**, 273.

Schubert, R. H. W. (1971). Status of the names *Aeromonas* and *Aerobacter liquefaciens* Beijerinck and designation of a neotype strain for *Aeromonas hydrophila* Stanier. Request for an Opinion. *Int. J. syst. Bact.* **21**, 87.

Schultes, L. M. & Evans, J. B. (1971). Deoxyribonucleic acid homology of *Aerococcus viridans. Int. J. syst. Bact.* **21**, 207.

Schütze, H. (1928). *Bacterium pseudotuberculosis rodentium.* Rezeptorenanalyse von 18 Stämmen. *Arch. Hyg. Bakt.* **100**, 181.

Schütze, H. (1932a). *B. pestis* antigens. I. The antigens and immunity reactions of *B. pestis. Br. J. exp. Path.* **13**, 284.

Schütze, H. (1932b). *B. pestis* antigens. II. Antigenic relationship of *B. pestis* and *B. pseudotuberculosis rodentium. Br. J. exp. Path.* **13**, 289.

Sedlák, J., Dlabač, V. & Motliková, M. (1965). The taxonomy of the Serratia genus. *J. Hyg. Epidem. Microbiol. Immun.* **9**, 45.

Sedlák, J., Puchmayerova-Šlajsova, M., Keleti, J. & Lüderitz, O. (1971). On the taxonomy, ecology and immunochemistry of genus Citrobacter. *J. Hyg. Epidem. Microbiol. Immun.* **15**, 366.

Seeliger, H. P. R. (1961). *Listeriosis.* Basel: Karger.

Segal, B. (1940). The utilization of acetyl methyl carbinol by *Staphylococcus albus* and *aureus. J. Bact.* **39**, 747.

Sevag, M. G. & Green, M. N. (1944). The role of carbohydrates in the development of pigment by *Staphylococcus aureus. J. Bact.* **48**, 496.

Sharpe, M. E. (1955). A serological classification of lactobacilli. *J. gen. Microbiol.* **12**, 107.

Sharpe, M. E. (1970). Cell wall and cell membrane antigens used in the classification of lactobacilli. *Int. J. syst. Bact.* **20**, 509.

Sharpe, M. E., Fryer, T. F. & Smith, D. G. (1966). Identification of the lactic acid bacteria. In *Identification Methods for Microbiologists*, part A, p. 65. Edited by B. M. Gibbs & F. A. Skinner. London: Academic Press.

Shattock, P. M. F. (1949). The streptococci of group D; the serological grouping of *Streptococcus bovis* and observations on serologically refractory group D strains. *J. gen. Microbiol.* **3**, 80.

Shaw, C. (1956). Distinction between Salmonella and Arizona by Leifson's sodium malonate medium. *Int. Bull. bact. Nomencl. Taxon.* **6**, 1.

Shaw, C. & Clarke, P. H. (1955). Biochemical classification of Proteus and Providence cultures. *J. gen. Microbiol.* **13**, 155.

Shaw, C., Stitt, J. M. & Cowan, S. T. (1951). Staphylococci and their classification. *J. gen. Microbiol.* **5**, 1010.

Sherman, J. M., Niven, C. F., Jr & Smiley, K. L. (1943). *Streptococcus salivarius* and other non-hemolytic streptococci of the human throat. *J. Bact.* **45**, 249.

Sherris, J. C., Shoesmith, J. G., Parker, M. T. & Breckon, D. (1959). Tests for the rapid breakdown of arginine by bacteria: their use in the identification of pseudomonads. *J. gen. Microbiol.* **21**, 389.

Shewan, J. M., Hobbs, G. & Hodgkiss, W. (1960). A determinative scheme for the identification of certain genera of Gram-negative bacteria, with special reference to the Pseudomonadaceae. *J. appl. Bact.* **23**, 379.

Shreeve, B. J., Ivanov, I. N. & Thompson, D. A. (1970). Biochemical reactions of different serotypes of *Pasteurella haemolytica. J. med. Microbiol.* **3**, 356.

Shuman, R. D., Nord, N., Brown, R. W. & Wessman, G. E. (1972). Biochemical and serological characteristics of Lancefield groups E, P, and U streptococci and *Streptococcus uberis. Cornell Vet.* **62**, 540.

Shuman, R. D. & Wellman, G. (1966). Status of the species name *Erysipelothrix rhusiopathiae* with request for an Opinion. *Int. J. syst. Bact.* **16**, 195.

Sierra, G. (1957). A simple method for the detection of lipolytic activity of micro-organisms and some observations on the influence of the contact between cells and fatty substrates. *Antonie van Leeuwenhoek*, **23**, 15.

Simmons, J. S. (1926). A culture medium for differentiating organisms of typhoid-colon aerogenes groups and for isolation of certain fungi. *J. infect. Dis.* **39**, 209.

Singer, J. & Bar-Chay, J. (1954). Biochemical investigation of Providence strains and their relationship to the Proteus group. *J. Hyg., Camb.* **52**, 1.

Singer, J. & Volcani, B. E. (1955). An improved ferric chloride test for differentiating Proteus-Providence group from other Enterobacteriaceae. *J. Bact.* **69**, 303.

Skadhauge, K. & Perch, B. (1959). Studies on the relationship of some alpha-haemolytic streptococci of human origin to the Lancefield group M. *Acta path. microbiol. scand.* **46**, 239.

Skerman, V. B. D. (1949). A mechanical key for the generic identification of bacteria. *Bact. Rev.* **13**, 175.

Skerman, V. B. D. (1959–67). *A Guide to the Identification of the Genera of Bacteria*, 1 edn, 1959; 2 edn, 1967. Baltimore: The Williams & Wilkins Co.

Slack, J. M. (1968). Subgroup on taxonomy of micro-aerophilic actinomycetes. Report on organization, aims and procedures. *Int. J. syst. Bact.* **18**, 253.

Slack, J. M., Landfried, S. & Gerencser, M. A. (1969). Morphological, biochemical, and serological studies on 64 strains of *Actinomyces israelii. J. Bact.* **97**, 873.

Ślopek, S. & Durlakowa, I. (1967). Studies on the taxonomy of *Klebsiella* bacilli. *Arch. Immun. Ther. exp* .**15**, 481.

Slotnick, I. J. & Dougherty, M. (1964). Further characterization of an unclassified group of bacteria causing endocarditis in man: *Cardiobacterium hominis* gen. et sp. n. *Antonie van Leeuwenhoek*, **30**, 261.

Small, N. (1968). Evaluation of PathoTec™ strips in diagnostic bacteriology. *Am. J. med. Technol.* **34**, 65.

Smibert, R. M. (1970). Cell wall composition in the classification of *Vibrio fetus. Int. J. syst. Bact.* **20**, 407.

Smith, D. G. & Shattock, P. M. F. (1962). The serological grouping of *Streptococcus equinus. J. gen. Microbiol.* **29**, 731.

Smith, G. R. (1961). The characteristics of two types of *Pasteurella haemolytica* associated with different pathological conditions in sheep. *J. Path. Bact.* **81**, 431.

Smith, H. W. (1953). Modifications of Dubos's media for the cultivation of *Mycobacterium johnei. J. Path. Bact.* **66**, 375.

Smith, I. W. (1963). The classification of 'Bacterium salmonicida'. *J. gen. Microbiol.* **33**, 263.

Smith, J. E. (1962). Characteristics of staphylococci from the nose of healthy dogs. *J. comp. Path. Ther.* **72**, 131.

Smith, J. E. & Thal, E. (1965). A taxonomic study of the genus *Pasteurella* using a numerical technique. *Acta path. microbiol. scand.* **64**, 213.

Smith, L. DS. & King, E. (1962*a*). *Clostridium innocuum*, sp. n., a spore-forming anaerobe isolated from human infections. *J. Bact.* **83**, 938.

Smith, L. DS. & King, E. O. (1962*b*). Occurrence of *Clostridium difficile* in infections of man. *J. Bact.* **84**, 65.

Smith, M. L. (1932). The effect of heat on sugar solutions used for culture media. *Biochem. J.* **26**, 1467.

Smith, N. R. (1947). The identification of sporeforming bacteria isolated from incompletely sterilized agar. *J. Bact.* **53**, 45.

Smith, N. R., Gibson, T., Gordon, R. E. & Sneath, P. H. A. (1964). Type cultures and proposed neotype cultures of some species in the genus *Bacillus. J. gen. Microbiol.* **34**, 269.

Smith, N. R., Gordon, R. E. & Clark, F. E. (1946). Aerobic mesophilic sporeforming bacteria. *U.S. Dep. Agric. Misc. Publ.* no. 559.

Smith, N. R., Gordon, R. E. & Clark, F. E. (1952). Aerobic sporeforming bacteria. *U.S. Dep. Agric. Agriculture Monograph*, no. 16.

Smith, P. B., Tomfohrde, K. M., Rhoden, D. L. & Balows, A. (1972). API system: a multitube micromethod for identification of Enterobacteriaceae. *Appl. Microbiol.* **24**, 449.

Smith, R. F., Rogers, R. R. & Bettge, C. L. (1972). Inhibition of the indole test reaction by sodium nitrite. *Appl. Microbiol.* **23**, 423.

Sneath, P. H. A. (1956). Cultural and biochemical characteristics of the genus *Chromobacterium. J. gen. Microbiol.* **15**, 70.

Sneath, P. H. A. (1957a). Some thoughts on bacterial classification. *J. gen. Microbiol.* **17**, 184.

Sneath, P. H. A. (1957b). The application of computers to taxonomy. *J. gen. Microbiol.* **17**, 201.

Sneath, P. H. A. (1960). A study of the bacterial genus *Chromobacterium. Iowa St. J. Sci.* **34**, 243.

Sneath, P. H. A. (1972). Computer taxonomy. In *Methods in Microbiology*, vol. 7A, p. 29. Edited by J. R. Norris & D. W. Ribbons. London: Academic Press.

Sneath, P. H. A. & Cowan, S. T. (1958). An electro-taxonomic survey of bacteria. *J. gen. Microbiol.* **19**, 551.

Sneath, P. H. A. & Johnson, R. (1972). The influence on numerical taxonomic similarities of errors in microbiological tests. *J. gen. Microbiol.* **72**, 377.

Sneath, P. H. A. & Johnson, R. (1973). Numerical taxonomy of *Haemophilus* and related bacteria. *Int. J. syst. Bact.* **23**, 405.

Sneath, P. H. A. & Sokal, R. R. (1962). Numerical taxonomy. *Nature, Lond.* **193**, 855.

Sneath, P. H. A., Whelan, J. P. F., Singh, R. B. & Edwards, D. (1953). Fatal infection by *Chromobacterium violaceum. Lancet*, ii, 276.

Snell, J. J. S. (1973). The distribution and identification of non-fermenting bacteria. *Publ. Hlth Lab. Serv Techn. Mon.* no. 4.

Snell, J. J. S. & Davey, P. (1971). A comparison of methods for the detection of phenylalanine deamination by Moraxella species. *J. gen. Microbiol.* **66**, 371.

Snell, J. J. S., Hill, L. R., Lapage, S. P. & Curtis, M. A. (1972). Identification of *Pseudomonas cepacia* Burkholder and its synonymy with *Pseudomonas kingii* Jonsson. *Int. J. syst. Bact.* **22**, 127.

Snell, J. J. S. & Lapage, S. P. (1971). Comparison of four methods for demonstrating glucose breakdown by bacteria. *J. gen. Microbiol.* **68**, 221.

Snell, J. J. S. & Lapage, S. P. (1973). Carbon source utilization tests as an aid to the classification of non-fermenting Gram-negative bacteria. *J. gen. Microbiol.* **74**, 9.

Snyder, M. L., Donnelly, D. & Nix, M. J. (1951). On some practical applications of impregnated, dried paper discs containing various reagents for the cultural differentiation of bacteria. *Am. J. med. Technol.* **17**, 105.

Sokal, R. R. (1965). Statistical methods in systematics. *Biol. Rev.* **40**, 337.

Sokal, R. R. & Sneath, P. H. A. (1963). *Principles of Numerical Taxonomy.* San Francisco: W. H. Freeman & Co.

Soltys, M. A. (1948). Anthrax in a laboratory worker, with observations on the possible source of infection. *J. Path. Bact.* **60**, 253.

Soule, M. H. (1932). Identity of *Bacillus subtilis*, Cohn 1872. *J. infect. Dis.* **51**, 191.

Spicer, C. C. (1956). A quick method of identifying Salmonella H antigens. *J. clin. Path.* **9**, 378.

Spray, R. S. & Johnson, E. J. (1946). The preparation of Loeffler's serum and similar coagulable mediums. *J. Bact.* **52**, 141.

Stableforth, A. W. & Jones, L. M. (1963). Report of the Subcommittee on taxonomy of the genus *Brucella. Int. Bull. bact. Nomencl. Taxon.* **13**, 145.

Stanbridge, T. N. & Preston, N. W. (1969). The motility of some Clostridium species. *J. gen. Microbiol.* **55**, 29.

Stanford, J. L. & Beck, A. (1969). Bacteriological and serological studies of fast growing mycobacteria identified as *Mycobacterium friedmannii. J. gen. Microbiol.* **58**, 99.

Stanford, J. L., Pattyn, S. R., Portaels, F. & Gunthorpe, W. J. (1972). Studies on *Mycobacterium chelonei. J. med. Microbiol.* **5**, 177.

Stanier, R. Y., Palleroni, N. J. & Doudoroff, M. (1966). The aerobic pseudomonads: a taxonomic study. *J. gen. Microbiol.* **43**, 159.

Starr, M. P. & Mandel, M. (1969). DNA base composition and taxonomy of phytopathogenic and other enterobacteria. *J. gen. Microbiol.* **56**, 113.

Steel, K. J. (1958). A note on the assay of some sulphydryl compounds. *J. Pharm. Pharmac.* **10**, 574.

Steel, K. J. (1961). The oxidase reaction as a taxonomic tool. *J. gen. Microbiol.* **25**, 297.

Steel, K. J. (1962a). The practice of bacterial identification. *Symp. Soc. gen. Microbiol.* **12**, 405.

Steel, K. J. (1962b). The oxidase activity of staphylococci. *J. appl. Bact.* **25**, 445.

Steel, K. J. (1963). Serological classification of *Pasteurella pseudotuberculosis* and *Pasteurella septica. Mon. Bull. Minist. Hlth*, **22**, 176.

Steel, K. J. (1965). Microbial identification. *J. gen. Microbiol.* **40**, 143.

Steel, K. J. & Cowan, S. T. (1964). Le rattachement de *Bacterium anitratum, Moraxella lwoffi, Bacillus mallei* et *Haemophilus parapertussis* au genre *Acinetobacter* Brisou et Prévot. *Annls Inst. Pasteur, Paris*, **106**, 479.

Steel, K. J. & Fisher, P. J. (1961). A fallacy of the nitrate reduction test. *Mon. Bull. Minist. Hlth*, **20**, 63.

Steel, K. J. & Midgley, J. (1962). Decarboxylase and other reactions of some Gram-negative rods. *J. gen. Microbiol.* **29**, 171.

Sterne, M. & Warrack, G. H. (1964). The types of *Clostridium perfringens. J. Path. Bact.* **88**, 279.

Stewart, D. J. (1965). The urease activity of fluorescent pseudomonads. *J. gen. Microbiol.* **41**, 169.

Stokes, E. J. (1958). Anaerobes in routine diagnostic cultures. *Lancet*, i, 668.

Stokes, E. J. (1960, 1968*a*). *Clinical Bacteriology*, 2 edn, 1960; 3 edn, 1968. London: Edward Arnold.

Stokes, E. J. (1968*b*). Quality control in diagnostic bacteriology. *Proc. R. Soc. Med.* **61**, 457.

Street, C. & Goldner, M. (1973). The recognition of *Streptococcus mutans. Can. J. publ. Hlth*, **64,** 48.

Stuart, C. A., Formal, S. & McGann, V. (1949). Further studies on B5W, an anaerogenic group in the Enterobacteriaceae. *J. infect. Dis.* **84**, 235.

Stuart, C. A. & Rustigian, R. (1943*a*). Further studies on one type of paracolon organism. *Am. J. publ. Hlth*, 33, 1323.

Stuart, C. A. & Rustigian, R. (1943*b*). Further studies on the Eijkman reactions of Shigella cultures. *J. Bact.* **46**, 105.

Stuart, C. A., van Stratum, E. & Rustigian, R. (1945). Further studies on urease production by Proteus and related organisms. *J. Bact.* **49**, 437.

Stuart, C. A., Wheeler, K. M. & McGann, V. (1946). Further studies on one anaerogenic paracolon organism, type 29911. *J. Bact.* **52**, 431.

Stuart, M. R. (1970). Some taxonomic aspects of *Listeria monocytogenes*. Thesis, University of Birmingham.

Stuart, M. R. & Pease, P. E. (1972). A numerical study on the relationships of *Listeria* and *Erysipelothrix*. *J. gen. Microbiol.* **73**, 551.

Stuart, R. D. (1959). Transport medium for specimens in public health bacteriology. *Publ. Hlth Rep., Wash.* **74**, 431.

Subcommittee on Taxonomy of staphylococci and micrococci [of the International Committee on Bacteriological Nomenclature] (1965). Recommendations. *Int. Bull. bact. Nomencl. Taxon.* **15**, 109.

Sulkin, S. E. & Willett, J. C. (1940). A triple sugar–ferrous sulfate medium for use in identification of enteric organisms. *J. Lab. clin. Med.* **25**, 649.

Sutter, V. L. & Foecking, F. J. (1962). Biochemical characteristics of lactose-fermenting *Proteus rettgeri* from clinical specimens. *J. Bact.* **83**, 933.

Swan, A. (1954). The use of a bile–aesculin medium and of Maxted's technique of Lancefield grouping in the identification of enterococci (group D streptococci). *J. clin. Path.* **7**, 160.

Szturm-Rubinsten, S. (1963). Les biotypes de *Shigella sonnei. Annls Inst. Pasteur, Paris*, **104**, 423.

Szturm-Rubinsten, S. & Piéchaud, D. (1962). Sur l'utilisation du lactose par les germes du groupe *Alkalescens–Dispar. Annls Inst. Pasteur, Paris*, **103**, 935.

Szturm-Rubinsten, S. & Piéchaud, D. (1963). Observations sur la recherche de la β-galactosidase dans le genre *Shigella. Annls Inst. Pasteur, Paris*, **104**, 284.

Talley, A. J. (1968). Bacteriophage for the recognition of Salmonella and Arizona. *Am. J. med. Technol.* **34**, 542.

Tarshis, M. S., Kinsella, P. C. & Parker, M. V. (1953). Blood media for the cultivation of *Mycobacterium tuberculosis.* VII. Comparison of blood agar–penicillin and Lowenstein–Jensen media under routine diagnostic conditions. *J. Bact.* **66**, 448.

Taylor, A. W. (1950). Observations on the isolation of *Mycobacterium johnei* in primary culture. *J. Path. Bact.* **62**, 647.

Taylor, C. B. (1945–6). The effect of temperature of incubation on the results of tests for differentiating species of coliform bacteria. *J. Hyg., Camb.* **44**, 109.

Taylor, C. B. (1951). The soft-rot bacteria of the coli-aerogenes group. *Proc. Soc. appl. Bact.* **14**, 95.

Taylor, C. E. D., Lea, D. J., Heimer, G. V. & Tomlinson, A. J. H. (1964). A comparison of a fluorescent antibody technique with a cultural method in the detection of infections with *Shigella sonnei. J. clin. Path.* **17**, 225.

Taylor, J. (1961). Host specificity and enteropathogenicity of *Escherichia coli. J. appl. Bact.* **24**, 316.

Taylor, J. (1966). Host–parasite relations of *Escherichia coli* in man. *J. appl. Bact.* **29**, 1.

Taylor, W. I. (1965). Isolation of shigellae. I. Xylose lysine agars; new media for isolation of enteric pathogens. *Am. J. clin. Path.* **44**, 471.

Taylor, W. I. & Harris, B. (1965). Isolation of shigellae. II. Comparison of plating media and enrichment broths. *Am. J. clin. Path.* **44**, 476.

Thirst, M. L. (1957*a*). Hippurate hydrolysis in Klebsiella–Cloaca classification. *J. gen. Microbiol.* **17**, 390.

Thirst, M. L. (1957*b*). Gelatin liquefaction: a microtest. *J. gen. Microbiol.* **17**, 396.

Thjøtta, Th. (1920). On the bacillus of Morgan No. 1 – a metacolon-bacillus. *J. Bact.* **5**, 67.

Thjøtta, Th. & Bøe, J. (1938). *Neisseria hemolysans*. A hemolytic species of *Neisseria* Trevisan. *Acta path. microbiol. scand.* Suppl. 37, 527.

Thom, A. R., Stephens, M. E., Gillespie, W. A. & Alder, V. G. (1971). Nitrofurantin media for the isolation of *Pseudomonas aeruginosa. J. appl. Bact.* **34**, 611.

Thomas, C. G. A. & Hare, R. (1954). The classification of anaerobic cocci and their isolation in normal human beings and pathological processes. *J. clin. Path.* **7**, 300.

Thompson, R. E. M. & Knudsen, A. (1958). A reliable fermentation medium for *Neisseria gonorrhoeae*: a comparative study. *J. Path. Bact.* **76**, 501.

Thornley, M. J. (1960). The differentiation of *Pseudomonas* from other Gram-negative bacteria on the basis of arginine metabolism. *J. appl. Bact.* **23**, 37.

Thornley, M. J. (1967). A taxonomic study of *Acinetobacter* and related genera. *J. gen. Microbiol.* **49**, 211.

Timakov, V. D., Petrovskaya, V. G., Bondarenko, V. M. & Khomenko, N. A. (1972). Genetic data concerning *Shigella flexneri* serotypes 5 and 6. *Int. J. syst. Bact.* **22**, 149.

Tittsler, R. P. (1938). The fermentation of acetyl-methyl-carbinol by the Escherichia–Aerobacter group and its significance in the Voges–Proskauer reaction. *J. Bact.* **35**, 157.

Tittsler, R. P. & Sandholzer, L. A. (1936). The use of semi-solid agar for the detection of bacterial motility. *J. Bact.* **31**, 575.

Todd, E. W. & Hewitt, L. F. (1932). A new culture medium for the production of antigenic streptococcal haemolysin. *J. Path. Bact.* **35**, 973.

Topley & Wilson's Principles of Bacteriology and Immunity (1929–64). Five edns: **1**, 1929; **2**, 1936; **3**, 1946; **4**, 1955; **5**, 1964. London: Edward Arnold.

Trabulsi, L. R. & Edwards, P. R. (1962). The differentiation of *Salmonella pullorum* and *Salmonella gallinarum* by biochemical methods. *Cornell Vet.* **52**, 563.

Traub, W. H. (1972). Bacteriocin typing of *Serratia marcescens* isolates of known serotype/-groups. *Appl. Microbiol.* **23**, 979.

Tsukamura, M. (1969). Numerical taxonomy of the genus *Nocardia*. *J. gen. Microbiol.* **56**, 265.

Tsukamura, M. (1971). Proposal of a new genus, *Gordona*, for slightly acid-fast organisms occurring in sputa of patients with pulmonary disease and in the soil. *J. gen. Microbiol.* **68**, 15.

Tsukamura, M. (1974). Differentiation of the '*Mycobacterium*' *rhodochrous*-group from nocardiae by β-galactosidase activity. *J. gen. Microbiol.* **80**, 553.

Tsukamura, M. & Mizuno, S. (1968). 'Hypothetical Mean Organisms' of mycobacteria. A study of classification of mycobacteria. *Jap. J. Microbiol.* **12**, 371.

Tucker, D. N., Slotnick, I. J., King, E. O., Tynes, B., Nicholson, J. & Crevasse, L. (1962). Endocarditis caused by a Pasteurella-like organism. Report of four cases. *New Engl. J. Med.* **267**, 913.

Tulloch, W. J. (1939). Observations concerning bacillary food infection in Dundee during the period 1923–38. *J. Hyg., Camb.* **39**, 324.

Tunnicliffe, E. A. (1941). A study of *Actinobacillus lignieresi* from sheep affected with actinobacillosis. *J. infect. Dis.* **69**, 52.

Turner, G. C. (1961). Cultivation of *Bordetella pertussis* on agar media. *J. Path. Bact.* **81**, 15.

Ulrich, J. A. (1944). New indicators to replace litmus in milk. *Science, N.Y.*, **99**, 352.

Ulrich, J. A. & Needham, G. M. (1953). Differentiation of *Alcaligenes faecalis* from *Brucella bronchisepticus* [sic] by biochemical and nutritional methods. *J. Bact.* **65**, 210.

Vallée, A., Thibault, P. & Second, L. (1963). Contribution a l'étude d'*A. lignieresii* et d'*A. equuli*. *Annls Inst. Pasteur, Paris*, **104**, 108.

van Loghem, J. J. (1944–5). The classification of the plague-bacillus. *Antonie van Leeuwenhoek*, **10**, 15.

Varney, P. L. (1961). A new closure for bacteriologic culture tubes. *Am. J. clin. Path.* **35**, 475.

Vaughn, R. H., Osborne, J. T., Wedding, G. T., Tabachnick, J., Beisel, C. G. & Braxton, T. (1950). The utilization of citrate by *Escherichia coli*. *J. Bact.* **60**, 119.

Vendrely, R. (1958). La notion d'espèce bactérienne à la lumière des découvertes récentes. La notion d'espèce a travers quelques données biochimiques récentes et le cycle L. *Annls Inst. Pasteur, Paris*, **94**, 142.

Vera, H. D. (1971). Quality control in diagnostic microbiology. *Hlth Lab. Sci.* **8**, 176.

Verhoef, J., van Boven, C. P. A. & Winkler, K. C. (1972). Phage-typing of coagulase-negative staphylococci. *J. med. Microbiol.* **5**, 9.

Véron, M. (1965). La position taxonomique des Vibrio et de certaines bactéries comparables. *C. r. hebd. Séanc. Acad. Sci., Paris*. **261**, 5243.

Véron, M. (1966). Taxonomie numérique des vibrions et de certaines bactéries comparables. II. – Corrélation entre similitudes phénétiques et la composition en bases de l'ADN. *Annls Inst. Pasteur, Paris*, **111**, 671.

Vickerstaff, J. M. & Cole, B. C. (1969). Characterization of *Haemophilus vaginalis*, *Corynebacterium cervicis*, and related bacteria. *Can. J. Microbiol.* **15**, 587.

Vörös, S. (1969). Les nucléases exocellulaires chez les bactéries Gram négatives en particulier les Enterobacteriaceae. *Annls Inst. Pasteur, Paris*, **116**, 292.

Vörös, S., Angyal, T., Németh, V. & Kontrohr, T. (1961). The occurrence and significance of phosphatase in enteric bacteria. *Acta microbiol. hung.* **8**, 405.

Voss, J. G. (1970). Differentiation of two groups of *Corynebacterium acnes*. *J. Bact.* **101**, 392.

Wahba, A. H. & Takla, V. (1962). A new chemical flocculation test for cholera vibrio identification. *Bull. Wld Hlth Org.* **26**, 306.

Walker, P. D. & Wolf, J. (1971). The taxonomy of

Bacillus stearothermophilus. In *Spore Research*, p. 247. Edited by A. N. Barker, G. W. Gould & J. Wolf. London: Academic Press.

Warner, G. S., Faber, J. E., Jr & Pelczar, M. J., Jr (1952). A serological study of certain members of the aerobic nonpathogenic neisseria group. *J. infect. Dis.* **90**, 97.

Washington, J. A., II, Yu, P. K. W. & Martin, W. J. (1971). Evaluation of accuracy of multitest micromethod system for identification of *Enterobacteriaceae. Appl. Microbiol.* **22**, 267.

Wayne, L. G., Dietz, T. M., Gernez-Rieux, C., Jenkins, P. A., Käppler, W., Kubica, G. P., Kwapinski, J. B. G., Meissner, G., Pattyn, S. R., Runyon, E. H., Schröder, K. H., Silcox, V. A., Tacquet, A., Tsukamura, M. & Wolinsky, E. (1971). A co-operative numerical analysis of scotochromogenic slowly growing mycobacteria. *J. gen. Microbiol.* **66**, 255.

Weaver, R. E., Tatum, H. W. & Hollis, D. G. (1972). Revision of King, E. O. (1964). Atlanta, Georgia: Center for Disease Control.

Weinberg, M. & Séguin, P. (1915). Flore microbienne de la gangrène gazeuse. *C. r. Séanc. Soc. Biol.* **78**, 686.

Welshimer, H. J. & Meredith, A. L. (1971). *Listeria murrayi* sp. n.: a nitrate-reducing mannitol-fermenting *Listeria. Int. J. syst. Bact.* **21**, 3.

Werkman, C. H. & Gillen, G. F. (1932). Bacteria producing trimethylene glycol. *J. Bact.* **23**, 167.

Wetmore, P. & Gochenour, W. S., Jr (1956). Comparative studies of the genus *Malleomyces* and selected *Pseudomonas* species. I. Morphological and cultural characteristics. *J. Bact.* **72**, 79.

Wetmore, P. W., Thiel, J. F., Herman, Y. F. & Harr, J. R. (1963). Comparison of selected *Actinobacillus* species with a hemolytic variety of *Actinobacillus* from irradiated swine. *J. infect. Dis.* **113**, 186.

Wetzler, T. F., Freeman, N. R., French, M. LV., Renkowski, L. A., Eveland, W. C. & Carver, O. J. (1968). Biological characterization of *Listeria monocytogenes. Hlth Lab. Sci.* **5**, 46.

Whitby, J. L. & Blair, J. N. (1970). A computer-linked data processing system for routine hospital bacteriology. In *Automation, Mechanization and Data Handling in Microbiology*, p. 23. Edited by A. Baillie & R. J. Gilbert. London: Academic Press.

White, F., Rattray, E. A. S. & Davidson, D. J. G. (1962). Serological typing of coagulase positive staphylococci isolated from the bovine udder. *J. comp. Path. Ther.* **72**, 19.

White, J. N. & Starr, M. (1971). Glucose fermentation endproducts of *Erwinia* spp. and other enterobacteria. *J. appl. Bact.* **34**, 459.

White, M. L. & Pickett, M. J. (1953). A rapid phosphatase test for *Micrococcus pyogenes* var. *aureus* for detection of potentially pathogenic strains. *Am. J. clin. Path.* **23**, 1181.

White, T. G. & Shuman, R. D. (1961). Fermentation reactions of *Erysipelothrix rhusiopathiae. J. Bact.* **82**, 595.

Whittenbury, R. (1963). The use of soft agar in the study of conditions affecting the utilization of fermentable substrates by lactic acid bacteria. *J. gen. Microbiol.* **32**, 375.

Whittenbury, R. (1964). Hydrogen peroxide formation and catalase activity in the lactic acid bacteria. *J. gen. Microbiol.* **35**, 13.

Whittenbury, R. (1965a). The differentiation of *Streptococcus faecalis* and *S. faecium. J. gen. Microbiol.* **38**, 279.

Whittenbury, R. (1965b). A study of some pediococci and their relationship to *Aerococcus viridans* and the enterococci. *J. gen. Microbiol.* **40**, 97.

Whittenbury, R. (1966). A study of the genus *Leuconostoc. Arch. Mikrobiol.* **53**, 317.

Wildhack, W. A. & Stern, J. (1958). The Peek-a-boo system – optical coincidence subject cards in information searching. In *Punched Cards: their Applications to Science and Industry*, 2 edn, p. 125. Edited by R. S. Casey, J. W. Perry, M. M. Berry & A. Kent. New York: Reinhold Publ. Corp.

Wilfert, J. N., Barrett, F. F., Ewing, W. H., Finland, M. & Kass, E. H. (1970). *Serratia marcescens*: biochemical, serological, and epidemiological characteristics and antibiotic susceptibility of strains isolated at Boston City Hospital. *Appl. Microbiol.* **19**, 345.

Wilkinson, A. E. (1962). Notes on the bacteriological diagnosis of gonorrhoea. *Br. J. vener. Dis.* **38**, 145.

Willcox, W. R., Lapage, S. P., Bascomb, S. & Curtis, M. A. (1973). Identification of bacteria by computer. Theory and programming. *J. gen. Microbiol.* **77**, 317.

Willers, J. M. N., Ottens, H. & Michel, M. F. (1964). Immunochemical relationship between Streptococcus MG, F III and *Streptococcus salivarius. J. gen. Microbiol.* **37**, 425.

Williams, C. O. & Wittler, R. G. (1971). Hydrolysis of aesculin and phosphatase by members of the order Mycoplasmatales which do not require sterol. *Int. J. syst. Bact.* **21**, 73.

Williams, O. B. & Morrow, M. B. (1928). The bacterial destruction of acetyl-methyl-carbinol. *J. Bact.* **16**, 43.

Williams, R. A. D. & Bowden, E. (1968). The starch-gel electrophoresis of glucose-6-phosphate dehydrogenase and glyceraldehyde-3-phosphate dehydrogenase of *Streptococcus faecalis*, *S. faecium*, and *S. durans*. *J. gen. Microbiol.* **50**, 329.

Williams, R. E. O. (1956). *Streptococcus salivarius* (vel *hominis*) and its relation to Lancefield's group K. *J. Path. Bact.* **72**, 15.

Williams, R. E. O. (1958). Laboratory diagnosis of streptococcal infections. *Bull. Wld Hlth Org.* **19**, 153.

Williams, R. E. O. & Corse, J. (1970). Phage-typing for coagulase negative staphylococci. *J. med. Microbiol.* **3**, P ix.

Williams, R. E. O. & Harper, G. J. (1946). Determination of coagulase and alpha-haemolysin production by staphylococci. *Br. J. exp. Path.* **27**, 72.

Williams, R. E. O. & Hirch, A. (1950). The detection of streptococci in air. *J. Hyg., Camb.* **48**, 504.

Williams, R. E. O., Hirch, A. & Cowan, S. T. (1953). *Aerococcus*, a new bacterial genus. *J. gen. Microbiol.* **8**, 475.

Williams, R. E. O. & Rippon, J. E. (1952). Bacteriophage typing of *Staphylococcus aureus*. *J. Hyg., Camb.* **50**, 320.

Williams, S. T. & Davies, F. L. (1967). Use of a scanning electron microscope for the examination of actinomycetes. *J. gen. Microbiol.* **48**, 171.

Williamson, D. H. & Wilkinson, J. F. (1958). The isolation and estimation of the poly-β-hydroxybutyrate inclusions of *Bacillus* species. *J. gen. Microbiol.* **19**, 198.

Willis, A. T. (1960). The lipolytic activity of some clostridia. *J. Path. Bact.* **80**, 379.

Willis, A. T. (1964). *Anaerobic Bacteriology in Clinical Medicine*, 2 edn. London: Butterworths.

Willis, A. T. (1969). *Clostridia of Wound Infection*. London: Butterworths.

Willis, A. T. & Gowland, G. (1962). Some observations on the mechanism of the Nagler reaction. *J. Path. Bact.* **83**, 219.

Willis, A. T., O'Connor, J. J. & Smith, J. A. (1966). Some observations on staphylococcal pigmentation. *Nature, Lond.* **210**, 653.

Wilson, G. S. (1933). Tuberculous bacillaemia. *Spec. Rep. Ser. med. Res. Coun.* no. 182.

Wilson, G. S. [printed Sir Graham] (1965). Guidance in preparing the typescript of scientific papers. *Mon. Bull. Minist. Hlth*, **24**, 280.

Wilson, G. S. & Atkinson, J. D. (1945). Typing of staphylococci by the bacteriophage method. *Lancet*, i, 647.

Wilson, G. S. & Smith, M. M. (1928). Observations on the Gram-negative cocci of the nasopharynx, with a description of *Neisseria pharyngis*. *J. Path. Bact.* **31**, 597.

Wilson, W. J. (1934). A blood agar tellurite arsenite selective medium for *B. diphtheriae*. *J. Path. Bact.* **38**, 114.

Wilson, W. J. & Blair, E. M. McV. (1941). A tellurite–iron–rosolic acid medium selective for *B. dysenteriae* (Flexner). *Br. med. J.* ii, 501.

Winslow, C.-E. A., Broadhurst, J., Buchanan, R. E., Krumwiede, C., Jr, Rogers, L. A. & Smith, G. H. (1917). The families and genera of the bacteria: preliminary report of the Committee of the Society of American Bacteriologists on characterization and classification of bacterial types. *J. Bact.* **2**, 505.

Winslow, C.-E. A., Broadhurst, J., Buchanan, R. E., Krumwiede, C., Jr, Rogers, L. A. & Smith, G. H. (1920). The families and genera of bacteria. Final report of the Committee of the Society of American Bacteriologists on characterization and classification of bacterial types. *J. Bact.* **5**, 191.

Winslow, C.-E. A. & Rogers, A. F. (1906). A statistical study of generic characters in the Coccaceae. *J. infect. Dis.* **3**, 485.

Wolf, J. & Barker, A. N. (1968). The genus *Bacillus*: aids to the identification of its species. In *Identification Methods for Microbiologists*, part B, p. 93. Edited by B. M. Gibbs & D. A. Shapton. London: Academic Press.

Wolf, J. & Chowdhury, M. S. U. (1971). The *Bacillus circulans* complex: biochemical and immunological studies. In *Spore Research*, p. 227. Edited by A. N. Barker, G. W. Gould & J. Wolf. London: Academic Press.

Wood, A. J., Baird, E. A. & Keeping, F. E. (1943). A primary division of the genus *Shigella* based on the trimethylamine test. *J. Bact.* **46**, 106.

Wood, M. (1959). The clotting of rabbit plasma by group D streptococci. *J. gen. Microbiol.* **21**, 385.

Wood, R. D. (1957). Hand-sorted punched cards in taxonomic research. *Brittonia*, **9**, 65.

Work, E. (1970). The distribution of diamino acids in cell walls and its significance in bacterial taxonomy. *Int. J. syst. Bact.* **20**, 425.

Wright, H. D. (1933). The importance of adequate reduction of peptone in the preparation of media for the pneumococcus and other organisms. *J. Path. Bact.* **37**, 257.

Wright, H. D. (1934*a*). A substance in cotton-wool inhibitory to the growth of the pneumococcus. *J. Path. Bact.* **38**, 499.

Wright, H. D. (1934*b*). The preparation of nutrient agar with special reference to pneumococci, streptococci and other Gram-positive organisms. *J. Path. Bact.* **39**, 359.

226

Young, V. M., Kenton, D. M., Hobbs, B. J. & Moody, M. R. (1971). *Levinea*, a new genus in the family Enterobacteriaceae. *Int. J. syst. Bact.* **21**, 58.

Yourassowsky, E., Hansen, W., Labbe, M. & van Molle, J. (1965). Problemes taxinomiques. Orientation mecanographique du diagnostic des espèces microbiennes. *Acta clin. Belg.* **20**, 279.

Zierdt, C. H. (1970). Synonymy of species of *Corynebacterium*: priority of *C. acnes*. *Int. J. syst. Bact.* **20**, 23.

Zierdt, C. H. (1971). Autolytic nature of iridescent lysis in *Pseudomonas aeruginosa*. *Antonie van Leeuwenhoek*, **37**, 319.

Zierdt, C. H. & Marsh, H. H., III (1971). Identification of *Pseudomonas pseudomallei*. *Am. J. clin. Path.* **55**, 596.

Zierdt, C. H., Webster, C. & Rude, W. S. (1968). Study of the anaerobic corynebacteria. *Int. J. syst. Bact.* **18**, 33.

Zinnemann, K. (1960). *Haemophilus influenzae* and its pathogenicity. *Ergebn. Mikrobiol. ImmunForsch. exp. Ther.* **33**, 307.

Zinnemann, K. (1973). The ups and downs of the influenza bacillus. *Univ. Leeds Rev.* **16**, 126.

Zinnemann, K., Rogers, K. B., Frazer, J. & Boyce, J. M. H. (1968). A new V-dependent *Haemophilus* species preferring increased CO_2 tension for growth and named *Haemophilus paraphrophilus*, nov. sp. *J. Path. Bact.* **96**, 413.

Zinnemann, K., Rogers, K. B., Frazer, J. & Devaraj, S. K. (1971). A haemolytic V-dependent CO_2-preferring *Haemophilus* species *Haemophilus paraphrohaemolyticus* nov. spec. *J. med. Microbiol.* **4**, 139.

Zinnemann, K. & Turner, G. C. (1962). Taxonomy of *Haemophilus vaginalis*. *Nature, Lond.* **195**, 203.

Zinnemann, K. & Turner, G. C. (1963). The taxonomic position of '*Haemophilus vaginalis*' [*Corynebacterium vaginale*]. *J. Path. Bact.* **85**, 213.

ZoBell, C. E. (1932). Factors influencing the reduction of nitrates and nitrites by bacteria in semisolid media. *J. Bact.* **24**, 273.

ZoBell, C. E. & Feltham, C. B. (1934). A comparison of lead, bismuth, and iron as detectors of hydrogen sulphide produced by bacteria. *J. Bact.* **28**, 169.

Zvirbulis, E. & Hatt, H. D. (1969). Status of names of bacterial taxa not evaluated in *Index Bergeyana* (1966). Addendum III. *Achromobacter* to *Lactobacterium*. *Int. J. syst. Bact.* **19**, 309.

Index

229